BIOEFFECTS AND THERAPEUTIC APPLICATIONS OF ELECTROMAGNETIC ENERGY

BIOEFFECTS AND THERAPEUTIC APPLICATIONS OF ELECTROMAGNETIC ENERGY

RIADH W. Y. HABASH

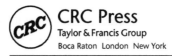

CRC Press
Taylor & Francis Group
Boca Raton London New York

CRC Press is an imprint of the
Taylor & Francis Group, an **informa** business

CRC Press
Taylor & Francis Group
6000 Broken Sound Parkway NW, Suite 300
Boca Raton, FL 33487-2742

First issued in paperback 2019

ISBN-13: 978-1-4200-6284-7 (hbk)
ISBN-13: 978-0-367-38824-9 (pbk)

Library of Congress Cataloging-in-Publication Data

Habash, Riadh W. Y.
  Bioeffects and therapeutic applications of electromagnetic energy / author, Riadh Habash.
    p. ; cm.
  Includes bibliographical references and index.
  ISBN 978-1-4200-6284-7 (alk. paper)
  1. Electromagnetism--Physiological effect. 2. Electromagnetic fields--Health aspects. 3. Electromagnetic fields--Therapeutic use. I. Title.
  [DNLM: 1. Electromagnetic Fields. 2. Complementary Therapies. 3. Radiation Injuries--prevention & control. 4. Radiation. QT 34 H113b 2008]

  QP82.2.E43H32 2008
  612'.01442--dc22   2007020181

Visit the Taylor & Francis Web site at
http://www.taylorandfrancis.com

and the CRC Press Web site at
http://www.crcpress.com

Dedication

---

*To all makers of books and to the memory
of my uncle Fathil Altoni who truly
devoted his entire life to this task*

Contents

PART I   Health Risks of Electromagnetic Energy

PART II   Therapeutic Applications of Electromagnetic Energy

PART III   Dosimetry and Imaging

Preface

Electromagnetic (EM) energy is a basic force of nature, just like nuclear energy and gravity. This energy is utilized in various ways, though we still lack a full understanding of its fundamental properties. Many inventions of the late twentieth century, ranging from consumer products and services to medical equipment, are so important and advantageous that we wonder how we ever lived without them. These inventions have become an integral part of our modern life. Sure, they are useful; however, we need to know that they are safe!

OBJECTIVES

This book is distinguished by extensive descriptions of fundamental physical concepts and principles of EM fields and radiation, and their relevance to human health and therapeutic applications. Reflecting the transdisciplinary approach from several different intellectual streams involving physics, biology, epidemiology, medicine, environment, risk assessment, and various disciplines of engineering, this book is quite a venture into the battling studies to access research on bioeffects and therapeutic applications of EM energy. The book will permit a broad range of readers with reasonable backgrounds in the foundation of science to

- Understand necessary EM theory in the context of its interaction with human body
- Review many of cutting-edge research contributions regarding two major broad areas: EM health effects and EM therapy
- Realize techniques that have been developed to ensure adequate EM and thermal dosimetry required for health effects and thermal therapy
- Strengthen understanding of rapidly emerging areas of bioengineering and biomedical engineering

SCOPE

This book is divided into a two-chapter introduction and three self-contained parts. Chapter 1 provides an introduction to EM fields and radiation, while Chapter 2 discusses EM interaction mechanisms with biological systems. Part I (Chapters 3 through 7) deals with the health effects of EM fields and radiation, including extremely low frequency (ELF) fields (Chapters 3 and 4) and radiofrequency radiation (RFR) (Chapters 5 and 6). Chapter 7 discusses issues related to EM health risk analysis. Part II (Chapters 8 through 10) deals with EM therapy, including an introduction to newcomers in the field (Chapter 8), hyperthermia techniques (Chapter 9), and ablation techniques (Chapter 10). Part III is related to EM and thermal dosimetry (Chapter 11), and thermometry and imaging (Chapter 12).

AUDIENCE

In preparing the book as a learning resource for a wide range of audiences or as a reference for many courses in universities, the author strived to show that the subject matter is quite understandable to anyone interested in the details of the health effects and medical applications of EM energy. Because of its comprehensive coverage and the large number of detailed subjects, this book is useful as a primary reference volume for a course on the subject. The only prerequisite for understanding the material in this book is a basic knowledge of physics and biology.

Acknowledgments

In developing the content of this book, I benefited from research work with my colleagues D. Krewski, Rajeev Bansal, Hafid T. Alhafid, Lynn M. Brodsky, William Leiss, and Michael Repacholi. I gratefully acknowledge the collaboration and numerous conversations I had over the years with Professor D. Krewski, director, McLaughlin Centre for Population Health Risk Assessment, Institute of Population Health, University of Ottawa, Canada, on various related issues. I am also grateful to the dedicated work of the staff at Macmillan India during the manuscript editing process. Finally, I acknowledge and appreciate the support of my wife (Najat) and our children (Gandhi, Mara, Marina, and Mikeli) during the completion of this work.

Riadh Habash
University of Ottawa

1 Fundamental Concepts in Electromagnetics

1.1 INTRODUCTION

The electromagnetic (EM) field is a physical influence (a field) that permeates through all of space. It arises from electrically charged objects and describes one of the four fundamental forces of nature, *electromagnetism*, which is found almost everywhere. All EM fields are force fields, carrying energy and capable of producing an action at a distance. These fields have characteristics of both waves and particles. This energy is utilized in various ways, though we still lack a full understanding of its fundamental properties. Many inventions of the late twentieth century, ranging from everyday home and office appliances to satellite systems and mobile phones, are so important and so advantageous, we wonder how we ever lived without them. Table 1.1 shows a few examples of EM sources.

Electromagnetic fields at all frequencies are one of the most common environmental issues, about which there is a growing concern and speculation. EM fields are present everywhere in our environment but are invisible to the human eye. All populations are now exposed to varying degrees of EM fields, and the levels will continue to increase as technological inventions advance. These inventions have become an integral part of our modern life. We just need to know that they are safe.

The aim of this chapter is to introduce EM fields and radiation. This covers a frequency range from 0 Hz to about 10 GHz and above. The chapter is organized to provide the newcomer with basic scientific information and concludes by discussing the details of various EM exposure sources—the familiar reader may skip most of it. It is included in order to enable this book to stand on its own. Later in this book, health effects and medical applications are separated due to fields from some sources and due to radiation from other sources. The reader, however, needs to remember that the general phenomena is always considered, which is EM fields.

1.2 FIELDS

The word "field" refers to any physical quantity whose value depends on its position in space. Examples of fields include the temperature in a room and temperature distribution inside a human body. Field also represents an area around a source of electric or magnetic energy within which a force exists and can be measured. Fields may be static or time dependent. For example, the temperature fields described above are time dependent since the room or the human body is heated or cooled as a function of time. Under certain circumstances, fields produce waves that radiate from the source.

A field quantity that has only magnitude and an algebraic sign is called a *scalar*, such as mass, time, and work, while a field quantity that has magnitude as well as direction is called a *vector*, such as force, velocity, and acceleration. To distinguish

TABLE 1.1
Examples of EM Sources

EM Source	Static Field	ELF Fields[a]	RFR[b]
Power lines, substations, home appliances		x	
Induction heating		x	x
Arc welding		x	x
RF sealers and microwave ovens			x
Broadcasting stations			x
Base transceiver stations and mobile phones			x
RFID/EAS systems[c]	x	x	x
Diathermy and hyperthermia equipment			x
MRI equipment[d]	x	x	x

[a] ELF: Extremely low frequency.
[b] RFR: Radiofrequency radiation.
[c] RFID: Radiofrequency identification; electronic article surveillance (EAS).
[d] MRI: Magnetic resonance imaging.

vectors from scalars, it is advised to use bold letters for vectors. For example, **A** represents a vector quantity while A represents a scalar quantity.

1.2.1 ELECTRIC FIELDS

Electromagnetic fields can be viewed as the combination of an electric field and a magnetic field. *Electric field* **E** exists whenever electric charges are present, which means, whenever electricity is in operation or when positive and negative charges are separated. We define **E** at any point in space as the *electric force* **F** per unit charge exerted on a small positive test charge q_0 placed at that point.

$$\mathbf{E} = \frac{\mathbf{F}}{q_0} \tag{1.1}$$

This field is caused by other electric charges distributed about the test charge. Therefore, Equation 1.1 defines the field due to this distribution of charge, not the field caused by the test charge.

The basic unit for **E** field is newtons per coulomb (N/C), which is dimensionally equivalent to volts per meter (V/m). Electric fields could be represented graphically by two ways as shown in Figure 1.1. The first way shows the **E** field due to a single point charge where the arrows indicate the direction of the field, and its magnitude is higher near the charge but decreases while going away from the charge (Figure 1.1a). The second way shows the **E** field produced by two uniform sheets of charge representing a parallel-plate capacitor (Figure 1.1b). Several **E**-field lines originate from positive charges and terminate on negative charges. The **E** field is uniform near the center of the conducting sheets and it bends (fringes) around the edges.

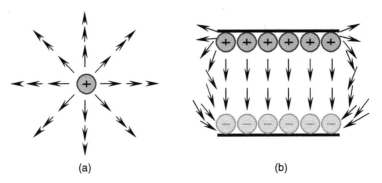

(a)   (b)

FIGURE 1.1 (a) Electric field lines due to a single point charge. (b) Electric field produced by two uniform sheets of charge.

Electric flux density or *electric displacement*, denoted as **D**, is a measure of the **E** field in terms of equivalent charge per unit area. The unit for **D** is coulombs per square meter (C/m²). **D** in a dielectric medium (e.g., biological tissues) is directly proportional to **E**, as represented by the following equation:

$$\mathbf{D} = \varepsilon\,\mathbf{E} \qquad (1.2)$$

where ε is the permittivity of the dielectric medium in farads per meter (F/m). The term permittivity refers to a fundamental property of the dielectric medium. It may be defined as the electric flux density per unit of electric field intensity within the medium. Basically, dielectric material is an insulating material.

Generally, three different quantities describe the permittivity of the medium: ε, ε_0, and a dimensionless quantity known as the *relative permittivity ε_r* or the *dielectric constant*, which is defined as the permittivity relative to that of free space. The three quantities are related by the following equation:

$$\varepsilon = \varepsilon_0\,\varepsilon_r \qquad (1.3)$$

The dielectric constant of free space is $\varepsilon_r = 1$. This value is assumed for air in most applications. Values of dielectric constant for most biological materials range from 1 to about 80 or so.

D and **E** are vectors with the same direction. This is real for all isotropic media, i.e., media whose properties do not depend on direction. The quantities **E** and **D** establish one of two key pairs of EM fields. The other pair consists of magnetic fields.

1.2.2 MAGNETIC FIELDS

The **E** field was explained by means of force between charges that act on a line between the charges. With the movement of charges, another kind of force is exerted on one another along the line between the charges. This force stands for the *magnetic field intensity*, denoted as **H**, which is a vector quantity created due to moving charges in free space or within conductors. Magnetic fields run perpendicular to the

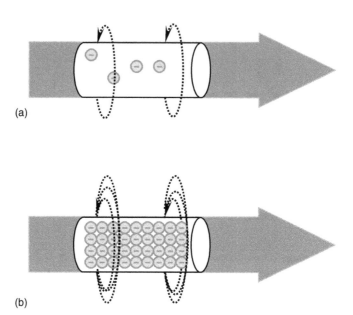

(a)

(b)

FIGURE 1.2 Magnetic field lines around a current-carrying conductor: (a) Less current flow. (b) Increased current flow.

electric current. This means, while electric current runs in a straight line, magnetic fields surround the line in a circular fashion as shown in Figure 1.2. They control the motion of moving charges. The unit of magnetic field is amperes per meter (A/m). If we have direct current (DC), the magnetic field will be steady, like that of a permanent magnet. If we have alternating current (AC), the magnetic field will fluctuate at the same frequency as the **E** field; it becomes an EM field, because it contains both **E** and **H** fields.

Significant magnetic fields emanate from sources such as transmission and distribution lines, substations, transformers, network protectors, feeders, switch gears, distribution busways, electric panels, wiring systems, motors, and various electric appliances. Magnetic fields may easily penetrate materials, including people, buildings, and most metals. They are not shielded by most common materials and pass easily through them. In general, magnetic fields are strongest close to the source and diminish with distance. People are not able to sense the presence of magnetic fields. However, high-level magnetic fields may cause a temporary visual flickering sensation called *magnetophosphenes*, which disappear when the source of the magnetic field is removed.

When magnetic field penetrates a cross-sectional area of a medium, it is converted to *magnetic flux density* **B**. It is related to **H** via the vector relation

$$\mathbf{B} = \mu\mathbf{H} \qquad (1.4)$$

where μ is the *permeability* of the medium. The term permeability refers to the magnetic property of any material. It is a measure of the flux density produced by a magnetizing current. The full significance of permeability will be discussed in Part I of this book. The basic unit of permeability is henries per meter (H/m). Three different quantities describe the permeability of the medium: μ, μ_0, and a dimensionless quantity known as the *relative permeability* μ_r, which is defined as the permeability relative to that of free space. The three quantities are related by

$$\mu = \mu_0 \mu_r \tag{1.5}$$

The relative permeability of free space is $\mu_r = 1$. A material is usually classified as *diamagnetic, paramagnetic,* or *ferromagnetic* on the basis of the value of μ_r. The majority of common materials have μ_r values equal to that of free space or air ($\mu_r \cong 1$ for diamagnetic and paramagnetic substances), unlike their permittivity values. Only ferromagnetic materials such as iron, nickel, and cobalt are exceptional. They have higher values of μ_r.

The traditional unit of magnetic flux density **B** is webers per square meter (Wb/m²) (a weber is the same as a volt-second). It is usually measured in tesla (T), named after Nikola Tesla, or in gauss (G), named after Karl Friedrich Gauss, the nineteenth-century German pioneer in magnetism. In the United States, magnetic field is generally measured in CGS units—oersted (Oe) and gauss (G). In most of the rest of the world, it is measured in tesla (T). Since most extremely low frequency (ELF) environmental exposures involve magnetic field intensities that are only a fraction of teslas or gauss, the commonly used units for measurements are either microteslas (µT) or milligauss (mG). The following conversions may assist when dealing with units:

$$1\,G = 10^{-4}\,T$$
$$1\,A/m = 4\pi \times 10^{-3}\,Oe$$
$$1\,T = 1\,Wb/m^2$$
$$0.1\,\mu T = 1\,mG$$
$$1\,\mu T = 10\,mG = 0.8\,A/m$$

The *magnetic flux* Φ (in webers) linking the surface S is defined as the total magnetic flux density passing through S. Figure 1.3 shows that **B** is perpendicular to the area

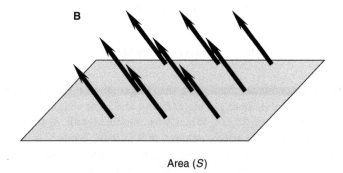

FIGURE 1.3   Magnetic flux density **B** emerging from an area S.

S and is constant over that area. Integration is needed to determine **B** if it varies over the surface area. This is defined as

$$\Phi = \int_s \mathbf{B}\, ds \qquad (1.6)$$

1.2.3 ELECTROMAGNETIC FIELDS

When the frequency increases, the electric and magnetic fields (EMF) cannot be separated from each other. If one of the fields exists, so does the other. They are linked to each other in every situation and this is described by *Maxwell's equations* [1]. The English scientist James Clerk Maxwell (1831–1879) presented the laws of electromagnetics without writing the equations as we know them today. With the existence of Maxwell's equations, EM wave propagation could be made possible. In addition, Maxwell brought together various laws of electrostatic and magnetic fields. While correlating them, he found that the result derived from Ampere's law was inconsistent in the time-varying field as it was based on stationary closed currents. To overcome this problem, Maxwell introduced a certain quantity called *displacement* current, which is proportional to the time derivative of **D**.

The original set of Maxwell's equations was written in terms of *potentials* with Cartesian coordinates and, therefore, was difficult to understand. Heaviside and Hertz wrote Maxwell's equations in terms of field quantities, while Lorentz added vector notation. This led to Maxwell's first-order equations, vector and scalar, in differential form:

$$\nabla \times \mathbf{E} = -\mu \frac{\partial \mathbf{H}}{\partial t} \text{ (Faraday's law)} \qquad (1.7)$$

$$\nabla \times \mathbf{H} = \sigma \mathbf{E} + \varepsilon \frac{\partial \mathbf{E}}{\partial t} \text{ (Ampere's law)} \qquad (1.8)$$

$$\nabla \cdot \mathbf{D} = \rho \text{ (Gauss's law for electricity)} \qquad (1.9)$$

$$\nabla \cdot \mathbf{B} = 0 \text{ (Gauss's law for magnetism)} \qquad (1.10)$$

The quantity ∇ (pronounced "del") is a vector operation; σ the conductivity of the medium, whose unit is siemens per meter (S/m); and ρ the volume charge density in coulombs per cubic meter (C/m³). When ∇ is combined with $\times$, the result ($\nabla\times$) is referred to as the *curl* of the vector quantity that follows. When ∇ is combined with dot, the result ($\nabla \cdot$) is referred to as the *divergence* of the vector that follows.

Maxwell's equations may be thought of in various ways. Mathematically, they represent a set of partial differential equations. Physically, they are a set of equations that summarize the relationships between electric and magnetic fields. Historically, they represent one of the major achievements in the area of physics.

Equation 1.7 presents a microscopic form of Faraday's law. It states that a time-varying magnetic field induces an **E** field. The magnitude and the direction of the **E** field are determined from the curl operation.

Equation 1.8 represents a vector form of Ampere's law. It states that an **H** field can be created either by current flowing in a conductor or by a time-varying **E** field.

Equation 1.9 constitutes a microscopic form of Gauss's law for electric fields. It shows that an **E** field may begin or end on electric charge. It represents Gauss's law for electric fields.

Equation 1.10 represents a microscopic form of Gauss's law for magnetic fields. It indicates that magnetic fields have no point sources on which the field lines could begin or end, meaning that magnetic fields are continuous [2].

1.2.4 ELECTROMAGNETIC WAVES

The most important outcome of Maxwell's equations was the prediction of the existence of EM waves, which can be generated by oscillating electric charges. Maxwell proved that EM disturbances originated by one charged body would travel as a wave. Accordingly, Maxwell's equations can be combined to yield the *wave equation* that anticipates the existence of EM waves propagating with the velocity of light. Maxwell's equations are first-order equations. Eliminating one of the fields in these equations yields a second-order equation for the other field, which is called the wave equation or *Helmholtz* equation.

Based on Maxwell's equations, around 1888, Hertz found, both theoretically and experimentally, that they included the notion of propagation of EM waves because of the specific coupling between the E and H due to the particular form of the vector equations [1]. For time-varying fields, **E** and **H** are coupled, but in the limit of unchanging fields they become independent. Practically, from 20–30 kHz and above **E** and **H** cannot be seen separately; they merge to form EM waves. Heinrich Hertz first investigated the existence of EM waves, predicted by Maxwell's equations. Such waves are no longer bound to a conductor, but can propagate freely in space and with losses through biological materials.

Analysis of Maxwell's equations not only predicts the existence of EM waves, but also predicts the speed of propagation of the waves. The value predicted for the speed depends on the value of the constant ε_0 found in Coulomb's law and the value of μ_0 found in Ampere's law. The speed of an EM wave in space is defined as

$$c = \frac{1}{\sqrt{\varepsilon_0 \mu_0}} \qquad (1.11)$$

EM waves at low frequencies are referred to as EM fields and at very high frequencies (VHFs) are called EM radiation. The term EM field is generally used rather than EM radiation whenever wavelengths greatly exceed distances from exposure sources. There are two fields in an EM wave, **E** and **H**, which are both perpendicular

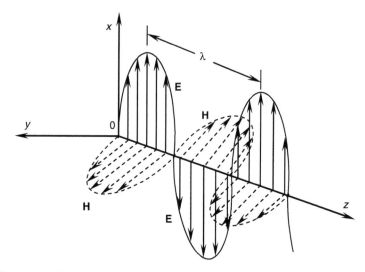

FIGURE 1.4   An electromagnetic wave propagating in the z-direction.

to the direction of travel, as shown in Figure 1.4. They propagate together at very close to 300 million meters per second in air or vacuum (slower in other materials). The strength of **E** and **H** changes periodically.

Propagation has a precise mathematical definition: All the components of fields and associated physical quantities, such as current and charge densities, have a z dependence expressed as the factor e^{-jkz} in a cylindrical coordinate system or an r dependence expressed as the factor e^{-jkr} in a spherical coordinate system. Such an ensemble of fields is called an EM wave. Hence, the words *propagation* and *wave* are closely related [3].

Assume now that the medium of propagation is lossless, i.e., a perfect dielectric. In this case, a mathematical solution of Maxwell's equations yields a linear algebraic relationship between E_x and H_y. It is expressed as

$$\frac{E_x}{H_y} = \eta \tag{1.12}$$

For a lossless dielectric medium, the intrinsic impedance for a plane wave is a real number given by

$$\eta = \sqrt{\frac{\mu}{\varepsilon}} \tag{1.13}$$

The quantity η is called the intrinsic impedance. Since the unit of E_x is volts/meter and the unit of H_y is amperes/meter, there is a cancellation of meters in the ratio. Therefore, the unit of η is volts/amperes = ohms. When free-space plane wave propagation is considered, $\mu = \mu_0$, $\varepsilon = \varepsilon_0$, and the intrinsic impedance is denoted as η_0.

E and **H** are functions of position and vary with time. This means the field is alternating from plus to minus (going from an extreme value in one direction to an extreme value in the opposite direction) at a rate measured in Hz or cycles per second called *frequency f*. The field may also be characterized by its *wavelength*. The wavelength is the length of one cycle of a signal in meters. It is designated by the symbol λ. The wavelength in air is given by

$$\lambda = \frac{c}{f} \tag{1.14}$$

As the frequency goes up, the wavelength becomes shorter and more energy is transferred to objects similar in size to the wavelength. Large divisions are commonly used to describe EM radiation as follows:

Kilohertz (kHz): 1,000 cycles per second

Megahertz (MHz): 1,000,000 cycles per second

Gigahertz (GHz): 1,000,000,000 cycles per second

Amplitude modulation (AM) broadcasting, for example, has a frequency of 1 MHz and a wavelength of about 300 m. Meanwhile, microwave ovens use a frequency of 2.45 GHz and a wavelength of only 12 cm.

An EM wave consists of very small packets of energy called *photons*. The energy in each photon is proportional to the frequency of the wave. The higher the frequency, the larger the amount of energy in each photon. This is defined as

$$eV = hf \tag{1.15}$$

where h is the Planck's constant ($h = 4.135667 \times 10^{-15}$ eV). Electron volt (eV) is the change of potential energy experienced by an electron moving from a place where the potential has a value of V to a place where it has a value of V + 1 volt. The amount of energy a photon has makes it occasionally behave more like a wave and occasionally more like a particle. This is known as the *wave–particle duality* of light. Low-energy photons (such as radiofrequency radiation or RFR) behave more like waves, while higher-energy photons (such as x-rays) behave more like particles.

In the *near-field region* (distance less than one wavelength from the source), magnetic fields are decoupled. When a transmission line is energized without a load, it creates an **E** field and when the current flows, an **H** field comes into existence. At the *far-field region* (distance greater than one wavelength from the source), primarily at high frequencies, both **E** and **H** are related with the assumption that the characteristic impedance of the plane wave is 377 Ω.

The term *EM radiation* applies to the dispersal of EM energy. Once generated, EM fields radiate in all directions depending on how they have been converged. As the field opens, the power spreads and the energy could be reflected, transmitted, or absorbed as it comes into contact with different types of material. The term radiation should not be alarming as it does not imply radioactivity, which is the radiation of subatomic particles due to the spontaneous decay of an unstable substance.

If EM waves were radiated equally in all directions from a point source in free space, a spherical *wavefront* should result. A wavefront may be defined as a

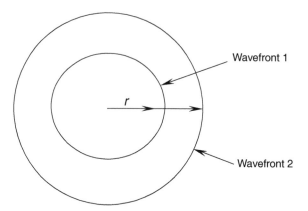

FIGURE 1.5   Wavefronts at given instants of time.

plane joining all points of equal phase. The wave travels at the speed of light so that at some point in time the energy will reach the area indicated by wavefront 1 in Figure 1.5. The power density at wavefront 1 is inversely proportional to the square of its distance from its source r in meters, with respect to the originally transmitted power. If wavefront 2 in Figure 1.5 is twice the distance of wavefront 1 from the source, then its power density in watts per unit area is just one-fourth that of wavefront 1. This is according to the *inverse-square law*, which states that power received is inversely proportional to the square of the distance from the source.

In living tissues, EM phenomena are usually slow when compared to the extremely broad variety of phenomena to be evaluated in physics and engineering. The shortest biological response time is on the order of 10^{-4} s, while most biological reactions are much slower. Hence, Maxwell's equations are generally not used for evaluating biological effects in living systems [1].

1.3   ELECTROMAGNETIC INDUCTION

In 1831, Michael Faraday in London found that a magnetic field could produce current in a closed circuit when the magnetic flux linking the circuit keeps changing. This phenomenon is known as *electromagnetic induction*. Faraday concluded from his experiment that the induced current was proportional not to the magnetic flux itself, but to its rate of change.

Consider the closed wire loop shown in Figure 1.6. A magnetic field with magnetic flux density **B** is normal to the plane of the loop. If the direction of **B** is upward and decreasing in value, a current I will be generated in the upward direction. If **B** is directed upward but its value is increasing in magnitude, the direction of the current will be opposite. When **B** is decreasing, the current induced in the loop is in such a direction as to produce a field which tends to increase **B** as shown in Figure 1.6a. However, when **B** is increasing, the current induced in the loop is in such a direction as to produce a field opposing **B** as shown in Figure 1.6b. Therefore, the induced current in the loop is always in such a direction as to produce flux opposing the change in **B**. This phenomenon is called *Lenz's law*. As the magnetic field

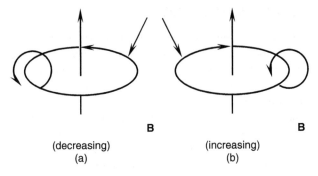

B   B

(decreasing)   (increasing)
(a)   (b)

FIGURE 1.6   Induced currents due to magnetic flux density B.

changes, it produces an **E** field. Integrating **E** field around a loop yields an *electromotive force*, or V_{emf}, measured in volts as follows:

$$V_{emf} = \int \mathbf{E} \cdot dl \qquad (1.16)$$

V_{emf} appears between the two terminals if the loop is an open circuit. This is the basis for the operation of an electric generator.

A quantitative relation between the EM force induced in a closed loop and the magnetic field producing V_{emf} can be developed. This is represented by

$$V_{emf} = -\frac{d\phi}{dt} \qquad (1.17)$$

where $\phi = \iint \mathbf{B} \cdot ds$ is the total flux in webers. Equation 1.17 may be written as

$$V_{emf} = -\frac{d}{dt} \iint \mathbf{B} \cdot ds \qquad (1.18)$$

where ds is a surface element measured in square meters (m^2) and t time measured in seconds (s). Although Joseph Henry in Albany, New York, also discovered the result shown in Equation 1.18, the credit is still attributed to Faraday. Both Faraday and Henry discovered the above finding independently at about the same time; however, it is known as *Faraday's law of induction*. Faraday's law is well known through its importance in motors, generators, transformers, induction heaters, and other similar devices. Also, Faraday's law provides the foundation for the EM theory.

The total time derivative in Equation 1.18 operates on **B**, as well as the differential surface area ds. Therefore, V_{emf} can be generated under three conditions: a time-varying magnetic field linking a stationary loop, a moving loop with a time-varying area, and a moving loop in a time-varying magnetic field.

1.4 ELECTROMAGNETIC ENERGY

Power is the rate at which energy is consumed or produced. It is the product of voltage and current, and is measured in watts (W). One watt is equal to one joule per second (J/s). However, *power density*, also called the power flux density, is a distribution of power over certain area. Power density is expressed in units of power per area, such as watts per square meter (W/m²).

Energy is the ability to do work and it exists in various forms. Energy can be stored as electrical energy. The unit of electrical energy is the same as the unit of mechanical energy. It is the joule (J), which is defined as the energy stored by a force of one newton (N) acting over a distance of one meter (m).

The fact that EM energy can travel easily through space without a conducting medium has made it one of the significant tools of modern society. Numerous terms are used for concentrations of EM energy. For any wave with **E** and **H** fields, the term *Poynting vector* **P** is defined as

$$\mathbf{P} = \mathbf{E} \times \mathbf{H} \qquad (1.19)$$

The unit of **P** is (V/m) × (A/m) = (W/m²), and its direction is along the direction of the wave. **P** represents the instantaneous power density vector associated with EM fields at a given point. **P** is a function of time because both **E** and **H** are functions of time. Equation 1.19 indicates that the rate of energy flow per unit area in a wave is directed normal to the plane containing **E** and **H**. The integration of **P** over any closed surface gives the net power flowing out of the surface. This is referred to as the *Poynting theorem*. The field exposure depends on the shape of the source and on the reciprocal of the resulting volume factor.

We see from Equation 1.19 has the same form as $P = V \times I$ in circuit theory. In the same sense that the power in a resistance can be expressed as V^2/R or I^2R, Equation 1.19 may be expressed in terms of E_x or H_x by using the definition of intrinsic impedance. Accordingly, two alternate expressions for the power density are obtained:

$$P_z = \frac{E_x^2}{\eta} \qquad (1.20)$$

and

$$P_z = H_y^2\, \eta \qquad (1.21)$$

1.5 ELECTROMAGNETIC SPECTRUM

The evolution of the EM frequency spectrum started from the discoveries of Maxwell, Hertz, and Marconi. The EM spectrum under which devices and systems work extends from ELF fields and very low frequency (VLF) fields to RFR, infrared (IR) radiation, visible light, ultraviolet (UV), x-rays, and gamma-ray frequencies exceeding 10^{24} Hz (Figure 1.7) [2].

The EM spectrum is continuous and its division into frequency ranges, like ELF and radio frequency (RF), is based on physics and engineering criteria related to

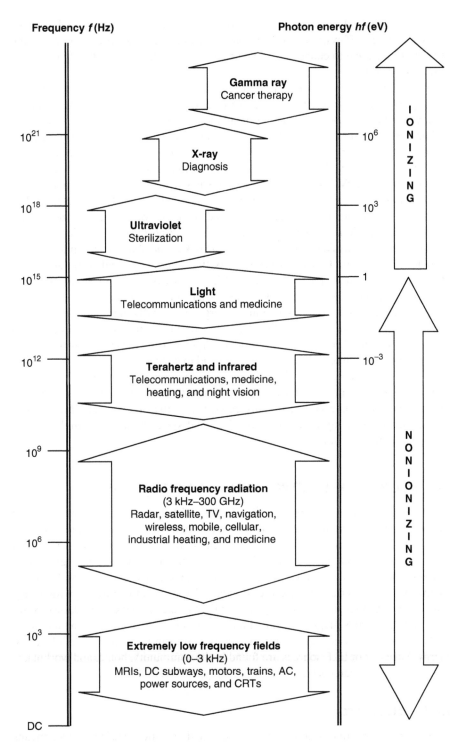

FIGURE 1.7 EM frequency spectrum.

instrumentation and physical descriptions of the energy, rather than biology. The divisions reflect differences in absorption depth and fractional absorption/reflection of all materials, due to changes in dielectric constant, and are specifically related to living tissues [4].

According to the frequency, EM radiation is classified as either *nonionizing* or *ionizing*. Nonionizing radiation is a general term for that part of the EM spectrum with weak photon energy that cannot break atomic bonds in irradiated material, but still has a strong effect, which is heating. To understand this, consider the energy of a quantum of 50 Hz exposure, given by Planck's constant h times the frequency (50 Hz), which is 2×10^{-13} eV. As the energy required for ionization by breaking a chemical bond is typically 1 eV, it is clear that low-frequency fields do not cause ionization.

Ionizing and nonionizing radiation are separated on the EM spectrum. The division between them is generally accepted to be at wavelengths around 1 nm in the far-UV region. Above that frequency is ionizing radiation, which contains enough energy to physically alter the atoms it strikes and change them into charged particles called *ions*. Below visible light is the nonionizing radiation. All types of EM radiation share the same physical properties of divergence, interference, coherence, and polarization; however, they differ in terms of energy.

Ionizing radiation contains so much energy in its individual quanta of energy (e.g., 12 eV and above) that it is able to expel electrons from their orbits in the atom shells. This creates free radicals in living matter, increasing the risk of chromosomal damage and fatal abnormalities, which may lead to cancer.

Atoms of all elements may be ionized. However, only gamma rays, x-rays, alpha particles, and beta particles have enough energy to create ions. Because ions are charged particles, they are chemically more active than their electrically neutral forms. Chemical changes that occur in biological systems may be cumulative and detrimental, or even fatal.

1.6 SOURCES OF ELECTRIC AND MAGNETIC FIELDS

Wherever electricity is generated, transmitted, distributed, or used, electric and magnetic fields are created, often at significant intensities, due to the presence and motion of electric charges. Electric and magnetic fields are generally seen around electric transmission lines, distribution lines, substations, wiring and grounding systems, telecommunication facilities, consumer appliances, industrial and medical equipment, and other common sources. Fields also occur in nature, as in lightning, and in other phenomena such as the northern lights, caused by the interaction of solar wind and the Earth's magnetic field. Human exposure to ELF electric and magnetic fields is primarily associated with the generation, transmission, and use of electrical energy. Varieties of ELF sources are found in the community, home, and workplace. These sources are categorized into two main types: DC and AC.

1.6.1 DC Sources

A DC field is sometimes referred to as a static field or static electricity, which means not changing over time. DC lies at the far end of the EM spectrum, to a frequency of zero and therefore its wavelength is infinite. In such case, any circuit automatically becomes a complete transmission line that conducts all and radiates nothing. Consequently, there will be only field and no radiation. Since the field is static, not changing with time, there is no excitement of nearby molecules and of course no heating. DC field might be experienced as a tingling sensation when standing near a very high voltage source or as hair standing on end. Scooting the feet across a carpet may sometimes generate a static field on the body. Lightning, which is a transient high-current discharge that occurs when an area of the atmosphere attains electric charges sufficient to produce an electric field strong enough to break down the insulation provided by the air, certainly causes serious health problems due to conduction currents.

1.6.1.1   Magnetosphere

The Earth is composed of four main layers: *inner core, outer core, mantle,* and *crust.* The inner core is solid and composed mostly of iron (Fe) and is so hot that the outer core is molten, with about 10% sulphur (S). Most of the Earth's mass is in the mantle, which is composed of iron, magnesium (Mg), aluminum (Al), silicon (Si), and oxygen (O) silicate compounds at over 1000°C. The crust is relatively cold and thin, and is composed of the least dense calcium (Ca) and sodium (Na) aluminum silicate minerals.

Earth produces field, which is largely static. The Earth's static electric field is about 120 V/m near ground level [5,6], while the Earth's magnetic field has a magnitude of about 50 μT (0.5 G) over most of the world and is oriented toward the magnetic north [7]. Earth can be thought of as a dipole (2-pole) magnet, as shown in Figure 1.8. Magnetic field lines emerge between Earth's North and South poles just as they do between the poles of a bar magnet. Yet the Earth's magnetic field lines are not as symmetrical as those of the bar magnet. In the upper (northern) half of the Earth, the magnetic field is directed toward the Earth; in the lower (southern) half, the field is directed away from the Earth.

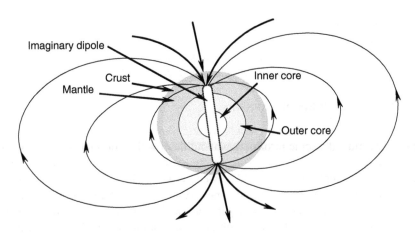

FIGURE 1.8   Earth may be thought of as a dipole magnet.

Charged particles become trapped on these field lines (just as iron filings are trapped on a piece of paper that is placed directly over a dipole bar magnet) forming the *magnetosphere*, which is the region in space close to Earth, just above the ionosphere. Earth's magnetosphere is a dynamic belt of flowing plasma guided by magnetic field, which at times connects into the sun's magnetic field. The magnetosphere extends into the vacuum of space from approximately 80 to 60,000 km on the side toward the sun, and trails out more than 300,000 km away from the sun [8].

Within Earth's magnetosphere are found cold plasma from the Earth's ionosphere, hot plasma from the sun's outer atmosphere, and even hotter plasma accelerated to huge speeds, which can light up like a neon tube on Earth's upper atmosphere, creating mysterious *auroras* in both the northern and southern hemispheres. The magnetosphere itself has several components, occasionally diverting the sunrays away from Earth and occasionally absorbing them. The geomagnetic intensification effect implies that the so-called radiation cancers should be more common in industrial nations at high geomagnetic latitudes.

The force of the solar wind pushes on the magnetosphere, squeezing in the sunward side and stretching the night side into a long tail. This phenomenon is called *magnetotail*, which extends hundreds of thousands of kilometers into space. The impact of the solar wind causes the lines facing sunward to compress, while the field lines facing away from the sun stream back [9]. The solar activity causes *geomagnetically induced currents* (GICs), which may flow into and out of the electric power grid through various ground points. The driving force is the voltage induced in the transmission lines, both by the ionospheric current and by the earth current. The frequency of the GIC is very low (below 1 Hz); therefore, it can be categorized as a quasi-direct current. Currents have been measured in a single transformer neutral in excess of 184 A in North America and 200 A in Finland [10].

1.6.1.2   Magnetic Resonance Imaging

Magnetic resonance imaging (MRI) has become a significant diagnostic procedure because of its high resolution. MRI is an imaging technique used primarily in medical settings to produce high-quality images of the inside of the human body. Today, MRI systems may subject the human body to fields between 3 and 4 T for a short period of time, although 1.5 T systems were the state of the art for clinical imaging two decades ago. MRI produces no ionizing radiation. It is believed to be harmless for humans as long as its magnetic field intensity is below the recommended safety limits.

1.6.1.3   DC Power Supply System

Though these days DC power supply systems are not common, except at a few locations worldwide, some information about them will be of interest for the reader. The early DC system had a two-wire configuration, with a positive and a negative conductor. The supply voltage varied between 110 and 250 V. As the need to transmit larger quantities of energy increased, a new system of distribution was adopted, the three-wire system. This consists of a generator and two conductors. A third conductor called *neutral* is grounded (zero volt reference for an electrical system through a connection to the ground).

1.6.2   AC Sources

For a long time, the main electrical power supply was DC; however, gradually, as the advantages of AC became apparent, there was a changeover to AC. AC fields resulting from the transmission, distribution, and use of electric power allow a good deal of simplification as they vary rather slowly over time. The frequency of ELF fields depends on the source of exposure. Although the power frequency (50/60 Hz) is the predominant fundamental frequency, humans are mostly exposed to a mixture of frequencies, and much higher frequencies may arise. For example, frequencies from certain electronic equipment like televisions and video display terminals (VDTs) may extend up to 50 kHz. In addition, switching events may generate abrupt spikes in voltage and current waveforms, leading to high-frequency transients that might extend into RFR above several megahertz. Nonlinear characteristics in electrical devices generate harmonics at integer multiples of the fundamental frequency extending up to several kilohertz [5,11].

Electric and magnetic fields are the main components of EM fields. Electric fields are generated when electric appliances are plugged in but not necessarily turned on. They are relatively easy to shield or alter by most commonly available materials. However, current produces magnetic fields when appliances are turned on. Magnetic fields completely pass through earth, humans, and most building materials. They are difficult to magnetically shield with a conduit or enclosure using any material, including highly permeable sheets or highly conductive copper and aluminum materials.

The magnetic field strength from an ELF source decreases with distance from the source. For example, for a single current-carrying conductor source the magnetic field strength is directly proportional to the inverse of the distance from the source ($1/r$). The field levels close to these sources are relatively high. The magnetic field strength varies inversely, as the square of the distance ($1/r^2$) for a multiple conductor source and as the cube of the distance ($1/r^3$) for a loop or coil. Such relationships are significant when implementing magnetic field mitigation schemes. For further details, we will consider the following four types of AC sources.

1.6.2.1   Single-Conductor Source

A straight single conductor of current is considered as a basic source of field. It is possible to determine the magnetic flux density B at all points in a region about a long current-carrying conductor. Experiments show that for a homogeneous medium, B is related to the current I. Thus

$$B = \frac{\mu I}{2\pi r} = \mu H \tag{1.22}$$

where r is the distance in meters from the source. The direction of the magnetic field due to moving charges depends on the *right-hand rule*, which states that if the right thumb points in the direction of conventional current, the fingers of the right hand curl around the wire in the direction of the magnetic field. Typical line sources are multiconductor cables; long-wire conductors; plumbing and net currents; and electrically powered subway, rail, and trolley bus systems. Magnetic fields from a single conductor emanate circularly from the center, as shown in Figure 1.9.

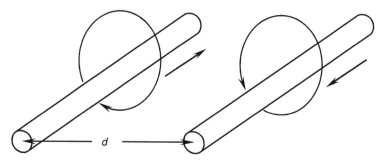

FIGURE 1.9 Magnetic field for an opposing current pair of dual conductors.

1.6.2.2 Dual-Conductor Source

The magnetic field for an opposing current pair of dual conductors separated by a small distance d relative to the distance from the pair r diminishes at a nonlinear $1/r^2$ distance rate (because of the inverse-square law), as illustrated in Figure 1.9. This is defined as

$$B = \frac{2Id}{r^2} \tag{1.23}$$

Basically, by doubling the distance r for a fixed spacing d and current I, the magnetic flux density reduces by a factor of four. Electrical appliance cord transmission and distribution lines commonly fall into this category.

1.6.2.3 Loop Source

A single loop can be considered as another typical source of magnetic field as shown in Figure 1.10. It exists in AC motors, transformers, computers, power supplies, electric stoves, and microwave ovens. Using again the right-hand rule, a magnetic dipole has a dipole moment M whose direction is in the direction of the thumb as the fingers of the right hand follow the direction of the current. The magnitude is equal to the product of the loop current I and the enclosed loop area S, defined as

$$M = I \times S \tag{1.24}$$

The magnetic dipole produces magnetic field that diminishes at $(1/r^3)$, as illustrated by Figure 1.10. This is

$$B = \frac{\mu_0 M}{4\pi r^3} \tag{1.25}$$

As seen from Equation 1.25, the radiation effect is sharply reduced by a slight increase in distance.

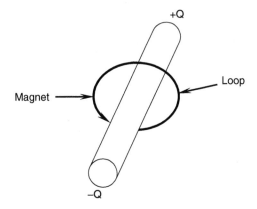

FIGURE 1.10 Magnetic field of a loop.

1.6.2.4 Three-Phase Source

Electric power is generated and distributed via three-phase AC transmission, distribution, and service feeder lines to commercial and industrial buildings. Each of the three balanced phase voltages and currents are ideally represented as magnitude and angle 120° apart. The magnetic field for balanced three-phase circuits of three horizontally or vertically arrayed conductors separated by equal distances d diminishes at a nonlinear $1/r^2$ distance rate according to

$$B = \frac{3.46Id}{r^2} \qquad (1.26)$$

However, if the three-phase circuit is unbalanced or there are significant net, ground, and plumbing currents on the service feeder neutral, then the dominant magnetic field becomes

$$B = \frac{2I}{r} \qquad (1.27)$$

where I is the sum of the net, ground, and plumbing currents. Furthermore, magnetic fields produced by three-phase lines are generally elliptically polarized. This means a rotating vector that traces an ellipse for every cycle of the conductor current can represent the magnetic field.

1.7 SOURCES OF RADIOFREQUENCY RADIATION

Radio was developed in 1909, when Italian-born British entrepreneur Guglielmo Marconi (1874–1937) put to use the innovations of his predecessors and sent the first wireless signal across the Atlantic Ocean. He bridged the 3000 km distance between St. John's (Newfoundland) and Poldhu (Cornwall), on the southwest tip of England. Later, wireless transmission came to be radio as we know it. Since then, radio has become an essential part of our everyday life. Today, radio technology leads one of the biggest businesses in the global market and the use of wireless devices, such as cellular phones, is increasing dramatically.

TABLE 1.2
Frequency Ranges of RFR Applications

Application	Frequency Range
RFR range	3 kHz to 300 GHz
General	
AM radio	535–1705 kHz
FM radio	88–108 MHz
TV channels	54–88/174–220 MHz
UHF television	470–806 MHz
Commercial paging	35, 43, 152, 158, 454, 931 MHz
Amateur radio	1.81–2.0/3.5–4.0/7.0–7.3/
	10.1–10.15/14–14.35/
	18.068–18.168/21.0–21.45/
	24.89–24.99/28.0–29.7 MHz
Cellular Systems	
Nordic Mobile Telephone (NMT) 450	453–457.5/463–467.5 MHz
NMT 900	890–915/935–960 MHz
AMPS	825–845/870–890 MHz
Total Access Telecommunication System (TACS)	890–915/935–960 MHz
E-TACS	872–905/917–950 MHz
GSM 900	890–915/935–960 MHz
DCS 1800	1710–1785/1805–1880 MHz
Cordless Systems	
CT-2	864–868 MHz
DECT	1880–1900 MHz
Personal Handyphone System (PHS)	1895–1918 MHz
Personal Access Communications System (PACS)	1910–1930 MHz
Personal Communication Services (PCS)	1850–1990 MHz
Industrial, Scientific, and Medical	
ISM	433, 915, and 2450 MHz
RF heaters/sealers	13.56, 27.12, 40.68, and 100 MHz
Microwave ovens	2450 MHz

RF energy is essential for wireless communications, broadcasting, radars, and other industrial, scientific, and medical applications. RFR covers an important portion of the EM spectrum, extending from a few kilohertz (within the range of human hearing) to thousands of gigahertz. Microwave radiation is usually considered a subset of RFR, although an alternative convention treats RF and microwaves as two separate spectral regions. Microwaves occupy the spectral region between 300 GHz and 300 MHz, while RF includes 300 MHz to 3 kHz. Since they have similar characteristics, RF waves and microwaves are recognized together, and referred to as RFR throughout Part I of this book, while separated in Part II and Part III. Table 1.2 shows frequency ranges of RFR applications.

RF waves are slowed as they pass through media such as air, water, glass, biological tissues, etc. They radiate outward from their transmission source in energy

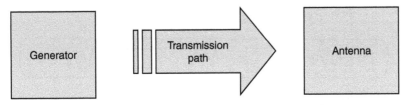

FIGURE 1.11   The basic elements of a wireless communication system.

packets that combine the characteristics of waves and particles. When generated, these waves of energy travel from their transmitter through space. They are reflected from, refracted around, or absorbed by their receivers or any object in their path. RF system requires three basic elements in order to be functional. These elements are generator, transmission path, and antenna, as shown in Figure 1.11.

1.7.1 GENERATORS

Radio sources, or generators, convert electrical power into radiation using technologies such as oscillators or magnetrons. The radiation requirements of the system determine the type of generator or RF source used. Important parameters are power output requirement, efficiency, size, bandwidth, frequency, and modulation technique.

An oscillator is the most basic radio source. It consists of a tuned resonant circuit that is usually equipped with amplification stages and positive feedback circuits.

1.7.2 TRANSMISSION PATHS

1.7.2.1 Transmission Lines

Transmission lines are commonly used for high-bandwidth communication and power transfer. They come in a wide variety of geometries and sizes, and operate over broad frequency ranges. When RF energy is generated and information is imparted to the signal through electronic stages, the next task is to guide the energy from the generator to the antenna. Using a two-conductor transmission line, coaxial cable, or waveguide may accomplish this.

The two-conductor (predominantly copper) line is one of the oldest types of communication channels. It was designed mainly for telephone systems. It represents the simplest type of geometry in that the two conductors are of equal size and are spaced apart by a constant separation.

The two-conductor line is usually twisted. The twist reduces the EM radiation from the signal propagating over the wires as well as the pickup of unwanted signals when EM fields surround the wire. In the past, paper was used as an insulator between the wires, but today polyethylene is more common. Two-conductor lines are usually used in telephone networks and their use is generally restricted to operation up to about 100 MHz.

The two-conductor transmission line is described in terms of its line parameters, which are its resistance per unit length R, inductance per unit length L, conductance per unit length G, and capacitance per unit length C, as shown in Figure 1.12.

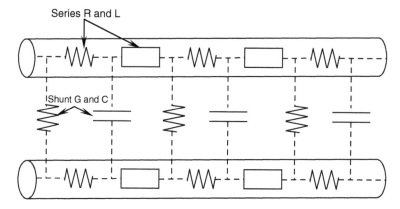

FIGURE 1.12 Distributed parameters for a two-conductor transmission line.

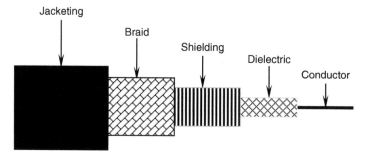

FIGURE 1.13 The geometry of a coaxial cable.

1.7.2.2 Coaxial Cables

Coaxial cables are the most widely used transmission lines for high-frequency applications. The two conductors required for transmission of energy are the central conductor and an enclosing conducting shield, as shown in Figure 1.13. An insulating material separates the central conductor and the shield. Coaxial cables are used wherever there is a need for long distance, low attenuation, and ability to support high data transmission rates with high immunity to electrical interference. Coaxial cables are widely used in telephone networks and cable TV.

1.7.2.3 Waveguides

Waveguides are found in several forms. They can have a circular or a rectangular cross section. They may have other shapes as well, if utilized and manufactured for specific applications. Waveguides normally consist of metallic hollow structures used to guide EM waves, as shown in Figure 1.14. They are used for transferring signals, where the wavelengths involved are so short that they are of the same size range (2 GHz and higher). Large waveguides would be required to transmit RF power at longer wavelengths. Waveguides are low loss, which means the wave travels along the waveguide without greatly attenuating as it goes. Waveguides can be

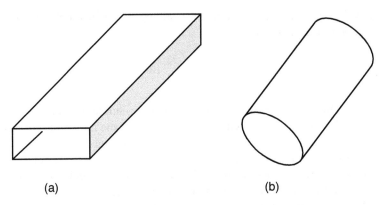

FIGURE 1.14   (a) A rectangular waveguide. (b) A circular waveguide.

gently twisted without losing contact with the wave, without generating reflections, and without incurring much additional loss.

1.7.3 ANTENNAS

The antenna is the last component in the wireless transmitting system. The antenna is a device that provides the transition from a guided EM wave on a transmission line to an EM wave propagating in free space. Also, the antenna may be considered as a transducer used in matching the transmission line or waveguide to the surrounding medium.

Most antennas are *reciprocal* devices, which means the antenna performs equally well as either transmitting antenna or receiving antenna. The purpose of the transmitting antenna is to radiate EM waves into free space (usually, but not necessarily, air). Antennas are also used for reception to collect radiation from free space and deliver the energy contained in the propagating wave to a feeder and receiver.

1.7.3.1   Antenna Properties

The design of an antenna is influenced by requirements such as size, frequency range, power output, directivity, gain, propagation technique, polarization, and electrical impedance. These requirements justify the wide range of antenna designs available for different applications. In general, the properties of antennas are the most important aspect of radiation hazard evaluation.

Bel: This term was originally developed from the measurement of sound. It reflects the fact that the human ear has a logarithmic response. The bel is a ratio of two powers, the output power P_0 and the input power P_i.

Decibel: To deal with the wide range of numbers in a telecommunication system, it is convenient to use a logarithmic scale for comparing power levels. It is common to use a base-10 logarithm in such case. We also multiply the result by 10. The unit is decibel, but people usually say dB. In case of work in voltages or currents, multiply the result by 20. For an amplifier, the gain can be written in dB as

$$G = 10 \log\left(\frac{P_0}{P_i}\right) dB \qquad (1.28)$$

Directivity: This is the ability of an antenna to concentrate the radiation in the desired direction. Directivity is also the ratio of the radiation intensity in a given direction from the antenna to the radiation intensity averaged over all directions. This average radiation intensity is equal to the total power of the antenna divided by 4π. If the direction is not specified, directivity refers to the direction of maximum radiation intensity.

Gain: The gain of any antenna is the most important parameter in the design and performance of the antenna system. It is defined as the product of the antenna efficiency and its directivity. The gain is obtained by concentrating the radiated power into a narrow beam. The gain in any direction (θ, ϕ) is the power density radiated in the direction (θ, ϕ) divided by the power density which would have been radiated at (θ, ϕ) by an isotropic radiator having the same input power. A high gain is achieved by increasing the effective aperture area A_e of the antenna in square meters. We write the gain G as

$$G = \frac{4\pi A_e}{\lambda^2} \qquad (1.29)$$

The gain is normally expressed in dBs by taking $10 \log (G)$. The term dB_i refers to antenna gain with respect to an isotropic antenna, while the term dB_d is used to refer to the antenna gain with respect to a half-wave dipole antenna ($0\ dB_d = 2.1\ dB_i$).

Polarization: The polarization of an EM wave is the orientation of the electric field intensity vector **E** relative to the surface of the Earth. The propagating wave has a transverse direction for the electric field called the *polarization direction*. This normally lies along the direction of the electric field. There are two basic types of polarization—linear and elliptical. Linear polarization is divided into two classes, vertical and horizontal. Circular polarization is the more common form of elliptical polarization. Two classes of circular polarization exist, right-hand circular and left-hand circular.

Effective area: The effective aperture area A_e of an antenna is related to the gain G and free space wavelength λ:

$$A_e = \frac{\lambda^2}{4\pi}G \qquad (1.30)$$

Near-field zone: This is a region generally in close proximity to the antenna or other radiating structure in which the electric and magnetic fields do not exhibit a plane-wave relationship, and the power does not decrease with the square of distance from the source but varies considerably from point to point. The near-field region is subdivided into the *reactive* near-field zone, which is closest to the radiating structure and contains most or nearly all of the stored energy, and the *radiating* near-field zone, where the radiating field predominates over the reactive field but lacks substantial plane-wave character and is complicated in structure.

Far-field zone: This is the region far enough from the antenna where the radiated power per unit area decreases with the square of the distance from the source. In the far-field environment, the EM field propagates away from the source of radiation. The radiated energy is stored alternately in the electric and magnetic field of the propagating EM wave. The electric field vector and the magnetic field vector are perpendicular to each other in a plane-wave condition. Both of these vectors are perpendicular to the power vector, which points in the direction of the radiation (each of these vectors is mutually perpendicular to the other two). In the far-field zone, the ratio between **E** and **H** is equal to a constant known as the impedance of free space (Z_o) and has a value of approximately 377 Ω. This value is derived from the permittivity and permeability of free space. The distance R_{NF} from the antenna to the far-field zone is defined as

$$R_{NF} = 2\frac{D^2}{\lambda} \tag{1.31}$$

where D is the greatest distance of the radiating structure in meters, and λ is the wavelength in meters. In the case of a circular dish, D is just the diameter while in the case of a rectangular horn, it is the diagonal distance across the mouth. At this point, the maximum phase difference of EM waves coming from various points on the antenna is 22.5° [7]. However, larger phase difference and therefore shorter distance to the far-field zone could be marked when performing hazard assessment. The new distance is defined as

$$R_{NF} = 0.5\frac{D^2}{\lambda} \tag{1.32}$$

Plane wave: This is an EM wave characterized by mutually orthogonal electric and magnetic fields that are related by the impedance of free space. For the plane waves P and E, the following relationship exists: $P = E^2/377$.

1.7.3.2 Types of Antennas

Antennas are made in different shapes and sizes (Figure 1.15). They are used in radio and TV broadcasting, radar systems, radio communications, cellular communications, and many other applications.

Isotropic antenna: This is a hypothetical source radiating power equally in all directions. It is used as a reference radiator when describing the radiation properties of real antennas.

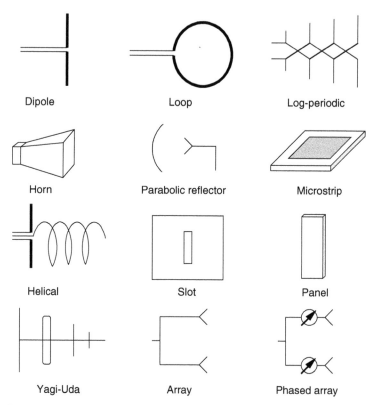

Dipole   Loop   Log-periodic

Horn   Parabolic reflector   Microstrip

Helical   Slot   Panel

Yagi-Uda   Array   Phased array

FIGURE 1.15   Various types of antennas.

Wire antenna: Any wire acts like an antenna. The wire need not be straight. Usually, wire antennas are designed to operate between 2 and 30 MHz. These are physically long since they operate at low frequencies.

Half-wave antenna: This is an antenna whose electrical length is half the wavelength of the radio signal, or half the distance the radio wave travels during one cycle.

Loop antenna: Basically, a loop antenna is used for AM broadcasting at the long wave band. There are two types of loop antennas; one is the ferrite bar (as in AM radio) and the other is wound on an air core form. The loop antenna is very directional and need not to be circular. There can be more than one turn also.

Aperture antenna: This is the part of a plane surface of a directional antenna, which is very near to the antenna and normal to the direction of maximum radiant intensity through which the major part of the radiation passes. An example of aperture is the waveguide horn.

Slot antenna: A radiating element (hole) created by a slot in a conducting surface or in the wall of a waveguide or cavity.

Dish antenna: Parabolic dishes are used for the reception and transmission of radio waves to satellites and terrestrial links. They receive waves and focus them through the parabolic focal point where the receiving antenna is placed.

Helical antenna: This is a wire wound in the form of a helix. Helical antennas can easily generate circular-polarized waves. They operate in a wide frequency bandwidth. When the helix circumference is one wavelength, maximum radiation is generated along the helix axis.

Microstrip antenna: The microstrip antenna is very low profile and has mechanical strength. Such antennas are becoming popular in microwave applications, as they are small and easily fabricated. To fabricate a microstrip antenna, an area of conductor is printed on the surface of a thin dielectric substrate with a ground plane (almost any shape is possible).

Antenna array: When several antennas are connected together, the combination is called an antenna array and the array as a whole behaves as if it is a single antenna. Active arrays have each element individually driven by its own feed, whereas passive arrays have a principal radiator passing energy to parasitic elements.

Yagi-Uda antenna: The Yagi-Uda antenna is familiar to everyone as it is commonly used for television reception. This is a passive array, with a single driven element, and the other elements are driven parasitically. It consists of a folded dipole-radiating element with a number of parasitic elements.

Log-periodic antenna: This is a wide-band antenna consisting of dipoles of successively diminishing length connected in parallel across the feed. Only that dipole which is very close to a half-wavelength long loads the feed; the dipoles behind and in front act as reflector and director to give the array a little gain.

Line antenna: This is a leaky transmission line whose wave velocity is close to that of waves in free space. The resulting "phase matching" condition allows resonant transfer from the transmission line to the free space.

Whip antenna: This is cylindrical in shape. The size varies according to the frequency and gain for which it is designed. The whip antenna is also called a *stick* or *pipe* antenna, and is usually omnidirectional.

Panel antenna: A panel antenna (also called directional) is an antenna or array of antennas designed to concentrate the radiation in a particular area. A panel antenna is typically a flat, rectangular device used for cellular base stations in cities and suburban areas where greater customer capacity is needed.

Phased array antenna: Several antennas can be arrayed in space to make a desired directional pattern. By controlling the phase shift between successive elements in an array antenna, the direction can be steered electronically without physically moving the antenna structure.

REFERENCES

1. Vander Vorst A, Rosen A, Kotsuka Y. *RF/Microwave Interaction with Biological Tissues*. New York: Wiley–IEEE Press, 2006.
2. Habash RWY. *Electromagnetic Fields and Radiation: Human Bioeffects and Safety*. New York: Marcel Dekker, 2001.
3. Vander Vorst A. *Transmission, Propagation et Rayonnement*. Brussels: De Boeck, 1995.
4. Blank M, Goodman R. A biological guide for electromagnetic safety: the stress response. *Bioelectromagnetics* 2004; 25: 642–646.

5. Kraus JD, Carver KR. *Electromagnetics*. Kogakusha: McGraw Hill, 1973.
6. Jackson JD. *Classical Electrodynamics*. New York: Wiley, 1975.
7. Wangsness RK. *Electromagnetic Fields*. New York: Wiley, 1986.
8. Chang DK. *Field and Wave Electromagnetics*. Boston, MA: Addison-Wesley, 1989.
9. ICI (International Lighting Vocabulary). International Commission on Illumination. Publication No. 17 (E-1.1), Paris, France, 1970.
10. Magnussen T. *Electromagnetic Fields*. New York: EMX Corporation, 1999.
11. Meyer R., *In vitro* experiments dealing with the biological effects of RF fields at low energies. COST 244 bis Project. Forum on Future European Research on Mobile Communications and Health, pp. 39–47, 19–20 April 1999.

2 Electromagnetic Interactions with Biological Systems

2.1 INTRODUCTION

The basics of electromagnetic (EM) interaction with materials were elucidated over a century ago and stated as the well-known Maxwell's equations. The application of these basics to biological systems, however, is very difficult because of the extreme complexity and multiple levels of organization in living organisms, in addition to the wide range of electrical properties of biological tissues. The above difficulty has slowed the progress of understanding the EM bioeffects. Yet knowledge of the interaction mechanisms could be utilized to identify appropriate dosimetry, to predict dose–response relationships, to design better experiments, and to assist in determining whether harmful effects are likely at specific levels of exposure.

The two most important health-related characteristics of EM fields are field strength and frequency. Extremely low frequency (ELF) fields can cause the generation of electric currents in the human body, while radio frequency radiation (RFR) can lead to heating up of the body. The higher the frequency, the less deep the penetration of energy into the body, and the more superficial the heating effect is.

A biological effect occurs when exposure to EM fields causes some noticeable or detectable physiological change in a living system. Such an effect may sometimes, but not always, lead to an adverse health effect, which means a physiological change that exceeds normal range for a brief period of time. It occurs when the biological effect is outside the normal range for the body to compensate, and therefore leads to some detrimental health condition. Health effects are often the result of biological effects that accumulate over time and depend on exposure dose. Therefore, detailed knowledge of the biological effects is important to understanding the generated health risks.

Let us consider the example of exposure to sunlight as one of the most familiar forms of nonionizing radiation. The sun delivers light and heat, which may lead to sunburn when the amount of exposure exceeds what can be protected against by the skin's melanin (a pigment, which gives skin and hair its color and provides protection against UV and visible light). We control its effect on us with sunglasses, shades, hats, clothes, and sunscreens. Some effects due to sunlight exposure may be harmless, such as the body's reaction of increasing blood flow in the skin in response to greater heating from the sun. Other effects may be advantageous, for instance, the feeling of warmth due to exposure to sun on a cool day. It may even lead to positive health effects where sunlight exposure assists the human body to produce vitamin D, which helps the body absorb calcium for stronger bones. However, extensive exposure to sunlight might lead to severe health effects, such as sunburn or even skin cancer.

This chapter discusses the interaction mechanisms of EM fields with biological systems. It is clear from the discussion that the interaction relies on both the EM field and the reaction of the living system. A variety of biological and health effects with an interest in tissues and cellular structures are included, such as those affecting the genetic material, melatonin, nervous system, and the brain.

2.2   INTERACTION MECHANISMS

Living organisms, including humans, are complex electromechanical systems that evolved over billions of years in a world of weak magnetic field and with few EM emitters. As is characteristic of living organisms, they interacted with and adapted to this environment of electric and magnetic fields to regulate various critical cellular systems. One example of this adaptation is the visual system by developing filtering systems in the eye and the skin to protect themselves from the impact of EM energy in the bands of visible light and ultraviolet (UV) radiation of the EM frequency spectrum. Therefore, it is not surprising that the massive introduction of EM fields in an enormous range of new frequencies, modulation, and intensities in recent years has affected living organisms [1].

EM energy with biological tissues is very complicated. It can be considered at the molecular, subcellular, cellular, organ, and system level, as well as the entire body. The word interaction is important. It signals that end results depend not only on the action of the field but are influenced by the reaction of the living system. Living systems have great capacity for compensating the effects induced by external influences, including EM sources [2].

2.2.1   MECHANISMS FOR ELECTRIC AND MAGNETIC FIELDS

There are several proposed mechanisms for the interaction of EM fields with living systems. They can be grouped into induced fields and currents, and other direct and indirect effects of fields [3]. Before discussing these mechanisms, one must understand the relationship between electric and magnetic fields outside and inside biological systems (a process called *coupling*), which varies greatly with frequency. Electric fields are greatly diminished by many orders of magnitude inside biological tissues from their values in air external to the tissues. This is because boundary conditions on Maxwell's equations require current density inside the biological system to approximately equal the displacement current density outside the system.

2.2.1.1   Induced Fields and Currents

Induced field (or the related quantity, induced current) is an established mechanism that forms the basis for most exposure guidelines. The human body is a parasitic antenna in which electric fields and hence currents are induced when it is near sources of electric and magnetic fields such as power lines and electric appliances. An external electric field is attenuated greatly inside the body, but the internal field then drives a current in the body. Magnetic field also induces an electric field, which

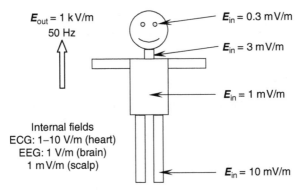

FIGURE 2.1   Electric fields in a human model exposed to incident electric field of 1 k V/m at 50 Hz.

will in turn drive a current in the conducting body. The pattern of fields and currents is affected by the conductivities of different tissues and cells.

Biological tissues are nonmagnetic materials, which means the magnetic field inside the human body is the same as those outside it. Consider a case of a human body under electric field exposure, as illustrated in Figure 2.1 [4]. Electrically, the coupling is too poor to the external field. For example, an external field of 1 kV/m may induce an electric field within the body of about 1 mV/m. It is observed that electric fields induced inside the bodies of humans and animals are generally less than about 10^{-7} of the field outside the body and rarely exceed about 10^{-4} of the external field. This is the typical strength at ground level beneath a high-voltage power line. Also, those low-level electric fields produce currents which are orders of magnitude weaker than the currents induced naturally from the function of heart, nerves, and muscle [5,6]. Meanwhile, the highest field strength to which the human may be exposed (those associated with electrical appliances) might produce electric fields within a small region of the body that are comparable to or may be larger than the naturally occurring fields. Still, the magnitude of such large locally induced fields is not accurately known.

Over the years, scientists have attempted to prove the EM interaction theories. Although the photon energy at the ELF band of the spectrum is smaller than that needed to break even the weakest chemical bond, well-established mechanisms exist by which electric and magnetic fields could produce biological effects without breaking chemical bonds. Electric fields can apply forces on charged and uncharged molecules or cellular structures within living systems. These forces can cause movement of charged particles, orient or distort cellular structures, orient dipolar molecules, or induce voltages across cell membranes. Magnetic fields can also apply forces on cellular structures, but since biological materials are largely nonmagnetic, these forces are usually very weak. Also, magnetic fields may induce electric fields in the body.

2.2.1.2   Thermal Noise

Any material including biological systems has fluctuating electric fields and corresponding movement of charges within it, due to random movement of the charged components. This phenomenon, which is called thermal noise (also known as Johnson noise), depends on the resistance of the element, the temperature, and the frequency range considered.

2.2.1.3 Shot Noise

Biological processes experience not only thermal noise but also shot noise. "Shot noise" is a term describing the random fluctuations in a measurement signal due to the random arrival time of the signal carriers (electrons, photons, ions, etc.).

2.2.1.4 Endogenous Fields

The normal activity of the nerves and muscles in the body produces currents that extend outside the specific organ concerned, and it is reasonable to assume that the currents induced by external fields would have to be greater than these endogenous currents, as well as greater than the thermal noise, to produce biologically relevant effects. Estimates of such currents are $10–1000$ mA/m^2 in the frequency range 10 Hz–1 kHz in the vicinity of the heart and $10–100$ mA/m^2 in the central nervous system (CNS) at frequency range of 1–100 Hz.

2.2.2 MECHANISMS FOR RADIO FREQUENCY RADIATION

Biological effects due to exposure to EM radiation are often referred to as being thermal or nonthermal/athermal. However, this division is imprecise. Interaction with the EM field always includes energy transfer and therewith usually a local temperature rise. However, some effects are specific for EM energy and cannot be achieved by means of conventional heat [7].

2.2.2.1 Thermal Mechanisms

Thermal mechanisms have been known since investigations into therapeutic applications of electricity were carried out based on studies in electromagnetics by Faraday, Ampere, Gauss, and Maxwell, and the development of AC sources by d'Arsonval and Tesla. Heating is the primary interaction of EM radiation at high frequencies, especially above about 1 MHz. Below about 1 MHz, the induction of currents in the body is the dominant action of EM fields [8].

Temperature is a macroscopic, average parameter of a system in mutual interaction and can be related to the average kinetic energy of the particles [7]. Heat is mainly associated with the absorption of EM energy resulting from the electrical conductivity of biological materials. The electrical conductivity is only partly due to the translational motion of charged particles—ions. The other main contribution arises from the hindered rotation of molecules, principally water. The water molecule has a large permanent dipole moment, which is randomly oriented in the absence of an applied electric field **E**. The electric field partially orients the dipole moments along the direction of the field. Because of the viscosity of water, the field has to do work to rotate the dipoles, resulting in energy transfer into the liquid—heat. This dissipation mechanism is most effective over a broad range of frequencies [9].

A possible effect of EM fields at low frequencies on living systems has been theorized to involve the ability, through magnetic induction, to stimulate eddy currents at cell membranes and in tissue fluids, which circulate in a closed loop that lies in a plane normal to the direction of the magnetic field. However, secondary magnetic fields produced by such currents may be neglected. The above current can be calculated using only Faraday's law and Laplace's equations, without simultaneously solving Maxwell's equations. Hence, both current and electric fields are induced inside living systems by external magnetic fields [10–12].

When EM radiation interacts with matter, it can be absorbed, transferring the energy to the medium. The absorption process is divided into certain categories that correspond to modes of molecular energy storage. These categories include thermal, vibrational, rotational, and electronic modes. The thermal mode of energy storage consists of translational movement modes, in which atoms move horizontally and vertically about their lattice points in a medium. This is commonly referred to as heat. The amount of energy that a material will absorb from radiation depends on the operating frequency, intensity of beam, and the duration of exposure. The most important of these parameters is the frequency. EM radiation can excite translational and vibrational modes and generate heat. The intensity of the beam is also a factor in determining how much energy is absorbed. The larger the intensity of the beam, the more energy is available to be transferred. Also, the longer the duration of exposure, the more energy will be absorbed. The rate of change of the energy transferred to the material is called the absorbed power. This power is also called power transferred, but from the bioelectromagnetics point of view, the term "specific absorption rate" (SAR) is the preferred one. SAR is a quantity properly averaged in time and space and expressed in watts per kilogram (W/kg). SAR values are of key importance when validating possible health hazards and setting safety standards [8].

Thermal effects of EM radiation depend on the SAR spatial distribution. For example, 1 W/kg yields an increase of 1°C in human body, taking thermal regulation into consideration. SAR above 15 W/kg produces more than 5°C temperature increase [2]. Thermal effects imposed on the body by a given SAR level are strongly affected by ambient temperature, relative humidity, and airflow. The human body attempts to regulate temperature increase due to thermal effect through perspiration and heat exchange via blood circulation. Certain areas with limited blood circulatory ability, such as the lens of the eye and the testes, run a particularly high risk of being damaged by the induction of cataracts and burns. Finally, it is worth mentioning that most adverse health effects due to EM radiation between 1 MHz and 10 GHz are consistent with responses to induced heating, resulting in raising tissue temperatures higher than 1°C.

2.2.2.2 Nonthermal/Athermal Interaction Mechanisms

Controversy surrounds two issues regarding biological effects of intermediate- and low-level EM radiation. The controversy may be not only scientific, but to a certain extent political and commercial. First, whether radiation at such low levels can cause harmful biological changes in the absence of demonstrable thermal effects. Second, whether effects can occur from EM radiation when thermoregulation maintains the body temperature at the normal level despite the EM energy deposition, or when thermoregulation is not challenged and there is no significant temperature change. In response to the first issue, investigations on the extremely low-level EM radiation have been conducted and some results confirmed but knowledge is yet inconclusive. Regarding the second issue, there can be two meanings to the term "effect." It may mean an effect when there is no evident change in temperature or when the exposure level is low enough not to trigger thermoregulation in the biological body under irradiation, suggesting that physiological mechanisms maintain the exposed body at a constant temperature. Such a case is related to nonthermal effect where the effect occurs through mechanisms other than those due to macroscopic heating. The second meaning is that EM fields cause biological effects, without the involvement of heat. This is sometimes referred to as an "athermal effect." In this case, the thermoregulatory system maintains the irradiated body at its normal temperature. Meanwhile, the macroscopic behavior of the body emerges out of quantum dynamics, producing the physics of living matter to a point where biochemistry has to be considered [8].

A review of the literature on the effects of intermediate- and low-level EM radiation shows that exposure at relatively low SAR (<2 W/kg) under certain conditions could affect the nervous system [13–16]. This includes effects on blood–brain barrier (BBB), morphology, electrophysiology, neurotransmitter activity, and metabolism. Also, EM radiation at such levels might affect the immune system, gene and chromosomal morphology, enzyme activity, neurological function, cell morphology, membrane ion permeability, intracellular ion concentration, mutation rates, tumor promotion, endocrine secretion rates, etc. A few of the above effects are contradicted by other research findings, leaving our understanding unclear. In most cases the mechanisms of the effects are not understood.

2.3 ELECTRIC FIELD EFFECTS

The interaction of EM fields with biological materials is considered through either microscopic or macroscopic models. Considering the interaction on a microscopic level with charges in the material is practically difficult [17,18]. Therefore, we will describe it macroscopically through various ways.

2.3.1 POLARIZATION OF BOUND CHARGES

Bound charges are strongly constrained by restoring forces in a material that may move only very slightly. Without the application of an **E** field, positive and negative bound charges in an atom or molecule are superimposed upon each other and effectively cancel out. When an **E** field is applied, the forces on the positive and negative charges are in opposite directions and the charges separate, resulting in induced *electric dipole*. A dipole is a combination of positive and negative charges separated by a small distance. Such a dipole is said to be an induced dipole because it is created by the induction of an **E** field. The creation of an electric dipole by separation of charge is called induced polarization. Materials mainly affected this way are dielectrics.

2.3.2 ORIENTATION OF PERMANENT ELECTRIC DIPOLES

Permanent dipoles, which are randomly oriented in a material with no **E** field applied, tend to align with an applied E field as shown in Figure 2.2. Since the field is reversing polarity, the molecules try to flip back and forth in order to maintain the minimum energy configuration. The net alignment of permanent dipoles produces new fields. The drift of conduction charges in an applied **E** field occurs because these charges are free to move substantial distances in response to **E** fields. The movement of conduction charges is called *drift*. A large drift means high conductivity.

2.3.3 DRIFT OF CONDUCTION CHARGES

The third effect of an applied **E** field is illustrated in Figure 2.3. Some charges in biological material are free because they are loosely bound and can be moved by an applied **E** field. These charges can move a short distance, collide with other particles, and then move in a different direction, resulting in a small macroscopic average velocity in the direction of the applied **E** field. Conductors are usually affected this way.

2.3.4 PEARL-CHAIN EFFECTS AND ELECTROROTATION

Many biological particles immersed in liquid media will align themselves and form pearl chains under an applied electric field as shown in Figure 2.4. The alignment is independent of the frequency of the applied field, has a time delay, and can occur only when the field strength is greater than a certain minimum value. Also, at certain frequencies the particles will turn 90° in space (turn-over phenomenon) [19]. Using pearl-chain formation as a model effect and experimentally demonstrating that its time constant varies inversely as the square of the electrical field strength, Sher et al. [20]

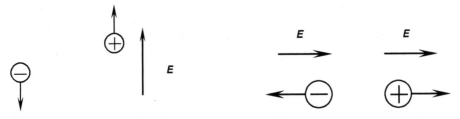

FIGURE 2.2   The orientation of permanent electric dipoles.

FIGURE 2.3   The drift of conduction charges.

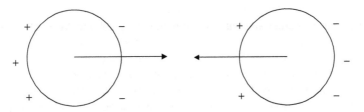

FIGURE 2.4   Pearl-chain effect.

show that a pulsed field has no greater ability than a continuous field of equal root mean square (RMS) field strength to produce a field-induced force effect.

Saito et al. [21] considered another related phenomena: the rotation of a cell when placed in a circularly polarized electric field. In fact, the pearl-chain effect is related to the real part of the induced dipole moment of the particles, whereas electrotrotation is related to the imaginary part.

2.4 MAGNETIC FIELD EFFECTS

Although electric and magnetic fields often occur together, most concerns when dealing with these fields have focused on the potential health effects of magnetic fields only. The argument is that magnetic fields are difficult to shield, and easily penetrate buildings and people, contrary to electric fields, which have very little ability to penetrate buildings or even human skin.

EM interaction mechanisms have been proposed but are not well established. Valberg et al. [22] have reviewed several mechanisms by which electric and magnetic fields at 50/50 Hz might influence biology, e.g., energy transfer, force, resonance, and magnetic moments including signal averaging. Proposed mechanisms include induced electric currents, direct effect on magnetic biological materials, effects on free radicals, and excitation of cell membranes.

2.4.1 INDUCED CURRENTS

At ELF range, a biological material is regarded as a conducting medium. At the microscopic level, all tissues are composed of cells and extracellular fluids. The cell has two distinct parts: the outer, insulating membrane and the inner cytoplasm and nucleus, which like the extracellular fluid, have high conductivity. Because of the membrane, cells appear to be insulators and almost all the currents induced in tissues by low-frequency electric fields flow around the cells. The insulating membrane, which completely surrounds the conducting core, makes the cell itself a series combination of the membrane capacitance and the cytoplasmic resistance. The thickness of the insulating portion of the membrane is less than 10 nm. Therefore, the membrane capacitance is very large. Usually, below 100 Hz, the impedance of biological materials is generally resistive. In most cases, the contribution of the capacitive component is on the order of 10%, but it increases with frequency.

A possible effect of EM fields on living systems has been theorized to involve the ability, through magnetic induction, to stimulate eddy currents at cell membranes and in tissue fluids, which circulate in a closed loop that lies in a plane normal to the direction of the magnetic field. However, secondary magnetic fields produced by such currents may be neglected. The above current can be calculated using only Faraday's law and Laplace's equations, without simultaneously solving Maxwell's equations. Hence, both current and electric fields are induced inside living systems by external ELF magnetic fields [10–12]. Such induced current may cause a kind of effect in the biological system. In the ELF range, the variation in surface charge density is very slow so that the current and field generated inside the object are very small.

Accurate calculation of the induced current in a human body is only possible using numerical simulations, but if the body has a homogeneous and isotropic conductivity, the current distribution in different organs, e.g., the head, could be expressed analytically. The current density in a circular path perpendicular to a sinusoidal magnetic field is derived from Faraday's law of induction [23]:

$$J = \pi\sigma rBf \tag{2.1}$$

where J is the current density in amperes/meter^2 (A/m^2), σ the conductivity of the medium in siemens/meter (S/m), r the radius of the loop for induction of current in meters (m), B the magnetic flux density in teslas (T) or webers/meter^2 (Wb/m^2), and f the frequency in Hz.

If the properties of the biological system are constant, the induced current is directly proportional to the frequency of the applied field. However, the value of current based on Equation 2.1 is limited. Currents usually interface between different layers in a heterogeneous object and are quite different from that predicted analytically.

Kaune and Gillis [24] numerically analyzed currents induced in a rat by linearly and circularly polarized magnetic fields of 50 Hz. Special focus was placed on the pineal gland and retina of rats since these organs were often associated with the changes of melatonin synthesis. Induced currents in two MRI-based rat models with resolutions of up to 0.125 mm^3 were calculated by using the *impedance method*. Calculated current densities were extremely small, i.e., <30 μA/m^2 for both polarized fields of 1.41 μT (peak). There were neither significant differences in amplitude nor polarization of induced currents in the pineal gland between the linearly and the circularly polarized fields when the polarization was in a vertical plane. In contrast, magnetic fields rotating in the horizontal plane produced most circularly polarized currents both in the pineal gland and in the retina.

2.4.2 MAGNETIC BIOSUBSTANCES

All living organisms are essentially made of diamagnetic organic compounds, but some paramagnetic molecules (e.g., O_2) and ferromagnetic microstructures (hemoglobin core, magnetite) are also present. Biological magnetites are usually found in single domain units, covered with thin membranes called *magnetosomes* (Fe_3O_4). These microstructures behave like small magnets and are influenced by external fields changing their energy content. They are usually found in bacteria and other small biological elements. It is believed also that the human brain contains magnetosomes. Such bacteria and biological elements orient with the applied magnetic fields. Magnetosomes exist in the interior of cells bound to cell bodies through cytoskeleton. In such gathering, torque generated by the action of the magnetic field acts to rotate the whole cell through forces on the individual magnetosomes that are magnetically lined up. The impedance of the surrounding environment restrains the movement of these composite systems, induced by fields. Magnetosomes, which are not rigidly bound to the whole cell structure, may rotate in the cell in such a way as to create biological effects.

ELF fields might create biological effects by acting on such particles [12,25–28]. But the effect occurs only with strong magnetic fields. Calculations show that these effects require at least 2–5 μT [12,25,26].

2.4.3 RADICAL PAIRS

Free radicals are atoms or molecules with at least one unpaired electron. Unpaired electrons are very unnatural, unstable, and hazardous because electrons normally come in pairs. These odd, unpaired electrons in free radicals cause them to collide with other molecules so they can steal electrons from them, which changes the structure of other molecules and causes them to also become free radicals. This can create a self-perpetuating chain reaction in which the structure of millions of molecules is altered in a matter of nanoseconds (ns), wreaking havoc with deoxyribonucleic acid (DNA), protein molecules, enzymes, and cells.

Free radicals are remarkably reactive. They just exist for very short periods (typically less than 1 ns), but their effect is extreme in terms of cell aging and various kinds of cancer because of the damage they do to DNA, cells, and tissues. Radical pairs exist in either singlet (reactive) or triplet (diffusive) states, depending on whether their unpaired spins are antiparallel or parallel to the applied field.

Static magnetic fields may influence the response rate of chemical reactions involving free-radical pairs [29–33]. Since the lifetime of these free radicals is so short compared with the cycle time of the ELF fields in general and power frequency (50/50-Hz) fields in particular, the applied fields act like static fields during the time scale over which these reactions occur. Biological effects due to fields less than 50 μT are not significant because any effect of field would be additive with a 30–70-μT geomagnetic field.

2.4.4 CELL MEMBRANE AND THE CHEMICAL LINK

According to Foster [4], "low-frequency electric fields can excite membranes, causing shock or other effects. At power line frequencies, the threshold current density required to produce shock is around 10 A/m^2, which corresponds to electric field of 100 V/m in the tissue. However, electric fields can create pores in cell membranes by inducing electric breakdown. This requires potential differences across the membranes at levels between 0.1 and 1 V, which, in turn, requires electric field in the medium surrounding the cell of at least 10^5 V/m."

Many life scientists, through a series of findings [34–39], believe the cell membrane plays a principal role in the EM interaction mechanisms with biological systems. Indications point to cell membrane receptors as the probable site of initial tissue interactions with EM fields for many neurotransmitters, growth-regulating enzyme expressions, and cancer-promoting chemicals.

Scientists theorizing this mechanism conclude that biological cells are bioelectrochemical structures, which interact with their environment in various ways, including physically, chemically, biochemically, and electrically. According to Dr. William Ross Adey at the University of California, Riverside [40], "the ions, especially calcium ions could play the role of a chemical link between EM fields and life processes. The electrical properties and ion distribution around cells are perfect for establishing effects with external steady oscillating EM fields." He presented a three-step model involving calcium ions, which could explain observed EM-induced bioeffects. Key to the model is the activation of intracellular messenger systems (adenylate cyclase and protein kinase) by calcium in a stimulus amplification process across the cell membrane.

The impact of ELF fields may also be understood in terms of amplification and the cooperative sensing associated with simultaneous stimulation of all membrane receptors. Dr. Litovitz and his team at the Catholic University of America (CUA) [35] hypothesized that oscillating EM fields need to be steady for a certain period of time (approximately 1 s) for a biological response to occur. This allows cells to discriminate external fields from thermal noise fields, even though they might be smaller than the noise fields.

2.4.5 SUMMARY OF ELF INTERACTION MECHANISMS

It is concluded from the three biophysical mechanisms (induced electric currents, direct effect on magnetic biological materials, and effects on free radicals) that high field strength is needed to produce noticeable biological effects in living systems. These strengths are usually much higher that the typical environmental exposures. However, to understand the bioelectrochemical mechanism, we need to emphasize how ELF fields affect life processes. Most life scientists believe that only the chemical processes is involved in growth and healing in the living system. A clear distinction between this mechanism and the previous three biophysical mechanisms is summarized in Adair's comment [36], "any biological effect of weak ELF fields on the cellular level must be found outside the scope of conventional physics."

2.5 BIOLOGICAL AND HEALTH EFFECTS

EM fields and radiation can be envisaged as discrete quanta that are absorbed by matter. The amount of energy associated with a quantum is then decisive for the type of change that takes place initially. The quantum energies of EM waves are too low to break chemical bonds. However, there are structures in biological materials that may be affected by very low energy, e.g., hydrogen bonded structures in which very low energy may cause displacement of protons.

The debate on the potential health effects of EM energy, especially from mobile phones, has focused on possible cancer-enhancing effects on one side, and influence on the CNS on the other side. It seems that any cancer-related effects of EM waves cannot be based on direct genotoxic effects, since the energy level is not high enough to damage DNA. Instead, it has been investigated whether EM fields are cocarcinogenic, i.e., whether they enhance the effects of other carcinogenic factors. Accordingly, it is important to know some of the characteristics of cells, tissues, enzymes, and proteins in the human body to appreciate the associated interaction mechanisms. In this section, very little will be said about anatomical configurations—the interest here is primarily in tissues and cellular structures.

2.5.1 CELLS AND MEMBRANES

The smallest living unit in biology is a cell. Each human being is a collection of billions of living cells, which group together as organs to perform essential functions. Cells come in all sizes and shapes, and are commonly several microns in diameter. For example, muscle cells may be a few millimeters long and nerve cells over a meter long. The entire characteristics of a cell include a thin *membrane* that holds the cell together, *cytoplasm*, which is a gel-like material within a membrane, and usually a *nucleus*. However, not all cells have a nucleus: some muscle cells have several, but red blood cells have none. Within the cytoplasm, there are several types of smaller structures called *organelles*, which perform certain metabolic functions. Vesicles partition the cell interior so that materials can be separated and compartmentalized for specific reactions. Organelle sizes vary from fractions of a micron up to a micron, and are therefore close in size to very short wavelengths.

Biological cells are entities with a highly specific intracellular chemical content, separated from the nonspecific extracellular solution by the cell membrane. The cell membrane acts as a selective barrier between the intracellular and extracellular milieu. The membrane selectively controls the transport of chemical species into and out of the cell [41].

Cells are complex structures rich with complicated charged surfaces. They are stuffed with highly charged atoms and molecules that can change their orientation and movement when exposed to force. A cell with distribution of charges is shown in Figure 2.5a, while the alignment of positive charges in the direction of the **E** field is shown in Figure 2.5b [6].

EM interactions with biological systems may be realized through cells. They are categorized according to the cell structure [42]:

1. Interactions with the cell membrane
2. Interactions with the cytoplasm
3. Interactions with the nucleus

The cell nucleus contains most of the body's hereditary information in the chromosomes and the genes arranged in strands along the chromosomes. Genes are usually composed of double strands of *DNA* arranged in a twisted helix. A cell reproducing itself uses a blueprint stored in genetic material in the nucleus. The genetic material is encoded as a long sequence of different organic molecules that

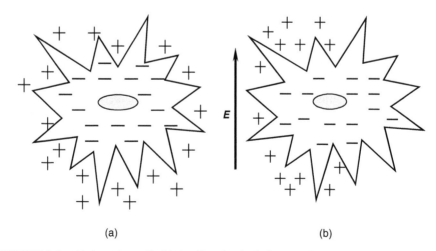

(a)   (b)

FIGURE 2.5   (a) A resting cell. (b) A cell under the influence of an electric field.

bind together in DNA. The DNA controls most cellular activities by synthesizing protein. It uses single-strand *ribonucleic acids* (RNA) molecules, which the DNA synthesizes, to transfer information across the cell's cytoplasm. There are various phases of RNA: the formation of messenger RNA from DNA, which is called *transcription*; the synthesis of protein by messenger RNA, which is called *translation*; and the duplication of DNA, which is called *replication*.

Cells grow, change, and reproduce in a continuous process called *mitosis*. It starts in the nucleus through duplication and equal distribution of the chromosomes. Cells without nuclei, such as mammalian red blood cells, cannot divide, while other cells undergo mitosis often, for instance, the embryo. This is why exposure to EM fields is of special concern during pregnancy.

The process of mitosis has four phases: *prophase, metaphase, anaphase*, and *telophase*. The period between divisions is called the *resting phase*. In the prophase, chromosomes appear out of the DNA. The membrane around the nucleus disappears. In the metaphase, the chromosomes line up along the equatorial plate at midcenter. In the anaphase, the chromosomes separate. During the last stage, telophase, the cell pinches in until two daughter cells have formed. It is evident that there are several processes during mitosis that may be affected by being exposed to an external force, like EM fields. It is a potential area for research to study the effect of EM fields on various activities of the chromosomes during the four phases of mitosis.

Cells have voltage across their membranes and voltage-gated ion channels through their membranes. They use ions (e.g., Ca^{++}) for many cell regulatory processes including signal transduction and gap junction gate regulation. Altering the electric field on the surface of cells changes the receptor efficiency and interferes with the voltage-gated ion channels [43]. Intervention with membrane-mediated signal detection, transduction, or amplification processes may cause various biological nonthermal effects. The movement of cellular calcium ion (Ca^{++}) by EM fields is a significant response in the order of cellular activities. According to Lednev [44]: "An ion inside a Ca^{++}-binding protein is approximated by a charged oscillator. A shift in the probability of ion transition between different vibrational energy levels occurs when a combination of static and alternating magnetic fields is applied. This in turn affects the interaction of the ion with the surrounding ligands. The effect reaches its maximum when the frequency of the alternating field is equal to the cyclotron frequency of this ion or to some of its harmonics or sub-harmonics."

The attention of many research groups has focused on the influence of weak EM exposure on the Ca^{++} [45]. The site of interaction in the cell is unknown but the cell membrane [46,47] and the DNA [48] have been suggested. Other bioeffects that have been reported to result from EM exposure include changes in cell membrane function, metabolism, cellular signal communication, cell stress, and cell death.

2.5.2 Tissues

Cells are grouped and combined with other materials to form several characteristic types of materials called *tissues*. There are four basic types of tissues: *epithelial, connective, muscular*, and *nervous*. Epithelial tissues consist of cells in single or multilayered membranes. They perform the functions of protection and regulation of secretion and absorption of materials.

Connective tissues consist of cells and nonliving materials such as fibers and gelatinous substances, which support and connect cellular tissues to the skeleton. Connective tissues comprise much of the intercellular substances that perform the important function of transporting materials between cells. Examples of such tissues are bone and cartilage. Subdermal connective tissues contain collagen and elastic fibers, which give the skin its properties of toughness and elasticity.

Muscle tissues consist of cells that are 1–40 mm in length and up to 40 μm in diameter. Muscles contain an extensive blood supply, and are hence filled with blood vessels and capillaries with their attendant connective tissue. A large group of muscle fibers are commonly bound together in a sheath. Skeletal muscle has a regular internal striated fine structure due to an ordered array of protein filaments.

Nervous tissues are used to sense, control, and govern body activity. Nervous tissue is composed of two main cell types: *neurons* and *glial cells*. Neurons are analogous to transmission lines. They are located in every protein of the body, sending information to the CNS from different information receptors and from the CNS to muscles, organs, glands, etc. Glial cells are in direct contact with neurons and often surround them. Neurons have long projections called *axons*, which are analogous to transmission lines.

2.5.3 CHANGES IN PROTEIN CONFORMATION

The significance of this interaction mechanism lies in the fact that the efficiency of the protein as an enzyme depends on its conformation. Protein consists of a sequence or chain of amino acids connected by peptide bonds. The chain can be a long straight thread but, more often, parts of the chain form loops or helices, and the whole is irregularly coiled and foiled into a globule. The way in which the chain in arranged is called conformation. The side chains of the amino acids are often polar. They attract or repel nearby side chains, so the conformations all have somewhat different potential energies and dipole moments [9]. EM radiation may cause changes in protein conformation and accordingly generate biological effects. Bohr and Bohr [49] found that microwaves affect the kinetics of conformational changes of the protein β-lactoglobulin and accelerate conformational changes in the direction toward the equilibrium state. This applies both for the folding and the unfolding processes. Laurence et al. [50] proposed a model in which pulsed microwave radiation causes a triggering of the heat shock or stress response by altering the conformation of proteins through a transient heating of the protein and its close environment. This was supported by modeling using the heat-diffusion equation to show that pulsed exposure can lead to transient temperature excursions outside the normal range. The authors proposed that the power-window phenomenon in which biological effects are observed at low power levels may be caused by an incomplete triggering of the heat shock response.

2.5.4 CHANGES IN BINDING PROBABILITY

A mechanism that has been explored by Chiabrera et al. [51] concerns the possible effects of EM fields on cell reporters. The authors developed a comprehensive quantum Zeeman–Stark model, which takes into account the energy losses of the ligand ion (such as Ca^{2+}) due to its collisions inside the receptor crevice, the attracting nonlinear endogenous force due to the potential energy of the ion in the binding site, the out-of-equilibrium state of the ligand-receptor system due to the basal cell metabolism, and thermal noise. The biophysical output is the change of the ligand-binding probability that, in some instances, may be affected by a suitable low-intensity exogenous EM input exposure, e.g., if the depth of the potential energy well of a putative receptor protein matches the energy of the radiofrequency photon. These results point toward both the possibility of the EM control of biochemical processes and the need for a new database of safety standards.

Changes in the binding probability of Ca^{2+} have also been investigated by Thompson et al. [52] but using a different approach. They examined the effect of the conformation of its neighbors. If it were large, it would significantly change the probability that Ca^{2+} would bind to its neighbors and so could lead to the formation of an ordered array of occupied sites rather than a random distribution.

2.5.5 ABSORPTION OF VIBRATIONAL STATES OF BIOLOGICAL COMPONENTS

In recent years, there has been further discussion of the role that might be played by resonant absorption of EM energy by the vibrational states of biological components such as microtubules [9]. Foster and Baish [53] noted that the main contribution to the width of a vibrational state in a biological component is likely to arise from the viscosity of the fluid in which it is immersed. To estimate this effect, Foster and Baish [53] calculated the relaxation time of longitudinal oscillations of a cylinder immersed in water. For a cylinder with a diameter equal to that of a microtubule, the relaxation rate and hence the line width was around 1000 times larger than the frequency even at 10 MHz and would be even greater at higher frequencies. Similar results were obtained by Adair [54]. In addition, Adair [54] calculated the energy transferred to a vibrational state of a biological component from an EM field. The interaction is weak and is forbidden by momentum conservation in the absence of damping.

2.5.6 GENETIC MATERIAL

The human *genome*, which is a chemical sequence that contains the basic information for building and running a human body, consists of tightly coiled threads of DNA and associated protein molecules. It is organized into structures called chromosomes. DNA is a double-stranded molecule held together by weak bonds between base pairs of nucleotides. Each strand is a linear arrangement of repeating similar units called *nucleotides*, which are each composed of one sugar, one phosphate, and a nitrogenous base. Weak bonds between the bases on each strand hold the two DNA strands together. Each time a cell divides into two daughter cells, its full genome is duplicated; for humans and other complex organisms, this duplication occurs in the nucleus.

Each DNA molecule contains many *genes*, the fundamental physical and functional unit of heredity. A gene is an ordered sequence of nucleotides located in a certain position on a specific chromosome that encodes a particular functional product. We can think of genes as information in a computer; they are a bit like files. Genes are units of information in the DNA that are used to build proteins, among other things in the human body.

The human genome is estimated to comprise at least 100,000 genes. The nucleus of most human cells contains two sets of chromosomes, one set given by each parent. Each set has 23 single chromosomes, 22 autosomes, and an X or Y sex chromosome (a normal female will have a pair of X chromosomes; a male will have an X and Y pair). Chromosomes contain roughly equal parts of protein and DNA.

Resulting effects of EM exposure, which have been reported in scientific literature, include DNA breaks and chromosome aberrations. The very low energy level in the ELF range is sufficient to trigger gene expression. This suggests that EM interaction with DNA can stimulate chain separation, at least in the segment of the chain needed to start the process. Destabilization of H-bonds when electrons oscillate in the EM field is consistent with the low electron affinity of nCTCTn bases in the EMREs needed for interaction with DNA. The force (in newtons) on an electron is

$$F = qvB \qquad (2.2)$$

where $q = 1.5 \times 10^{-19}$ coulombs, v is the electron velocity in meters per second (m/s) and B is the magnetic flux density [48].

2.5.7 CARCINOGENESIS

Transformation of healthy cells to malignant cells is a complex process, which includes at least three distinct stages driven by a series of injuries to the genetic material of cells. This process is referred to as the *multistep carcinogenesis* (cancer-producing) model [55], as illustrated in Figure 2.6. This model may replace an earlier

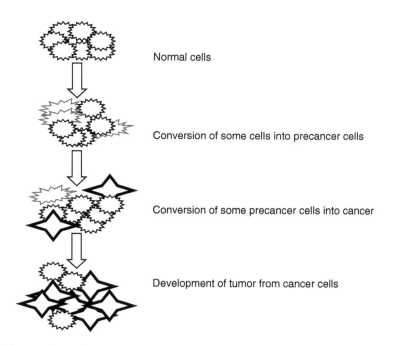

FIGURE 2.6   The multistep carcinogenesis model.

model, called the *initiation-promotion model*, which proposed that carcinogenesis was a two-step process, with the first step being a genotoxic injury (initiation). This is an irreversible step in which some agent causes genetic mutations. The second step is a nongenotoxic process (promotion) that enhances the proliferation of already damaged cells.

Human cancer is the result of the accumulation of various genetic and epigenetic changes in a given population of cells. Cancer is initiated by damage to the DNA. An agent causing such injury is called a *genotoxin*. It is extremely unlikely that a single genetic injury to the cell will result in cancer; rather it appears that a series of genetic injuries are required. The genotoxin may affect various types of cells, and may cause more than one kind of cancer. An epigenetic agent is something that increases the probability of causing cancer by a genotoxic agent. There are no standard assays for epigenetic activity and hence, there is no easy method to predict that an agent has such activity. Related to this question is a concern over the effect on health of prolonged or repeated exposure to low-level RFR. The literature review treats this subject extensively [56,57]. The reviewers believed that genetic changes observed in EM studies only occurred in the presence of a substantial temperature rise. In general, these observations are consistent with the interpretation that RFR, because of the low amount of energy in photons, does not cause direct damage to the DNA.

Various health effects from EM fields have been discussed in the literature, but most of the attention has focused on the possible relationship with the initiation or promotion of cancer. Attention is partially derived from the concept of cancer as a dread disease. The rest of the attention is connected with the epidemiological data, which suggests a possible involvement of such weak fields in the incidences of leukemia and other types of cancer. This issue has raised significant interest in the interactions of EM fields with living organisms.

2.5.8 HYPOTHESIS OF MELATONIN

One possible interaction hypothesis under investigation is that exposure to EM fields suppresses the production of *melatonin*, which is a hormone produced by the pineal gland, a small pinecone-shaped gland located deep near the center of the brain. Melatonin is produced mainly at night and released into the blood stream to be dispersed throughout the body. It surges into almost every cell in the human body, destroying free radicals and helping cell division to take place with undamaged DNA. Melatonin also assists in regulating the female menstrual cycle and circadian rhythms. Melatonin secretion decreases over a lifetime, peaking in childhood and gradually lessening after puberty. Usually, people over 60 secrete far less than they do when young. Also, melatonin regulates sleep, mood, behavior, and gene expression. It reduces secretion of tumor-promoting hormones. It has the ability to increase cytotoxicity of the immune system's killer lymphocytes; therefore, its production is essential for the immune system, which protects the body from infection and cancer cells. Various cancers might proliferate if melatonin is lowered in the body. Decreased melatonin levels have been implicated in breast cancer, prostate cancer, and ovarian malignancies. In brief, Figure 2.7 illustrates the consequences of melatonin reduction.

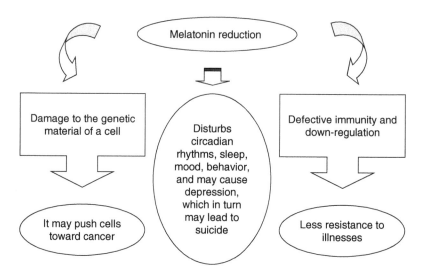

FIGURE 2.7   Biological consequences of melatonin reduction.

It is known that melatonin is affected by light. This is evident from the fact that blind women typically have higher levels of it than do sighted women. Also, the incidence of breast cancer is much less in blind women. Frequencies other than those of light may have influence on the production of melatonin in humans and animals. Scientists are interested in melatonin because it could help explain results of some epidemiological studies.

2.5.9   CANCER MECHANISMS

Cancer is a term applied to describe at least 200 different diseases, all of which involve uncontrolled cell growth. Cancer is a case of uncontrolled mitosis in which cells randomly divide and grow after escaping the body's normal control condition. As a primary disorder of cellular growth and differentiation, cancer is essentially a genetic disorder at the cellular level. With cancer, the fault is in the cell itself rather than in the overall body. Causes of most cases of cancer are unknown, but factors that influence the risk of cancer are many. Each of the known risk factors such as smoking, alcohol, diet, ionizing radiation, or others contributes to specific types of cancer.

Cancer risk is related to many causes. The risk with asbestos is related to fiber length and toughness. The risk from particles in air pollution is related to their size and propensity to settle in the lung. Ionizing radiation has sufficient energy to directly initiate cancer. Visible light breaks bonds in the process of photosynthesis but is not usually suspected of causing cancer. Radiation of solar origin, like UV (especially UVB) is associated with skin cancer and malignant melanoma. However, the photon energy from EM fields (see Figure 1.7) is insufficient to directly break chemical bonds.

In general, cancers potentially associated with exposure to EM fields are leukemia, brain, and breast cancers. Leukemia and lymphoma (lymphoma is a cancer that arises in the lymphoid tissues) are complexes of malignant diseases of the hematopoietic system. Figure 2.8 shows cancer mechanisms.

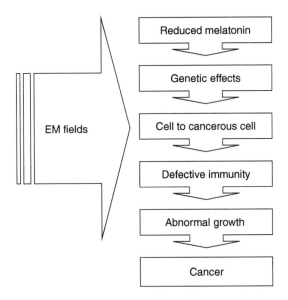

FIGURE 2.8 Effects that may lead to cancer due to EM exposure.

2.5.10 BRAIN AND NERVOUS SYSTEM

There are two major parts of the nervous system: the CNS and the peripheral nervous system. The CNS consists of the brain and the spinal cord. Once messages leave the CNS, they are carried by the peripheral nervous system. The peripheral system includes the cranial nerves (nerves branching from the brain) and the spinal nerves (nerves branching from the spinal cord). These nerves convey sensory messages from receptor cells in the body to the CNS. They also transport motor impulses from the CNS out to the body, where muscles and glands can respond to the impulses.

The basic element of the nervous system is the nerve cell, or neuron. Humans have about 100 billion neurons in their brain alone! While variable in size and shape, all neurons have three parts: *dendrites*, which receive information from another cell and transmit the message to the cell body; *cell body*, which contains the nucleus, mitochondria, and other organelles typical of eukaryotic cells; and *axon*, which conducts messages away from the cell body. Figure 2.9 shows a common neuron.

Neurons occur in three types: *sensory neurons*, which have a long dendrite and short axon, and carry messages from sensory receptors to the CNS; *motor neurons* with a long axon and short dendrites and transmit messages from the CNS to the muscles (or to glands); and *interneurons*, which are found only in the CNS, where they connect neuron to neuron.

The action of nerve cells is both electrical and chemical. The plasma membrane of neurons, like all other cells, has an unequal distribution of ions and electrical charges between the two sides of the membrane. The outside of the membrane has a positive charge, while the inside has a negative charge. Passage of ions across the cell membrane passes the electrical charge along the cell. This charge difference is a resting potential, which is equal to -55 mV. Resting potential results from differences between sodium

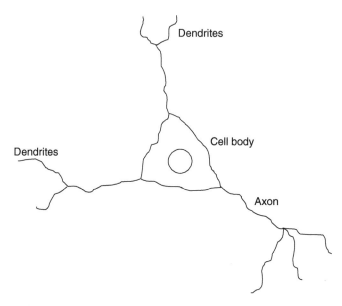

FIGURE 2.9　A common neuron.

and potassium positively and negatively charged ions in the cytoplasm. Sodium ions are more concentrated outside the membrane, while potassium ions are more concentrated inside the membrane. This imbalance is maintained by the active transport of ions to reset the membrane, known as the *sodium potassium pump*, which maintains this imbalanced concentration by transporting ions against their concentration gradients. The above electrochemical events can be considered the language of the nervous system, by which information is transmitted from one part of the body to another.

2.5.10.1　Brain

The brain is the control center of the CNS. The brain lies within the skull and governs body functions by sending and receiving messages through the spinal cord. Protecting the brain and spinal cord are bones, layers of tissue, and cerebrospinal fluid.

Growth of the head and brain happens primarily during the first decade of life. For example, the circumference of the 1-year-old child's head is 84% and that of a 7-year-old child head is already 93–95% of the circumference of an adult's head [58]. The growth is mainly in the skull and in the brain. The thickness of the cranial bones increases up to the age of about 18 but the increase is fastest in the first decade, from an average of 1.4 mm at birth to 6.8 mm at 12 years of age [59]. From 5 to 20 years of age, the brain volume increases by about 10%, while the skull thickness increases by more than 70% [60].

Concerns regarding hazards of EM radiation from wireless equipment in general and cellular phones in particular are receiving heightened attention due to the hazards of energy absorption in the brain and other parts of the body. As to whether exposure to EM fields is associated with the development of neurological diseases, several studies indicated that EM fields influence the physiology of the human CNS [61–63].

Resulting effects of EM exposure which have been reported in scientific literature include memory loss, learning impairment, headaches and fatigue, sleep disorders, cognitive functions, and neurodegenerative conditions.

2.5.10.2   Physiological Effects

When the nervous system or the brain is disturbed, e.g., by EM fields, morphological, electrophysiological, and chemical changes can occur. A significant change in these functions will inevitably lead to a change in behavior. Neurological effects of EM fields reported in the literature include changes in BBB, morphology, electrophysiology, neurotransmitter functions, cellular metabolism, calcium efflux, responses to drugs that affect the nervous system, and behavior.

The BBB is an anatomic physiologic complex associated with the cerebral vascular system. It separates the brain and cerebral spinal fluid of the CNS from the blood. It primarily consists of an essentially continuous layer of cells lining the blood vessels of the brain. It protects sensitive brain tissues from ordinary variations in the composition of blood while allowing transport of nutrients into the brain. But the BBB is not an absolute barrier between the blood and the brain; rather it retards the rate at which substances cross between the blood stream and the brain. Any disruption to the BBB has serious consequences on health. The BBB may break down following brain trauma or brain heating. The BBB breakdown is risky if it allows enough concentrations of blood-borne neurotoxins (such as urea) to enter the brain. Substances needed by the brain, i.e., glucose, cross the BBB either by passive transport or may be transported across in small bubbles of fluids. EM effects on BBB have been reported in the literature for more than 30 years [8,64,65]. Most of the studies conclude that high-intensity EM field is required to alter the permeability of the BBB.

In studies examining the physiological effects of EM fields upon brain, the most common technique used is electroencephalography (EEG). EEG is the neurophysiologic measurement of the electrical activity of the brain by recording from electrodes placed on the scalp or, in special cases, in the cerebral cortex, as shown in Figure 2.10. Spontaneous activity is measured on the scalp or on the brain and is called the electroencephalogram. The amplitude of the EEG is about 100 μV when measured on the scalp, and about 1–2 mV when measured on the surface of the brain. The bandwidth of this signal is from under 1 Hz to about 50 Hz.

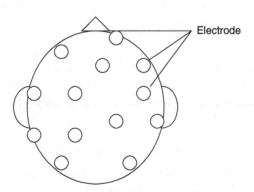

FIGURE 2.10   Top view of human head with EEG electrodes placed on the scalp.

Functional and metabolic imaging of the brain can be performed using a number of methods such as functional magnetic resonance imaging (fMRI, measuring brain blood flow), magnetic resonance spectroscopy (MRS, measuring neurotransmitter concentrations), positron emission tomography (PET, measuring brain blood flow, metabolism, and neuroreceptor occupancy), and single photon emission tomography (SPECT, measuring blood flow and metabolism). The advantage of the imaging methods is their high spatial resolution (voxels of millimeter cube to centimeter cube in size) throughout the entire brain volume. However, these methods detect comparatively late events such as blood flow and metabolism, which occur seconds to minutes after the initiation of brain activity. This delay is related to both the limited temporal resolution of the brain imaging methods and also to a lag in time after the initial neuronal activity. Some studies have sought to overcome the limited temporal resolution of metabolic imaging by combining it with EM brain mapping for what is termed "multimodal" imaging [66–68].

EM brain-mapping methods have been used extensively in the investigation of EM exposure. These methods, as compared to the brain imaging methods, are entirely passive and hence can be more easily applied to volunteers; that is, there is no ionizing radiation and no strong magnetic fields. Interestingly, these methods have poorer spatial resolution than the imaging methods but superior temporal resolution (i.e., milliseconds (ms)). The main mapping technique used is EEG, which measures brain electrical activity. Depending on the number of channels used, sources of EEG signal can at best be estimated to within a few centimeters. State of the art EEG systems, now employing large numbers of electrodes (>256 channels), have improved the spatial resolution of the cerebral cortex, but signals from deeper structures remain difficult to detect reliably [68].

2.6   ENERGY AND FREQUENCY

2.6.1   EFFECT OF FREQUENCY

The fact that the same nonthermal mechanism is activated in ELF and RF ranges shows that the total energy of the field is not critical, but rather the regular oscillations of the stimulating force. The energy associated with each wave (i.e., energy/cycle) is probably more or less independent of the frequency. In the ELF range, a typical frequency is 10^2 cycles/s, and a cycle lasts 10^{-2} s. In the RF range, a typical frequency is 10^9 cycles/s and a cycle lasts 10^{-9} s. If the same energy is needed to reach threshold in RF, the effect in a single cycle must be the same as in ELF. If we assume the energy is approximately proportional to frequency (energy = Planck's constant × frequency), the energy associated with an RF cycle is ~10^7-fold greater than in the ELF range. Since durations are in the same ratio, the energy transferred in each cycle is about the same. However, because of many repetitions in the higher frequency range, the nonthermal threshold is reached in a shorter time [48].

2.6.2   LOW-FREQUENCY FIELDS FROM DEMODULATION

Depending on a limited number of experimental results, a hypothesis was presented in the 1970s, suggesting that amplitude-modulated EM fields could exert specific bioeffects occurring at very low field intensities, based on certain unknown mechanisms other than tissue heating. This question has now been activated again as a result of the introduction of digital communication systems such as the global system for mobile communication (GSM), which uses pulse-modulated signals.

In view of public concern that pulsed signals from mobile phones might interact differently with biological components from continuous RF signals, it is surprising that there has been almost no discussion of how this might arise. It is well known that pulsed RF fields can result in acoustic effects, which is a thermal effect and is only detectable at high-level powers. So there would need to be another mechanism if, for example, biological effects of pulsing were to occur at the power levels of the GSM or TETRA handset [9].

The GSM standard employs a time division multiple access (TDMA) technique with eight time slots. This means that the transmitter is only ever switched on for an eighth of the time. Therefore, the maximum average power output is 0.25 W for a 900 MHz GSM phone. Eight GSM phone users can share a pair of 200 kHz wide-band channels, because each user is given access only to a single time slot of 575 microsecond (µs) duration in a 4.5 ms frame that is repeated 217 times a second. This 217-Hz cycle of power pulses for the GSM and 17.5 Hz for TETRA is in the range of the normal bioelectrical functions both in and between cells, so it may induce low-frequency power surges causing biological effects [69].

In addition, demodulation of these signals would lead to the presence of electric fields at 217 or 17.5 Hz and their harmonics, as well as fields at frequencies relating to the digital stream (tens of kHz). Now, the ICNIRP public exposure guidelines for low-frequency electric fields (4–100 Hz) of 2 mV/m (for tissue of resistivity 1 Ωm) is less than the corresponding guideline at 1 GHz of around 100 V/m. Accordingly, even weak demodulation of mobile phone signals at these fields produces low-frequency electric fields above the protection guidelines [9].

2.7 CONCLUDING REMARKS

Living organisms are complex electrochemical systems that evolved over billions of years in a world with a reasonably weak magnetic field and with few EM energy sources. As is characteristic of living systems, they interacted with and adapted to this environment of EM fields. In recent years there has been a massive introduction of equipment that emits EM fields in an enormous range of new frequencies, modulations, and intensities. The question of how these EM fields, static or low to high frequency interact with biological systems is a complicated subject and of great interest. Scientists with decades of practical experience are actively working to explain how EM fields interact with biological systems and cause biological effects. The explanation may go beyond the belief that EM properties of cells and tissues are prime pillars of EM interaction mechanisms by considering models for the scientific apprehension of life processes in biological systems. Collaboration among experts in biological sciences and engineering is required for reliable EM biological effects studies and successful medical applications.

REFERENCES

1. Frey AH. Evolution and results of biological research with low-intensity nonionizing radiation. In: Marini AA, Editor. *Modern Bioelectricity*. New York: Marcel Dekker, pp. 788–837, 1988.
2. Vander Vorst AV. RF/microwave radiation protection. *TUTB Newslett* 2003; 21: 12–15.
3. Swanson J, Kheifets L. Biophysical mechanisms: a component in the weight of evidence for health effects of power-frequency electric and magnetic fields. *Radiat Res* 2006; 165: 470–478.
4. Foster KR. Electromagnetic field effects and mechanisms. *IEEE Eng Med Biol* 1995; 15: 50–55.
5. King RWP. The interaction of power line electromagnetic fields with the human body. *IEEE Eng Med Biol* 1998; 17: 57–78.
6. Magnussen T. *Electromagnetic Fields*. New York: EMX Corporation, 1999.
7. Ponne CT, Bartels PV. Interaction of electromagnetic energy with biological material— relation to food processing. *Radiat Phys Chem* 1995; 45: 591–607.
8. Habash RWY. *Electromagnetic Fields and Radiation: Human Bioeffects and Safety*. New York: Marcel Dekker, 2001.
9. Challis LJ. Mechanisms for interaction between RF fields and biological tissue. *Bioelectromagnetics* 2005; 25: S98–S105.
10. Anderson LE, Kaune WT. Electric and magnetic fields at extremely low frequencies. In: Suess MJ, Benwell-Morison DA, Editors. *Nonionizing Radiation Protection*. European Series 25. World Health Organization Regional Publications, Geneva, Switzerland, pp. 175–243, 1989.
11. Tenforde TS. Biological interactions and potential health effects of extremely low frequency magnetic fields from power lines and other common sources. *Annu Rev Public Health* 1992; 13: 173–195.
12. Moulder JE. Biological studies of power-frequency fields and carcinogenesis. *IEEE Eng Med Biol* 1995; 15: 31–40.
13. Lai H. Research on the neurological effects of nonionizing radiation at the University of Washington. *Bioelectromagnetics* 1992; 13: 513–525.
14. Dimbylow PJ. FDTD calculations of SAR for a dipole closely coupled to the head at 900 MHz and 1.9 GHz. *Phys Med Biol* 1993; 38: 351–358.
15. Dimbylow PJ, Mann JM. SAR calculations in an anatomically realistic model of the head for mobile communication transceivers at 900 MHz and 1.8 GHz. *Phys Med Biol* 1994; 39: 1527–1553.
16. Martens L, DeMoerloose J, DeWagter C, DeZutter D. Calculation of the electromagnetic fields induced in the head of an operator of a cordless telephone. *Radio Sci* 1995; 30: 283–290.
17. Hurt WD. Multiterm Debye dispersion relations for permittivity of muscle. *IEEE Trans Biomed Eng* 1985; 32: 50–54.
18. Robert P. *Electrical and Magnetic Properties of Materials*. Norwood, MA: Artech House, 1988.
19. Hu CJ, Barnes FS. A simplified theory of pearl chain effects. *Radiat Environ Biophys* 1975; 12: 71–75.
20. Sher LD, Kresch E, Schwan HP. On the possibility of nonthermal biological effects of pulsed electromagnetic radiation. *Biophys J* 1970; 10: 970–979.
21. Saito M, Schwan HP, Schwarz G. Response of nonspherical biological particles to alternating electric fields. *Biophys J* 1955; 5: 313–327.
22. Valberg PA, Kavet R, Rafferty CN. Can low-level 50/50 Hz electric and magnetic fields cause biological effects? *Radiat Res* 1997; 148: 2–21.

23. Reilly JP. Peripheral nerve stimulation by induced electric currents: exposure to time-varying magnetic fields. *Med Biol Eng Comp* 1989; 3: 101–109.
24. Kaune WT, Gillis MF. General properties of the interaction between animals and ELF electric fields. *Bioelectromagnetics* 1981; 2: 1–11.
25. Kirschvink JL, Kobayashi-Kirschvink A, Diaz-Rioci JC, Kirschvink SJ. Magnetite in human tissue: a mechanism for the biological effect of weak ELF magnetic fields. *Bioelectromagnetics* 1992; 13: S101–S113.
26. Adair PK. Constraints of thermal noise on the effects of weak 50 Hz magnetic fields acting on biological magnetite. *Proc Natl Acad Sci USA* 1994; 91: 2925–2929.
27. Vaughan TE, Weaver JC. Energetic constraints on the creation of cell membrane pores by magnetic particles. *Biophys J* 1995; 71: 515–522.
28. Vaughan TE, Weaver JC. Molecular change due to biomagnetic stimulation and transient magnetic fields: mechanical interference constraints on possible effects by cell membrane pore creation via magnetic particles. *Bioelectrochem Bioenerg* 1998; 45: 121–128.
29. Blankenship RE, Schaafsma TJ, Parson WW. Magnetic field effects on radical pair intermediates in bacterial photosynthesis. *Biochim Biophys Acta* 1977; 451: 297–305.
30. Cozens FL, Scaiano JC. A comparative study of magnetic field effects on the dynamics of geminate and random radical pair processes in micelles. *J Am Chem Soc* 1993; 115: 5204–5211.
31. Scaiano JC, Mohtat N, Cozens L, McLean J, Thansandote A. Application of the radical pair mechanism to free radicals in organized systems: can the effect of 50 Hz be predicted from studies under static fields? *Bioelectromagnetics* 1994; 15: 549–554.
32. Walleczek J. Magnetokinetic effects on radical pairs: a paradigm for magnetic field interactions with biological systems at lower than thermal energy. In: Blank M, Editor. *Advances in Chemistry Series: Electromagnetic Fields. Biological Interactions and Mechanisms.* Washington: American Chemical Society, pp. 395–420, 1995.
33. Brocklehurst B, McLauchlan KA. Free radical mechanism for the effects of environmental electromagnetic fields on biological systems. *Int J Rad Biol* 1995; 59: 3–24.
34. Byus CV, Pieper SE, Adey WR. The effects of low-energy 50 Hz environmental electromagnetic fields upon the growth-related enzyme ornithine decarboxylase. *Carcinogenesis* 1987; 8: 1385–1389.
35. Litovitz TA, Krause D, Mullins JM. Effect of coherence time of the applied magnetic field on ornithine decarboxylase activity. *Biochem Biophys Res Comm* 1991; 178: 852–855.
36. Adair PK. Constraints on biological effects of weak extremely low frequency electromagnetic fields. *Phys Rev Lett* 1991; A43: 1039–1048.
37. Cain CD, Thomas DL, Adey WR. 50-Hz magnetic field acts as co-promoter in focus formation of C3H10T1/2 cells. *Carcinogenesis* 1993; 14: 955–960.
38. Kolomytkin O, Yurinska M, Zharikov S, Kuznetsov V, Zharikova A. Response of brain receptor systems to microwave energy exposure. In: Frey AH, Editor. *Nature of Electromagnetic Field Interactions with Biological Systems.* Austin, TX: RG Landes, pp. 195–205, 1994.
39. Eichwald C, Walleczek J. Magnetic field perturbations as a tool for controlling enzyme-regulated and oscillatory biochemical reactions. *Biophys Chem* 1998; 74: 209–224.
40. Adey WR. Cell membranes: the electromagnetic environment and cancer promotion. *Neurochem Res* 1988; 13: 571–577.
41. Rubinsky B. Cryosurgery. *Annu Rev Biomed Eng* 2000; 02: 157–187.
42. Meyer R. *In vitro* experiments dealing with the biological effects of RF fields at low energies, COST 244 bis project. *Forum on Future European Research on Mobile Communications and Health*, pp. 39–47, 19–20 April 1999.
43. Cherry N. *Criticism of the Health Assessment in the ICNIRP Guidelines for Radio-Frequency and Microwave Radiation (100 kHz–300 GHz).* New Zealand: Lincoln University, 2000.

44. Lednev VV. Possible mechanism for the influence of weak magnetic fields on biological systems. *Bioelectromagnetics* 1992; 12: 71–75.

45. Koch BCL, Sommarin M, Persson BR, Salford LG, Eberhardt JL. Interaction between weak low frequency magnetic fields and cell membranes. *Bioelectromagnetics* 2003; 24: 395–402.

46. Lednev VV. Possible mechanisms for the effect of weak magnetic fields on biological systems: correction of the basic expression and its consequences. In: Blank M, Editor. *Electricity and Magnetism in Biology and Medicine*. San Francisco, CA: San Francisco Press, pp. 550–552, 1993.

47. Blanchard JP, Blackman CF. Clarification and application of an ion parametric resonance model for magnetic field interaction with biological systems. *Bioelectromagnetics* 1994; 15: 217–238.

48. Blank M, Goodman R. Comment: a niological guide for electromagnetic safety: the stress response. *Bioelectromagnetics* 2004; 25: 542–545.

49. Bohr H, Bohr J. Microwave enhanced kinetics observed in ORD studies of a protein. *Bioelectromagnetics* 2000; 21: 58–72.

50. Laurence JA, French PW, Lindner RA, McKenzie DR. Biological effects of electromagnetic fields—mechanisms for the effects of pulsed microwave radiation on protein conformation. *J Theor Biol* 2000; 205: 291–298.

51. Chiabrera A, Bianco B, Moggia E, Kaufman JJ. Zeeman–Stark modeling of the RF EMF interaction with ligand binding. *Bioelectromagnetics* 2000; 21: 312–324.

52. Thompson CJ, Yang YS, Anderson V, Wood AW. A cooperative model for Ca^{++} efflux windowing from cell membranes exposed to electromagnetic radiation. *Bioelectromagnetics* 21: 455–464.

53. Foster KR, Baish JW. Viscous damping of vibrations in microtub. *J Biolog Phys* 2000; 25: 255–260.

54. Adair PK. Vibrational resonances in biological systems at microwave frequencies. *Biophys J* 2002; 2: 1147–1152.

55. Moulder JE. Power lines and cancer FAQs. In: *Electromagnetic Fields and Human Health*. Medical College of Wisconsin, Milwaukee, Wisc, USA, 1999.

56. Elder JA. Radiofrequency radiation activities and issues: a 1985 perspective. *Health Phys* 1987; 53: 507–511.

57. Michaelson SM, Lin JC. *Biological Effects and Health Implications of Radiofrequency Radiation*. New York: Plenum Press, 1987.

58. Prader A, Largo RH, Molinari L, Issler C. Physical growth of Swiss children from birth to 20 years of age. First Zurich longitudinal study of growth and development. *Helv Paediatr Acta* 1989; 43(Suppl 52): 1–25.

59. Koenig WJ, Donovan JM, Pensler JM. Cranial bone grafting in children. *Plast Reconstr Surg* 1995; 1: 1–4.

60. Simonson TM, Kao SC. Normal childhood developmental patterns in skull bone marrow by MR imaging. *Prediatr Radiol* 1992; 22: 556–559.

61. Cook MR, Graham C, Cohen HD, Gerkovich MM. A replication study of human exposure to 50-Hz fields: effects on neurological measures. *Bioelectromagnetics* 1992; 13: 251–285.

62. Graham C, Cook MR, Cohen HD, Gerkovich MM. Dose response study of human exposure to 50 Hz electric and magnetic fields. *Bioelectromagnetics* 1994; 15: 447–453.

63. Grasson M, Legros JJ, Scarpa P, Legros W. 50 Hz magnetic field exposure influence on human performance and psychophysiological parameters; two double-blind experimental studies. *Bioelectromagnetics* 1999; 20: 474–486.

64. Lin JC. The blood–brain barrier, cancer, cell phones, and microwave radiation. *IEEE Microw Mag* 2001; 2: 25–30.

65. Lin JC. Microwave radiation and leakage of albumin from blood to brain. *IEEE Micro Mag* 2004; 4: 22–27.
66. Goldman RI, Stern JM, Engel J Jr., Cohen MS. Simultaneous EEG and fMRI of the alpha rhythm. *Neuroreport* 2002; 13: 2487–2492.
67. Oakes TR, Pizzagalli DA, Hendrick AM, Horras KA, Larson CL, Abercrombie HC, Schaefer SM, Koger JV. Functional coupling of simultaneous electrical and metabolic activity in the human brain. *Hum Brain Map* 2005; 21: 257–270.
68. Cook CM, Saucier DM, Thomas AW, Prato FS. Exposure to ELF magnetic and ELF-modulated radiofrequency fields: the time course of physiological and cognitive effects observed in recent studies (2001–2005). *Bioelectromagnetics* 2006; 27: 613–627.
69. Habash RWH, Brodsky LM, Leiss W, Krewski DK, Repacholi M. Health risk of electromagnetic fields. Part II: Evaluation and assessment of radio frequency radiation. *Crit Rev Biomed Eng* 2003; 31: 197–254.

Part I

Health Risks of Electromagnetic Energy

3 Guidelines and Measurement for Electric and Magnetic Fields

3.1 INTRODUCTION

Just as coal enabled the industrial revolution, *electricity* is the unseen fuel of modern life. The use of electricity results in the production of electric and magnetic fields (EMF). There are two types of EMF classified according to the frequency range: ELF fields and VLF fields. ELF fields are defined as those having frequencies up to 3 kHz while VLF fields cover the frequency range 3–30 kHz. Because of the quasi-static nature of the EM fields at these frequencies, electric and magnetic fields act independently of one another and are measured separately. Electric fields created by voltage and measured in volts per meter are present whenever an electric appliance is plugged in. The appliance need not be turned on for electric fields to be detected. Magnetic fields, induced by alternating current and measured using the derived quantity magnetic flux density in Tesla or Gauss, are present when the appliance is turned on. The strength of EMF decreases as we move away from their sources. EMF exposure is commonly found in and around our homes and offices [1].

Electric and magnetic fields can occur separately or together, and accordingly it is possible for humans to be exposed to just one of these fields or both of them. For example, when a power cord is plugged into a socket outlet it creates an electric field along the cord. When the lamp is turned on, the flow of current through the cord creates a magnetic field; and the greater the current, the stronger the magnetic field. In the meantime, the electric field is still present.

It is possible for humans to be exposed to various levels of EMF. Power transmission lines, for example, generate both strong electric and magnetic fields. However, distribution lines generate weak electric fields but can generate strong magnetic fields, depending on the number of houses they supply.

Although electric and magnetic fields often occur together, most of the concern has focused on the potential health effects of magnetic fields. The basis for this concern is that magnetic fields are difficult to shield, and easily penetrate buildings and people, contrary to electric fields, which have very little ability to penetrate buildings or even human skin. Because the use of electricity is ubiquitous and plays a vital role in a society's economic capability, the possibility of harm from EMF to electric utility customers and workers deserves attention.

Whether or not there are health consequences associated with the EMF emanating from the generation, distribution, and utilization of electricity is a controversial issue, in which the tension between risks versus indispensable advantage comes into play. This is a common debate when complex environmental issues with considerable health and economic outcomes are scientifically analyzed. There are also economic consequences; for example, electrical utilities sometimes have had to redirect high-voltage power lines around populated areas and even stop their construction. The real estate industry is also increasingly concerned with issues related to EMF exposure. These include equipment interference, potential liability, property valuation, premises abandonment, and tenant concerns about potential health effects. Concerns about hazards have often pushed manufacturers to improve products by providing better shielding, which has a positive impact on the EM compatibility and performance of the product itself. The cost–benefit ratio for making such improvements is always a concern, but at the same time it is useful to note that endangering public trust is very important too.

This chapter provides a review of potential health risks associated with exposure to EMF. The review considers exposure guidelines, dosimetry, and field measurement surveys.

3.2 EXPOSURE GUIDELINES

Several decades of research in the area of bioelectromagnetics have led to a scientific consensus on the safety of EM fields. Expert committees reflect this consensus when developing exposure guidelines. For the purpose of this book, "safety standard" is a standard specifying measurable field values that limit human exposure to levels below those deemed hazardous to human health [2]. These standards consist of regulations, recommendations, and guidelines that would not endanger human health. The development of safety standards presupposes a few procedures, including (1) systematic review of the scientific literature, (2) identification of the health hazards and risk assessment, and (3) selection of maximum permissible exposure (MPE) values that produce an environment free from hazard.

Hazard can be an object or a set of circumstances that could potentially harm a person's health. Risk is the likelihood, or probability, that a person will be harmed by a particular hazard [3]. The more clearly the hazard is understood, the sooner a safety procedure can be established. In the end, safety is a social choice that people, governments, and organizations make. It assumes that the cost–benefit ratio is favorable, and that an option for minimizing exposure exists.

In relation to EM human health effects, most scientific information obtained from cellular and animal studies provides the foundation for assessing potential risks to humans. Studies in humans provide direct information regarding health effects and help validate animal studies. Epidemiological studies are more likely to provide information regarding the nature of the effect rather than provide detailed exposure-response or dose-response information. When extrapolating data from animals to develop exposure limits for humans, adjustments are usually needed to account for several potential limitations in the process [4].

The results from these studies permit the identification of MPE values indicating that below a threshold, an EM field level is safe according to available scientific knowledge. The permissible level is not an exact line between safety and hazard. However, no adverse effects exist below this defined limit and possible health risk increases with higher exposure level. Often, the MPE level is coupled with a "safety

TABLE 3.1

Maximum Permissible Exposure Values for Electric and Magnetic Fields

Year: Standard	Magnetic Field Safety Level	
1992: ANSI/IEEE	205 μT	
1993: NRPB	50 Hz, 1600 μT	
	60 Hz, 1330 μT	
1998: ICNIRP	General Public	Occupational
	83.3 μT	420 μT
1999: The Swedish Standard	Video Display Terminals	
	ELF (5 Hz–2 kHz): ≤0.2 μT	
	VLF (2 kHz–400 kHz): ≤0.025 μT	
1999: Safety Code 6	General Public	Occupational
	2.75 μT	6.15 μT
2002: ARPANSA	General Public	Occupational
	3 kHz–100 kHz: 6.1 μT	3 kHz–100 kHz: 31.4 μT

Note:　0.1 μT = 1 mG.

or uncertainty factor." This would imply that a safety limit in a standard is set just below the injury threshold (many times lower) for a sensitive individual. The incorporation of a suitable safety factor provides protection for both occupational and residential environments. This is because people in occupational settings can carry out risk analysis and risk management more accurately, whereas the public environment is less controlled and usually individual members of the public are unaware of their exposure. Moreover, the public may be regularly exposed and may not adequately be expected to take precautions to reduce or avoid the exposure.

Many institutions and organizations throughout the world have recommended safety limits for EMF exposure. These include the Institute of Electrical and Electronic Engineers (IEEE) [5–8], the National Radiological Protection Board (NRPB) of the United Kingdom [9–11], the International Commission on Nonionizing Radiation Protection (ICNIRP) [12–14], the Swedish Radiation Protection Institute [15], Health Canada [16], and the Australian Radiation Protection and Nuclear Safety Agency (ARPANSA) [17]. Table 3.1 shows various MPE values for EMF exposure [18–20].

Most of the exposure guidelines use a two-tier standard, indicating a basic restriction in terms of *current density* (J) and corresponding investigation levels or reference levels in terms of external field strengths. The exposure limits range from a few microteslas up to 1600 μT. The levels for those occupationally involved in various electrical industries are set higher than those for the general public.

3.2.1　Institute of Electrical and Electronics Engineers

The first formal standards project was initiated in 1960 when the American Standards Association (now the American National Standards Institute, or ANSI) approved the Radiation Hazards Standards project. This project, under the cosponsorship of the Department of the Navy and the Institute of Radio Engineers (now the IEEE), included the establishment of Committee C95, which published its first standard in 1966 [21]; revisions of the standard were published in 1974 [22] and 1982 [23]. In 1988, the C95 committee continued its work as Standards Coordinating Committee 28 (SCC28) under the sponsorship of the IEEE Standards Board (now the IEEE Standards Association Standards Board, or SASB) and established the ANSI/IEEE C95.1-1991 standard [5–8,24].

The ANSI/IEEE C95.1-1991 standard recommends that exposure averaged over any six-minute period and over a cross section of the human body should not exceed 0.614 kV/m for the electric field and 163 A/m (205 μT) for the magnetic field. The ANSI/IEEE standard is designed to keep the induced current in human body at least a factor of ten below the lowest reported stimulation thresholds for electrically excitable cells.

A document by the International Commission for Electromagnetic Safety (ICES) (IEEE C95.6-2002) [25] that covers human exposure to EMF (0–3 kHz) has been released. Recommendations are given to prevent harmful effects in human beings exposed to ELF fields. The recommendations are intended to apply to exposures of the general public, as well as to individuals in controlled environments. They are not intended to apply to the purposeful exposure of patients by or under the direction of practitioners of the healing arts and may not be protective with respect to the use of medical devices or implants. The basic restrictions and MPE values are derived to avoid (1) painful stimulation of sensory neurons, (2) muscle excitation that might lead to injuries while performing potentially hazardous activities, (3) excitation of neurons within the brain, (4) cardiac excitation that might lead to fibrillation, and (5) magneto-hydrodynamic effects.

3.2.2 NATIONAL RADIOLOGICAL PROTECTION BOARD

The NRPB provides information and advice to officials in the United Kingdom responsible for the protection from radiation hazards either in the population as a whole or within population subgroups. The recommended NRPB guidelines [9–11] are the same for occupational and public environments. The basic restriction specified by the NRPB is an induced current density of 10 mA/m^2 in the head and trunk while the investigation levels for EMF exposure at 50 Hz are 12 kV/m and 1600 μT, respectively [26].

3.2.3 INTERNATIONAL COMMISSION ON NONIONIZING RADIATION PROTECTION

The ICNIRP's mission is to coordinate knowledge of protection against various nonionizing exposures in the development of internationally accepted recommendations. The ICNIRP guidelines [12–14] specify "basic restrictions" and "reference levels." Basic restrictions on exposure to magnetic fields are based on established adverse health effects. For magnetic fields below 100 kHz, the physical quantity used to specify the basic restrictions is current density induced inside the body. Reference levels are values that are provided for practical exposure assessment purposes to determine whether the basic restrictions are likely to be exceeded. Compliance with the reference levels is designed to ensure compliance with the relevant basic restriction [14].

In 1999, the Council of the European Union issued recommendations concerning exposure of the general public to EM fields. The restrictions are based on the ICNIRP guidelines [27] for the general public (with a basic restriction of 2 mA/m^2). However, many European states have introduced lower precautionary-based exposure limits, such as Italy (2 µT) in 1998 and Switzerland (1 µT) in 1999. The above exposure limits are significantly below those designed to protect against acute effects.

3.2.4 SWEDISH STANDARDS

Sweden has been a leader in developing recommended visual ergonomic and EM emission standards for computer displays. Two prominent measurement and emission guidelines for monitors have emerged during the past few years. One, known as MPR-II, prescribes limits on EMF emissions in the ELF and VLF ranges, as well as electrostatic fields. Many major manufacturers of computer displays have embraced the Swedish guidelines. Nevertheless, the Swedish Confederation of Professional Employees (TCO), which represents over a million workers, requested more restrictive limits and test protocols. TCO published its own series of guidelines: TCO'90, TCO'92, TCO'95, and TCO'99, which in reality are a copy of MPR-II with some adjustments [15]. In addition, recent TCO guidelines include guidelines for energy consumption, screen flicker, luminance, and keyboard use.

3.2.5 RESTRICTIONS

Most of the above exposure guidelines are based on recognized and reproducible interactions between EMF and the human body. The observed effects were all acute effects of EMF exposure on excitable tissue, such as nerve and muscle. The basic restriction in all exposure guidelines has, to date, been specified in terms of induced current density as the principal measure of interaction of EMF with the body rather than the more directly relevant internal electric field. The use of current density originated for the pragmatic reason that data were more readily available in terms of current density than electric field. The data used in the early days to determine the thresholds for nerve and muscle tended to be investigated using injected currents, with the current density being calculated from the injected current on the basis of the geometry without requiring conductivity information [26]. Other investigators suggested the use of internal electric field as a basic restriction in future EMF exposure guidelines [28–30].

3.3 MEASUREMENT TECHNIQUES

To realize electric and magnetic fields, a common lamp is a good example for consideration. Electric fields are present when the lamp is plugged in, while magnetic fields are created when the lamp is plugged in and turned on, as illustrated in Figure 3.1.

3.3.1 FREQUENCY AND OBJECT SIZE

Electric and magnetic fields near a source are characterized by frequency. Therefore, any measurement of ELF fields should likely be frequency weighted. This means it

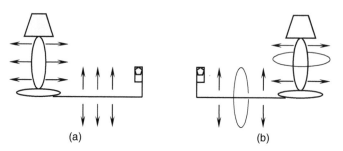

FIGURE 3.1   (a) Lamp off. (b) Lamp on.

should read the product of electric or magnetic field strength times the frequency. This frequency weighting should extend up to about 1000 Hz and then sensitivity should decrease at higher frequencies. To understand this, consider an external electric field of 20 kV/m at 50/60 Hz. This will produce high current inside the body. This current is proportional to field strength times the frequency. At 100/120 Hz (twice the frequency), only half as much field strength (10 kV/m) is necessary to produce the same current inside the body.

Another matter to be considered has to do with how magnetic fields (and not electric fields) induce current in the body. The current per area induced is proportional to field strength, frequency, conductivity, and length of the body. That is why children exposed to magnetic fields experience less current per area than do adults, and lab rats experience about 1/10 as much. The multiplication by body length does not apply to electric fields; as a result, both children and adults would experience the same current when exposed to them. A reasonably strong magnetic field (about 500 mG) and electric field (about 2 kV/m) exist in nature, but these fields are static ($f = 0$); hence they produce no current inside the body.

As discussed in previous chapters, the nature of electric fields is different from that of magnetic fields. Therefore, different measuring procedures are necessary to assess emission levels for each type of field. In fact, there are standard procedures that have already been fixed for the measurement of both electric and magnetic fields.

3.3.2   Electric Field Measurements

Electric fields exist between objects that are at different electric potentials, or voltages. For example, if a 9 V battery is connected to two metal plates at a given distance apart, an electric field will exist between them and is given by voltage divided by the distance, or 9 V/m. The measurement and calculation of such fields are quite complex. Although several techniques of measurement are available, the common one is the root-mean-square (RMS) average—taking the maximum field strength reading in three planes and extracting the square root of the sum of the squares of the individual readings. If the field is oscillating at a constant frequency, an electric field meter can be set such that it has the maximum sensitivity at that frequency. However, if the field is composed of different frequencies, as is the case of video display terminal (VDT) and other appliances, there will be a need for a limited number of frequencies to be measured. The range of frequencies, which is allowed in the RMS average, is called the *bandwidth* of the instrument.

Electric field measurements are performed with displacement current sensors that operate on the basis of measuring displacement current that flows between two closely spaced electrodes immersed inside the electric field. The sensors are placed on a nonmetallic tripod to prevent the influence of the operator's body on the measured field value. Commercially available meters are sufficient for measurement near power lines and other sources. They are not suitable for measurements in laboratories because of their size. Yet, smaller meters are also available [6]. To avoid the error of field perturbation caused by the body of the person holding the meter during measurement, a horizontal distance of at least 2.5 m should be maintained between the person and the meter.

3.3.3 MAGNETIC FIELD MEASUREMENTS

Magnetic fields in the environment come from a number of sources. The level of these fields is called *background level*. The background level of schools, hospitals, homes, and workplaces is always increasing due to the rapid increase in the use of electricity. The background field must be considered while measuring the magnetic field from a particular source. Before any assessment of emissions from the source is possible, it is important to define the background field in the place. To do that, the source under measurement must be turned off and readings in the surrounding area must be taken. If the background field is relatively high (i.e., above 5 mG), the contribution of the assigned appliance to the environment may be unmeasurable. Because of this fact, the Swedish specification MPR-II requires the background levels to be no greater than 0.4 mG for the measurement to be valid.

Differences among magnetic field meters are considerable. A good meter shows the strength of the field, its direction, and polarization of the magnetic field. The meter should measure fields in one direction at a time and display the maximum field strength at that location. However, a person under the exposure of the field is receiving the field from all directions.

To determine the maximum magnetic flux density at a particular location, the meter should be rotated through all possible angles so that the field can intersect with the sensor in such a way as to display the maximum reading. This means the maximum flux density in three orthogonal planes (B_x, B_y, and B_z) is measured and the resultant B_r, which is equal to the square root of the sum of the squares of the individual reading, is extracted [31].

To measure the polarization of the magnetic field, the user must adjust the orientation of the meter until the reading reaches a maximum (B_{max}). The field is linearly polarized when $B_r = B_{max}$, and circularly polarized when $B_r = 1.41 B_{max}$. The degree of polarization B_d is expressed by the axial ratio between the major and minor axes of the field ellipse. It is given by [1]

$$B_d = \sqrt{(B_r/B_{max})^2 - 1} \qquad (3.1)$$

Meters must be calibrated before use. The calibration of these instruments must be traceable to a particular standard. Portable calibrators are usually available. Users must follow the recommendations of both the calibrator and the meter manufacturer.

3.3.4 SIMPLIFIED METERS

To eliminate concerns, homes and offices should be checked using a simplified ELF-magnetic field meter, available from several vendors at a low price. One such device is the Gauss meter. Gauss is a common unit of measurement of AC magnetic field strength. Still, some engineers prefer Tesla as a unit of measurement (e.g., 1 μT = 10 mG). Inside the Gauss meter there is a coil of thin wire, typically with thousands of turns. As the magnetic field emanates through the coil it induces a current, which is amplified by the electronic circuitry inside the Gauss meter. If the Gauss meter has an induction coil with approximately 40,000 turns, a relatively low magnetic field strength of 1 mG would induce enough current to be read directly with a voltmeter. It is more practical, however, to build a Gauss meter with fewer turns and through operational amplification circuitry to increase the voltage or current and then calibrate the meter to read either in Gauss or milligauss.

It is necessary to take three perpendicular readings, one for each axis. It is better to always take the readings in the same order. For example, take the first reading in the x-axis direction. For the second reading, rotate the meter 90° and take the y-axis reading. For the third reading, rotate the meter 90° and take the z-axis reading. Once the readings are completed, it is possible to calculate a single combined reading by squaring the reading for each axis, adding the three squared numbers, and then taking the square root of the sum. For example, suppose the observed x, y, and z readings from the Gauss meter are 5, 6, and 7 mG, respectively. To find the combined field strength, carry out the following calculation:

$$\text{Square root of total} = \sqrt{25+36+49} = 10.488 \text{ mG}$$

It is not necessary to be so precise as to actually use the formula, especially if the highest reading on one axis is much stronger than the rest. For example, readings of 3, 0.4, and 0.5 mG would result in combined field strength of about 3.067 mG. Thus, just by using the dominant axis reading, the result is nearly the same as carrying out the calculation. In case the readings for each axis are close to each other, the combined reading can be as much as 73% more than any one axis.

Niple et al. [32] developed a portable meter for measuring low frequency currents in the human body. Contact currents flow when the human body provides a conductive path between objects in the environment with different electrical potentials. The range of currents the meter detects is approximately 0.4–800 μA. Figure 3.2 shows a contact current model with a meter. The meter measures the voltage between four different points on the human body. Ideally, these are the two wrists and two ankles, although almost any points can be chosen. With these voltages and

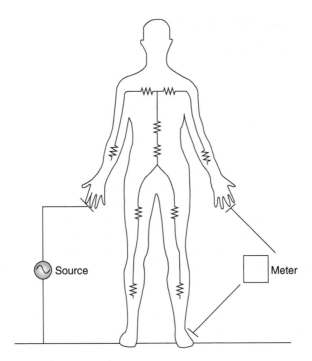

FIGURE 3.2   Contact current model.

information on the impedance of the body between the points, calculations of currents can be made.

3.4   MEASUREMENT SURVEYS

Engineering contributions in the field of EM risk have made it possible to assess the field strength or power density due to exposure from an EM source and check its compliance with exposure guidelines. Theoretical calculations are adequate in some situations; but measurements often prove more conclusive and less expensive, particularly at multiple-source sites. Therefore, theoretical calculations, particularly computational methods, are often not enough to assess compliance with safety limits. For this reason, EM measurements are usually performed to assure compliance with relevant guidelines to prevent overexposure conditions that could pose short- and long-term health problems. Measurements are also needed when the calculated fields are close to the threshold for overexposure or when fields are likely to be distorted by reflection from various objects [1]. In addition, assessment of EMF exposure levels for the general public and those associated with particular occupations provides the required background information for epidemiological assessment of disease risk. Major difficulties with respect to exposure assessment include the lack of knowledge about a relevant metric and the relevant induction period, the incomplete characterization of exposure sources, and the inability to combine exposures from different sources into one metric [33].

3.4.1   SOURCES OF EMF EXPOSURE

3.4.1.1   Residential Areas

Any residential or occupational site is subject to coincident exposure from many EMF sources external and internal to the site itself. External sources include high-voltage transmission lines, distribution lines, underground cables, substations, transformers, wiring and grounding systems, and transportation systems. In the workplace, sources of EMF include ground pathways, building wiring, and electrical devices such as computers, fax machines, copy machines, fluorescent lights, printers, scanners, telephone switching systems, motors, induction heaters, electronic article surveillance (EAS), demagnetizers, security systems, and metal detectors. In homes, there are two immediate sources of EMF. The first type includes internal wiring, meters, service panels, subpanels, and grounding systems. The second type includes electrical appliances such as electric blankets, electric waterbed heaters, hair dryers, electric shavers, television (TV) sets, VDTs, stereo systems, air conditioners, fluorescent lights, refrigerators, blenders, portable heaters, washers and dryers, coffee makers, vacuum cleaners, toasters, and other household appliances.

EMF exposures within residences vary from over 150 µT and 200 V/m a few centimeters from certain appliances to less than 0.02 µT and 2 V/m in the center of many rooms. Appliances that have the highest magnetic fields are those with high currents or high-speed electric motors (e.g., vacuum cleaners, microwave ovens, electric washing machines, dishwashers, blenders, can openers, electric shavers) [34]. Background magnetic fields are in general between 0.1 and 0.3 µT.

In residential areas, maintaining a distance from visible ELF–EMF sources may be relatively easy, but avoiding fields generated by concealed wiring is much more difficult. Furthermore, because concrete cannot block ELF–EMF and because the floor of one apartment serves as the ceiling of another, ELF–EMF from wiring in an apartment may reach the residents of adjacent apartments [35–37]. Apartment residents may therefore be at greater risk of exposure to ELF–EMF than residents of detached houses [38].

3.4.1.2   Power Lines and Cables

Underneath overhead power lines, the average magnetic flux density can be up to 30 µT for multiconductor 765 kV lines and 10 µT for 380 kV lines. Around power plants, average fields may be as high as 40 µT. Certain occupational environments may encounter magnetic fields of up to 130 milliteslas (mT). Actual magnetic fields depend on distance, voltage, current, and wire arrangement. However, actual electric fields are affected only by distance, voltage, and wire arrangement.

Exposures from arc welders and electrical cable splicers may exceed 100 µT and 5000 V/m. Exposure to power-frequency EMF is poorly correlated in occupational settings. Electric trains can also be a major source of exposure, as magnetic fields at seat height in passenger cars can be as high as 60 µT [39].

3.4.2   SITE SURVEYS

Safety regulations stipulate field limits in occupational and public environments, and thus there is a need for field measurement surveys. Such surveys are usually performed for one or more of the following reasons: (1) to evaluate a space where electrical devices are being greatly affected by electrical installation systems or other electromagnetic interference (EMI) sources, (2) to evaluate the impact of power lines or other electrical facilities and to provide guidance in the installation of further structures, (3) to assess the exposure conditions in homes or offices to assure compliance with relevant safety standards, and (4) to prevent overexposure conditions that may pose short- and long-term health problems.

A complete survey of any site requires measurements of personal exposure and background fields. Before any assessment of emissions from the EMF source is possible, it is important to define the background field. This is accomplished by turning off the source under measurement and taking readings from the surrounding area. If the background field is relatively high (above 0.5 μT), the contribution of the assigned appliance to the environment may be undetectable.

The instruments used to measure EMF are well developed, especially those designed to measure magnetic fields. Besides simple handheld survey meters, there are now portable personal meters that are able to record and illustrate the various characteristics of field exposure. There are three common types of field survey: spot, contour, and dosimetric. A spot survey, suitable for residential and small commercial sites, collects data in spots such as the center of an area or other selected points and arranges these data in a table format, referenced to a layout of the surveyed area. A contour survey is suitable for most commercial applications and assessment of outdoor areas, especially near power lines. In that sense, the mapping wheel is a suitable tool to conduct this survey. A dosimetric survey collects field data at a fixed point in an area (residential or workplace) in timed increments over a defined period (hours or days). It is useful to monitor the variation of fields and record the peaks in certain areas over various periods of time.

An important step in the process of measurement is to classify the area under investigation either as occupational or public. Such distinction is necessary before measurements are carried out, to ensure that proper exposure levels are used for evaluation and comparison.

Various measurement surveys have been conducted in North America [40–44], Europe [45–55], and Japan [56] (Table 3.2). In North America, power systems operate at a frequency of 60 Hz. However, utilities in Europe, Asia, and other places in the world supply users with 50 Hz of electrical power. This means that North American systems are associated with higher currents and accordingly higher magnetic fields. Nevertheless, levels of EMF vary from location to location, country to country, or continent to continent due to the power system used as well as the type of appliances and wiring practices.

3.4.3   ELECTRIC APPLIANCES

Electric and magnetic fields from particular appliances may vary greatly, depending on the way they are designed and manufactured. Surveys were conducted to measure

TABLE 3.2
Summary of EMF Measurement Surveys

Author	Country	Type of Study	Results
Zaffanella, 1993	USA	Residential Spot (900 homes)	Median field: 0.06 μT (28% > 0.1 μT; 11% > 0.2 μT; 2% > 0.5 μT).
Zaffanella and Kalton, 1998	USA	24-hour personal	Average field: 0.09 μT (44% > 0.1 μT; 14% > 0.2 μT; 2.5% > 0.5 μT, less than 1% >0.75 μT.
Kaune et al., 2000	USA	Occurrence of magnetic field events with 2–200 kHz (156 homes)	Homes located in rural surroundings had less transient events (3.3 nT and 33 nT) than homes in suburban/urban areas.
Kelsh et al., 2003	USA (California and New York)	Personal and survey; garment workers (three different sites)	Mean personal measurements at the waist for sewing ranged from 0.18 to 3.1 μT and survey measurements ranged from 0.10 to 2.7 μT.
Deadman et al., 1999	Canada (five provinces)	24-hour average exposure of children	Geometric mean (GM): 0.085 mT (15% > 0.2 mT). GM: 12.3 V/m. Quebec had the highest levels of fields; Alberta had the lowest. Electric heating, air conditioning, and housing type appeared to be useful predictors of magnetic field exposures.
Juutilainen et al., 1989	Finland (Kupio)	Residential (37 homes)	24-hour GM: 60 nT.
Preece et al., 1996	UK (Avon)	Spot and personal (50 homes)	Mean: 0.011–0.023 μT; Overall mean (0.017 ± 0.003) μT with the power "on." Mean: 0.008–0.015 μT: Overall mean (0.012 ± 0.002) μT with power "off."
Vistnes et al., 1997	Norway (Oslo)	Personal (65 school children living 28–325 m away from a 300 kV line)	24-hour GM: 15 nT.
Clinard et al., 1999	France (French dwellings)	Residential	GM < 0.010 μT for both indoor and outdoor measurements (only 5% > 0.12 μT).
Brix et al., 2001	Germany (Bavaria)	Personal (1952 people)	For 50 Hz: Mean = 0.101 μT; individual medians = 0.047 μT. For people living next to railway lines (16.66 Hz): Mean = 0.156 μT; median = 0.102 μT.
Tardón et al., 2002	Spain (Oviedo; Barcelona)	Environmental (50 schools)	Median: 0.015 μT in Oviedo, 0.016 μT in Barcelona. Average exposure, however, was higher in Barcelona (mean 0.057 μT) than in Oviedo (mean 0.017 μT). In playgrounds, the median level was 0.0095 μT and the maximum was 0.46 μT.

Reference	Country	Setting	Description
Forssen et al., 2002	Sweden (Stockholm)	Personal (97 adults and children)	For adults living close to power lines, the level of exposure at work was exceeded by the residential exposure. For subjects living >100 m from the line, the situation was the opposite. Even if the subjects were highly exposed (≥0.2 μT) at work/school, they spent 71% of their total time in fields <0.1 μT if the level of exposure at home was low (0.1 μT).
Yoshitomi, 2002	Japan	Residential (apartment electrical wiring)	Whole areas of several bedrooms were continuously exposed to 0.4–1.5 μT. The sources of these fields were 300 A, 100 V service drop wires and a service panel box on an exterior wall.
Ptitsyna et al., 2003	Russia and Switzerland	Occupational (Russian DC and Swiss AC powered 16.67 Hz electric trains)	Levels of quasi-static magnetic fields (0.001–0.03 Hz) were in the range 40 μT. Maximum levels of 120 μT were found in DC powered locomotives. At frequencies lower than 15 Hz, the average magnetic field generated by Swiss AC powered locomotives was 10 times greater than fields observed in Russian DC powered trains.
Jesús et al., 2004	Spain	Urban environment	The values of the spot measurements taken in the streets were all below the ICNIRP reference level, although 30% surpassed 0.2 μT.
Moriyama and Yoshitomi, 2005	Japan	Residential (apartment electrical wiring)	ELF magnetic fields were measured in a room with dimensions of $6.70 \times 4.40 \times 2.84$ m. The building consisted of 256 apartments. Magnetic fields were greater than 0.4 μT in 38% (floor level), 13% (0.5 m), 0% (1.00 m), 8% (1.50 m), 41% (2.00 m), and 40% (2.50 m) of the horizontal plane areas. The maximum value found in the floor space was 1.8 μT.
Szabó et al., 2006	Hungary	Occupational sewing machine operators	The average duration of the measurement periods was 449 min (range 420–470). The average arithmetic mean exposure for all women was 0.76 μT (range 0.06–4.27). The average of maximum values was 4.30 μT (range 0.55–14.80). Women working with older sewing machines experienced higher exposure than women working on newer sewing machines.
Szabó et al., 2007	Hungary	Residential; spot; exposure from transformer stations	The mean home and bed personal exposure above transformers was 0.825 and 1.033 μT, respectively.
Kaune et al., 2000	USA (Washington, DC, and Maryland)	Appliances (72 TV sets used by children to watch TV and 34 TV sets used to play video games)	GM: 0.0091 μT (ELF) and 0.0016 μT (VLF), respectively, for children watching TV programs. GM: 0.023 μT (ELF) and 0.0038 μT (VLF), respectively, for children playing video games.
Kaune et al., 2002	USA	Electric appliances headsets; home sewing machines	Fields near headsets at less than 60 Hz<0.01 μT. Home sewing machines produced magnetic fields >2.8 over ambient levels at the front surfaces of the lower abdomens of mothers.

fields from common appliances such as TV sets, hair dryers, stereo headsets, and sewing machines. Exposure levels were small compared to ambient levels [57]. Measured magnetic fields in proximity to the above electrical appliances were elevated over the ambient when these devices were in use [58]. Magnetic field measurements are the highest from electrical appliances in occupational settings. Szabó et al. [54] characterized occupational 50 Hz magnetic field personal exposure among female sewing machine operators. They measured the full shift of 51 seamstresses, who worked in two shifts (6–14 and 14–22 h) according to their normal work routine. The average duration of the measurement periods was 449 min. The average arithmetic mean exposure for all women was 0.76 μT while the average of maximum values was 4.30 μT. Women working with older sewing machines experienced higher exposure than women working on newer sewing machines. They concluded that women working as sewing machine operators experience higher than average occupational magnetic field exposure compared to other working women.

3.5   DOSIMETRY

The relationship between environmental exposures and electrical quantities induced in the body is often termed dosimetry [29]. A few research laboratories have conducted extensive computations of induced electric field and current density in heterogeneous models of the human body in uniform EMF [59–67].

Contact current may affect pluripotent progenitor cells in the bone marrow, the target cells for leukemia in adults and children. Small voltages present within the residence due to residential grounding practices drive the contact current. Children may have differential sensitivity because of their smaller body dimensions and cartilaginous growth plates at the ends of their bones, both of which produce increased current density (and thus electric fields) in bone marrow compared to adults. In addition, children have active marrow in their hands and feet, both locations with small cross sections [68–70].

Dawson et al. [63] created a model of a 5-year-old child by scaling the adult model purely for size but without adding voxels with marrow properties to the bones (such as the hand, wrist, and ankles) where children have red (blood-producing) marrow and adults do not. They noticed that electric fields in a model of child with anatomically correct marrow distribution would be higher, and the fields in an adult model exposed to 10 μA are roughly 25–50% of the values for the 5-year-old, depending on body location (the lower body impedance of an adult is more than offset by larger cross-sectional area).

Kowalski et al. [71] calculated current density threshold for exciting the motor cortex area of the brain by means of the finite element method (FEM). Their values were 6 and 2.5 A/m^2 at 2.44 kHz and 50 Hz, respectively.

Kang and Gandhi [67] used the widely accepted three-dimensional (3D) impedance method to calculate the electric fields and current densities induced in a human model for an assumed but representative EAS device. It was shown that the two compliance testing methods give substantially different results for the induced 1-cm^2 averaged current densities as required by the ICNIRP guidelines [12–14] or the 5-mm cube averaged electric fields required for compliance testing against the proposed IEEE guidelines [5–8]. The method of treating such exposures as multifrequency exposures gives induced current density or electric current that may be up to twice as large as compared to the approximate but simpler method of treating the highest of the pulses as a half sinusoid of the same duration and frequency. The authors suggest following the accurate method based on multifrequency analysis.

3.6 FIELD MANAGEMENT

The ultimate demand of the user is always to achieve field management, which includes engineering changes to reduce, avoid, or eliminate certain fields or field characteristics. The process of field management requires techniques with tremendous energetic extent. It involves the level of field, which depends on the field strength, frequency, direction, and type of field source.

3.6.1 MITIGATION TECHNIQUES FOR POWER LINES

It is basically known, for example, that reduction of magnetic fields generated from power lines relies on many options, including allocating larger rights-of-way (ROW), using cancellation techniques, and replacing overhead power lines with underground cables.

3.6.1.1 Underground Cables

Underground power transmission lines combined with compaction may substantially reduce their exposure, especially electric fields. The reduction of magnetic field is not due to the burying itself, but because underground power lines use plastic or oil for insulation rather than air. This allows the conductors to be placed closer together and therefore enables better phase cancellation. However, when high-voltage cables are buried in the ground, they must be kept at least 15–30 cm apart to limit mutual heating and they must be placed deep enough to provide clearance for activities on the ground surface (the depth increases with voltage). For cables operating at 33 kV and above, trenches wider than 1 m have to be excavated and the swathe of land required for a number of cables, necessarily spaced, can be as much as 30 m wide. Consequently, high-voltage underground cables over long distances are expensive and involve extensive work during installation and maintenance. For example, the capital cost of installing an underground cable is greater than that for an equally rated overhead power line. The ratio ranges from about 2:1 at 11 kV to 20:1 or more at 400 kV and above.

It should also be noted that magnetic fields at the center of an underground cable corridor might be much higher than those from overhead lines. This is due to the fact that ground-level magnetic fields from cables fall much more rapidly with distance than those from corresponding overhead power lines, but can actually be higher at small distances from the cable. According to Swanson and Renew [72], the magnetic fields under overhead lines on the ROW were about 24 μT and more than 100 μT for the buried line. At 30 m away, fields were about 4 μT for the overhead line and less than 1 μT for the buried line.

Accordingly, using underground cables remains an unreal choice for power utilities and the preferred choice by users. To realistically proceed with the advantages of this option, planned development to avoid hazards and pitfalls of existing power systems is required from the utilities. Offering guidance in new network construction may avoid much of the massive economic impact inevitable in mitigating suspected hazards associated with past and present technologies.

3.6.1.2 Rights of Way

The term rights of way as used in this book covers use that will encumber real property by granting a right to use and alter the landscape through construction of overhead power and communication lines or buildings (power plant, substation, radio tower, etc.). Generally, such uses are for a relatively long period of time, i.e., 10 years or longer.

It is important to know that the highest magnetic field strength from high-voltage power lines on the ROW during peak usage could be lower than the median measurement of magnetic field from many appliances. However, the duration of exposure from power lines is typically much longer than the duration of exposure to magnetic field from appliances. Here indeed lies the reason for public concern. Because of this lasting exposure, there is a demand to enlarge the ROW, although such action involves financial and land rights acquisition difficulties. Authorities in many countries now require power utilities to have more land around overhead power lines. Another solution could be to increase the height of the towers, so that the height of conductors above the ground will reduce the field intensity at the edge of the ROW.

3.6.1.3 Cancellation Techniques

It is well known that currents oscillating together at the same amplitude, frequency, and direction can add to each other. This fact is called *in phase* and it creates the highest magnetic fields. Likewise, fields that are precisely opposing each other achieve a significant cancellation. This means the phase current in a given conductor is opposed by current flowing in the opposite conductor. Such a case is called *out of phase*. This technique is workable for both single-phase systems and three-phase systems. Cancellation techniques could be successful to a great extent if the phase currents are balanced, a state that is practically difficult, if not impossible, to achieve. In that sense, other procedures may be considered.

3.6.2 Reducing the Level of ELF Exposure

Importantly for the user, there appear to be general procedures and suggestions to reduce the levels of electric and magnetic fields in homes and workplaces. Following are a few suggestions to minimize the level of ELF fields, as a procedure before resorting to various shielding techniques, except when shielding is the most effective and least expensive alternative [73]:

1. Determine sources of ELF fields. For example, a tri-axis Gauss meter could be used to determine the levels and locations of magnetic fields.
2. Use bundled and twisted power cable drops to reduce field generation.

3. Keep the drop, meter, service panels, and subpanels away from normally occupied rooms.
4. Fix up a thorough ground rod. Never provide a separate ground for subpanels. Affix an insulated bushing at the water meter to keep current imbalances from returning on the metal water pipes. Prevent metal-sheathed cabling from contacting water pipes, electrical conduits, or appliances by providing a separate ground path.
5. Keep high-load wiring from the main panel to a subpanel or to high-current appliances away from frequently used spaces.
6. Avoid separating hot and neutral wires, and ensure there is always a supply and return current in all wiring runs.
7. Place high-load appliances such as electric dryers and electric hot water heaters away from bedrooms, kitchens, etc.
8. Avoid using devices such as alarm clocks or electric blankets near the bed.
9. As a last solution, use shielding techniques to reduce the level of fields. Shielding ELF fields requires either diverting the fields around the area considered sensitive to the magnetic fields or to contain fields within the source producing them.

3.6.3 MITIGATION OF ELECTRIC FIELDS

As discussed in Chapter 1, if the charges exist in a medium that permits the charges to move, the medium is considered conductive and the field can be adjusted in magnitude and direction with the movement of the charges. At ELF fields, air has a conductivity of less than 10^{-9} siemens (S), while metals have conductivity greater than 10^7 S. The human body has a conductivity that ranges from 0.01 to 1.5 S [6]. Owing to the huge difference in conductivity, placing any grounded metallic surface between the electric field source and user will eliminate the electric field. The metal surface can be an inexpensive mesh chicken wire screen.

Cancellation techniques are applicable for electric fields. This can be achieved by placing together two conductors carrying charges to and from an electrical appliance. For plug-in appliances, a switched-off appliance has a larger electric field than a switched-on appliance. This is because most of the switches break only one of the conductor circuits.

Although cancellation techniques are the only practical electric field management technique for specific cases, shielding is the usual and easier technique to apply. In this case, both the user and equipment can be shielded, simply by placing a metal shroud around the object. Therefore, management of electric fields is not that difficult a task compared to the management of magnetic fields. While both cancellation and shielding techniques are applicable to electric and magnetic fields, shielding could be the best solution.

3.6.4 MITIGATION OF MAGNETIC FIELDS

In general, there are two basic magnetic field mitigation methods: passive and active. They may be used either separately or together as necessary.

3.6.4.1 Passive Shielding Techniques

Passive magnetic shielding is divided into two basic types based upon the selection of the shielding material: ferromagnetic and conductive. A ferromagnetic material shield is constructed with high-permeability (μ) material, especially annealed ferromagnetic Mumetal alloy (composed of 80% nickel and 15% iron, with the balance being copper, molybdenum, or chromium, depending on the recipe being used), which exhibits high magnetic conductivity. The relative permeability (μ_r) of Mumetal ranges between 350,000 and 500,000, depending on the composition and annealing process.

Mumetal either surrounds or separates the victims from the magnetic sources. All shielding materials work by diverting the magnetic flux to them, so although the field from a magnet will be highly reduced by a shield plate, the shield plate will itself be attracted to the magnet. Closed shapes are most effective for magnetic shielding, such as cylinders with caps and boxes with covers.

The electrical properties of ferromagnetic materials are complex functions of magnetic fields and frequencies. They have high saturation characteristics, which can be adjusted to achieve source shielding. Conducting material shields depend on the eddy current losses that occur within highly conductive materials (copper and aluminum). When a conductive material is subjected to an ELF field, eddy currents are induced within the material that flow in closed circular paths perpendicular to the inducing field. According to Lenz's law, these eddy currents oppose changes in the inducing fields; hence the magnetic fields produced by the circulating eddy currents attempt to cancel the larger external fields near the conductive surface, thereby generating a shielding effect. It is often effective but expensive to shield with multiple layers composed of highly conductive aluminum/copper plates and highly permeable Mumetal sheets.

Practically, shielding design depends on the following factors:

1. Maximum predicted worst-case magnetic field intensity and the Earth's geomagnetic (DC static) field at that location.
2. Type of material and properties such as conductivity, permeability, induction, and saturation, which are functions of material thickness.
3. Number of shield layers and spacing between sheet materials and layers.

Small, fully enclosed shields for VDTs, electronic equipment, and electrical feeders follow simple formulas that guide the design engineer through the process to a functional, but not necessarily optimal, design. After assembling a prototype, the design engineer measures the *shielding factor* (SF) and modifies the design by adding materials and layers to achieve the maximum shielding requirements. This is a very iterative design process, from the concept to final product.

Shielding factor is the ratio between the unperturbed magnetic field B_0 and the shielded magnetic field B_i. It is defined as

$$SF = \frac{B_0}{B_i}$$

or

$$SF = 20 \log 10 \left(\frac{B_0}{B_i} \right) dB \qquad (3.2)$$

For example, if the field before shielding is 500 mG and the field measured inside the shield is 10 mG, the SF is then 500/10 or 50 times. SF is usually expressed in decibels. The ratio in decibels for the above example is 34 dB.

Unfortunately, magnetic shielding is more of an art than a science, especially when shielding very large areas and rooms from multiple, high-level magnetic field sources. Currently, there are no reliable design formulas or field simulation programs that offer design engineers practical guidelines for shielding large exposed areas from multiple, high-level magnetic field sources.

3.6.4.2 Active Shielding Techniques

The use of active cancellation loops involves a system that senses the magnetic field in the region to be shielded and, through a feedback system, imposes a current on additional conductors such that it reduces the magnetic field in the region. Active shielding is therefore a technique that works best for full-room shielding of affected instrumentation once strong local sources have been moved or passively shielded. Design changes for power line mitigation include opposite phasing (or revising conductor arrangements to reduce fields), creating balanced currents, or other engineering design changes. For electrical equipment rooms, rearranging and moving electrical components is often the first step to consider since it is more cost-effective than installing magnetic field shields.

3.6.5 PROTECTION FROM VDTs

The source of electric fields in the VDT is the power supply and deflection coils. These components can create a surface potential of several kilovolts, depending upon humidity, temperature, air velocity, and ion concentration in the air. Reduction of the electrostatic potential and the electric fields is usually achieved by placing a conductive surface coating on the screen, which is connected to the power ground, together with metallic shielding of the power supply. Sometimes, the cathode ray tube (CRT)-type VDT may include a metal cage around all the internal components or a metal foil on the inside of the cabinet to shield electric fields.

There have been public debates about whether exposure from VDTs poses health problems. As yet, there is no conclusive evidence to settle the matter once and for all. Some simple precautions could be followed to reduce the exposure:

1. Use a low-emission VDT.
2. Most fields do not extend from the front of the screen of the VDT but from the inductive components located near the inside rear or sides of the equipment. Accordingly, avoid sitting or working at places where you expose

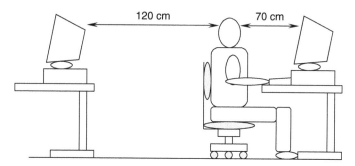

120 cm   70 cm

FIGURE 3.3   Minimum recommended distances between users and computers.

yourself to the emission from the backs and sides of other computers. If you find you are close to any VDT (less than 120 cm), you should change your work environment to enhance your safety (Figure 3.3).

3. Keep the computer screen as far away from you as you can manage (at least 70 cm) since magnetic field strength diminishes rapidly the farther you move from the VDT.

4. VDT users should be aware of ergonomic problems, which can be improved by the use of antiglare screens and proper eyeglasses (avoid wearing metal objects, which concentrate fields while using a computer).

5. Do not place a bed on the other side of the wall from a computer, as building materials cannot shield magnetic fields.

6. Before you use a new computer, leave it turned on for a few days in an empty ventilated room to allow for chemical outgassing.

7. Turn off the computer when it is not in use.

8. A notebook with liquid crystal display (LCD), which requires much less power and a narrow range of frequencies, could be a substitute to the desktop computer. The notebook emits virtually no fields. However, it has been found that high fields emanate from the keyboard.

REFERENCES

1. Habash RWY. *Electromagnetic Fields and Radiation: Human Bioeffects and Safety.* New York: Marcel Dekker, 2001.
2. Erdreich LS, Klauenberg BJ. Radio frequency radiation exposure standards: considerations for harmonization. *Health Phys* 2001; 80: 430–439.
3. WHO. *WHO Handbook on Establishing a Dialogue on Risks from Electromagnetic Fields.* Geneva: World Health Organization, 2002.
4. Dourson ML, Stara JF. Regulatory history and experimental support of uncertainty (safety) factors. *Regul toxicol pharmacol* 1983; 3: 224–238.
5. IEEE. Safety levels with respect to human exposure to radio frequency electromagnetic fields, 3 kHz to 300 GHz. *IEEE Standard C95.1-1991*, 1992.
6. IEEE. Standard for safety levels with respect to human exposure to radio frequency electromagnetic fields, 3 kHz to 300 GHz. *IEEE Standard C95.1-1991*, 1999.

7. IEEE. Recommended practice for determining the peak spatial-average specific absorption rate (SAR) in the human head from wireless communications devices. *IEEE Standard 1528-2003*, 2003.

8. IEEE. Standard for safety levels with respect to human exposure to radio frequency electromagnetic fields, 3 kHz to 300 GHz. *IEEE Standard C95.1-2005*, 2006.

9. NRPB. Board statement on restrictions on human exposure to static and time-varying electromagnetic fields. National Radiological Protection Board. Doc NRPB, 4(5), Chilton, Didcot, Oxon, UK, 1993.

10. NRPB. ICNIRP guidelines for limiting exposure to time-varying electric, magnetic, and electromagnetic fields (up to 300 GHz). Advice on aspects of implementation in the UK. National Radiological Protection Board. Doc NRPB, 10(2), Chilton, Didcot, Oxon, UK, 1999.

11. NRPB. Review of the scientific evidence for limiting exposure to electromagnetic fields (80–300 GHz). National Radiological Protection Board. Doc NRPB, 15(2), Chilton, Didcot, Oxon, UK, 2004.

12. ICNIRP. Guidelines for limiting exposure to time-varying electric, magnetic, and electromagnetic fields (up to 300GHz). *Health Phys* 1998; 74: 494–522.

13. ICNIRP. Responses to questions and comments on ICNIRP. *Health Phys* 1998; 75: 438–439.

14. ICNIRP. General approach to protection against non-ionizing radiation. *Health Phys* 2002; 82: 540–548.

15. TCO'99. Certification, display (CRT), TCO Report No. 1, Stockholm, Sweden, 1999.

16. Safety Code 6. Limits of human exposure to radiofrequency electromagnetic fields in the frequency range from 3 kHz to 300 GHz. Environmental Health Directorate, Health Protection Branch, Health Canada, Canada, 1999.

17. ARPANSA. Maximum exposure levels to radiofrequency fields—3 kHz–300 GHz. Radiation Protection Series No. 3. Australian Radiation Protection and Nuclear Safety Agency, Australia, 2002.

18. Habash RWY. Electromagnetics—the uncertain health risks. *IEEE Potentials* 2003; 22: 23–26.

19. Habash RWY. Foreseeable health risk of electric and magnetic field residential exposure. *Energy Environ* 2003; 14: 473–487.

20. Habash RWH, Brodsky LM, Leiss W, Krewski DK, Repacholi M. Health risk of electromagnetic fields. Part II: Evaluation and assessment of electric and magnetic fields. *Crit Rev Biomed Eng* 2003; 31: 154–195.

21. ASA. Safety levels of electromagnetic radiation with respect to personnel. *USASI Standard C95.1-1966*, 1966.

22. ANSI. Safety levels of electromagnetic radiation with respect to personnel. *ANSI Standard C95.1-1974*, 1974.

23. ANSI. Safety levels with respect to human exposure to radio frequency electromagnetic fields, 300 kHz to 300 GHz. *ANSI Standard C95.1-1982*, 1982.

24. Osepchuk JM, Petersen RC. Historical review of RF exposure standards and the International Committee on Electromagnetic Safety (ICES). *Bioelectromagnetics* 2003; 24: S7–S16.

25. IEEE. Standard for safety levels with respect to human exposure to electromagnetic fields, 0–3 kHz. *IEEE Standard C95.6-2002*, 2002.

26. Renew DC, Glover ID. Basic restrictions in EMF exposure guidelines. *Health Phys* 2002; 83: 395–401.

27. CEC. Council recommendations on the limitation of exposure of the general public to electromagnetic fields (0 Hz to 300 GHz). *J Eur. Comm* 1999; L199: 59–70.

28. Bailey WH. Health effects relevant to the setting of EMF exposure limits. *Health Phys* 2002; 83: 376–386.

29. Stuchly MA, Dawson TW. Human body exposure to power lines: relation of induced quantities to external magnetic fields. *Health Phys* 2002; 83: 333–340.

30. Reilly JP. Neuroelectric mechanisms applied to low frequency electric and magnetic field exposure guidelines—Part I: Sinusoidal waveforms. *Health Phys* 2002; 83: 341–355.

31. Silva MH, Hummon, Rutter D, Hooper C. Power frequency magnetic fields in the home. *IEEE Trans Power Delivery* 1989; 4: 465–478.

32. Niple JC, Daigle JP, Zaffanella LE, Sullivan T, Kavet R. A portable meter for measuring low frequency currents in the human body. *Bioelectromagnetics* 2004; 25: 369–373.

33. Ahlbom A. Neurodegenerative diseases, suicide and depressive symptoms in relation to EMF. *Bioelectromagnetics* 2001; S5: S132–S43.

34. Preece AW, Kaune WT, Grainger P, Golding J. Magnetic fields from domestic appliances in the UK. *Phys Med Biol* 1997; 42: 67–76.

35. Yoshitomi K. Measurement and reduction of power frequency magnetic fields in a residential area. *Trans Instit Elect Info Commun Engin B* 2002; J85-B: 538–546.

36. Adams J, Bitler JS, Riley K. Importance of addressing National Electrical Code (R) violations that result in unusual exposure to 60 Hz magnetic fields. *Bioelectromagnetics* 2004; 25: 102–106.

37. Moriyama K, Yoshitomi K. Apartment electrical wiring: A cause of extremely low frequency magnetic field exposure in residential areas. *Bioelectromagnetics* 2005; 26: 238–241.

38. Schuz J, Grigat JP, Stormer B, Rippin G, Brinkmann K, Michaelis J. Extremely low frequency magnetic fields in residences in Germany. Distribution of measurements, comparison of two methods for assessing exposure, and predictors for the occurrence of magnetic fields above background level. *Radiat Environ Biophys* 2000; 39: 233–240.

39. Chadwick P, Lowes F. Magnetic fields on British trains. *Ann Occup Hygiene* 1998; 5: 331–335.

40. Zaffanella L. Survey of residential magnetic field sources. Volume 1: Goals, Results and Conclusions, Volume 2: Protocol, Data Analysis, and Management, TR-102759-V1, TR-102759-V2, EPRI, Palo Alto, CA, 1993.

41. Zaffanella LE, Kalton GW. Survey of personal magnetic field exposure phase II, EMF RAPID Engineering Project #6, Enertech for Oak Ridge National Laboratory EMF Research Program, U.S. Department of Energy, 1998.

42. Deadman J-E, Armstrong BG, McBride ML, Gallagher R, Thériault G. Exposures of children in Canada to 60–Hz magnetic and electric fields. *Scand J Work Environ Health* 1999; 25: 368–375.

43. Kaune WT, Bracken TD, Senior RS, Rankin RF, Niple JC, Kavet R. Rate of occurrence of transient magnetic field events in U.S. residences. *Bioelectromagnetics* 2000; 21: 197–213.

44. Kelsh MA, Bracken TD, Sahl JD, Shum M, Kristie LE. Occupational magnetic field exposures of garment workers: results of personal and survey measurements. *Bioelectromagnetics* 2003; 24: 316–326.

45. Juutilainen J, Saali K, Eskelinen J, Matilainen P, Leinonen A-L. Measurements of 50 Hz magnetic fields in Finnish homes, Research Report IVO–A–02/89 Helsinki: Imatran Voima Oy, Finland, 1989.

46. Preece AW, Grainger P, Golding J, Kaune W. Domestic magnetic field exposure in Avon. *Phys Med Biol* 1996; 41: 71–81.

47. Vistnes AI, Ramberg GB, Bjornevik LR, Tynes T, Haldorsen T. Exposure of children to residential magnetic fields in Norway: is proximity to power lines an adequate predictor of exposure? *Bioelectromagnetics* 1997; 18: 47–57.

48. Clinard F, Milan C, Harb M, Carli P-M, Bonithon-Kopp C, Moutet J-P, Faivre J, Hillon P. Residential magnetic field measurements in France: comparison of indoor and outdoor measurements. *Bioelectromagnetics* 1999; 20: 319–326.

49. Brix J, Wettemann H, Scheel O, Feiner F, Matthes R. Measurement of the individual exposure to 50 and 16 2/3 Hz magnetic fields within the Bavarian population. *Bioelectromagnetics* 2001; 22: 323–332.

50. Tardón A, Velarde H, Rodriguez P, Moreno S, Raton M, Muñoz J, Fidalgo AR, Kogevinas M. Exposure to extremely low frequency magnetic fields among primary school children in Spain. *J Epidemiol Community Health* 2002; 56: 432–433.

51. Forssén UM, Ahlbom A, Feychting M. Relative contribution of residential and occupational magnetic field exposure over twenty-four hours among people living close to and far from a power line. *Bioelectromagnetics* 2002; 23: 239–244.

52. Ptitsyna NG, Kopytenko YA, Villoresi G, Pfluger DH, Ismaguilov V, Iucci N, Kopytenko EA, Zaitzev DB, Voronov PM, Tyasto, MI. Waveform magnetic field survey in Russian DC and Swiss AC powered trains: a basis for biologically relevant exposure assessment. *Bioelectromagnetics* 2003; 24: 546–556.

53. Jesús M. Paniagua, Antonio Jiménez, Montaña Rufo, Alicia Antolín. Exposure assessment of ELF magnetic fields in urban environments in Extremadura (Spain). *Bioelectromagnetics* 2004; 25: 58–62.

54. Szabó J, Mezei K, Thuróczy G, Mezei G. Occupational 50 Hz magnetic field exposure measurements among female sewing machine operators in Hungary. *Bioelectromagnetics* 2006; 27: 451–457.

55. Szabó J, Jánossy G, Thuróczy G. Survey of residential 50 Hz EMF exposure from transformer stations. *Bioelectromagnetics* 2007; 28: 48–52.

56. Moriyama K, Yoshitoni K. Apartment electrical wiring: a cause of extremely low frequency magnetic field exposure in residential area. *Bioelectromagnetics* 2005; 26: 238–241.

57. Kaune WT, Miller MC, Linet MS, Hatch EE, Kleinerman RA, Wacholder S, Mohr AH, Tarone RE, Haines C. Children's exposure to magnetic fields produced by U.S. television sets used for viewing programs and playing video games. *Bioelectromagnetics* 2000; 21: 214–227.

58. Kaune WT, Miller MC, Linet MS, Hatch EE, Kleinerman RA, Wacholder S, Mohr AH, Tarone RE, Haines C. Magnetic fields produced by hand held hair dryers, stereo headsets, home sewing machines, and electric clocks. *Bioelectromagnetics* 2002; 23: 14–25.

59. Gandhi OP. Some numerical methods for dosimetry: extremely low frequencies to microwave frequencies. *Radio Sci* 1995; 30: 161–177.

60. Dawson TW, DeMoerloose J, Stuchly MA. Comparison of magnetically induced ELF fields in humans computed by FDTD and scalar potential FD codes. *Applied Computational Electromagnetic Society* 1996; 11: 63–71.

61. Dawson TW, Caputa K, Stuchly MA. Influence of human model resolution of computed currents induced in organs by 60 Hz magnetic fields. *Bioelectromagnetics* 1997; 18: 478–490.

62. Dawson TW, Caputa K, Stuchly MA. High-resolution organ dosimetry to human exposure to low-frequency electric fields. *IEEE Trans Power Delivery* 1998; 13: 366–376.

63. Dawson TW, Caputa K, Stuchly MA, Kavet R. Induced electric fields in the human body associated with 60 Hz contact currents. *IEEE Trans Biomed Eng* 2001; 48: 1020–1026.

64. Dawson TW, Stuchly MA. High resolution organ dosimetry for human exposure to low frequency magnetic fields. *IEEE Trans Magn* 1998; 34: 1–11.

65. Dimbylow PJ. Induced current densities from low-frequency magnetic fields in a 2 mm resolution, anatomically realistic model of the body. *Phys Med Biol* 1998; 43: 221–230.
66. Dimbylow PJ. Current densities in a 2 mm resolution anatomically realistic model of the body induced by low frequency electric fields. *Phys Med Biol* 2000; 45: 1013–1022.
67. Kang G, Gandhi OP. Comparison of various safety guidelines for electronic article surveillance devices with pulsed magnetic fields. *IEEE Trans Biomed* Eng 2003; 50: 107–113.
68. Kavet R, Zaffanella L, Daigle J, Ebi K. The possible role of contact current in cancer risk associated with residential magnetic fields. *Bioelectromagnetics* 2000; 21: 538–553.
69. Sastre A, Kavet R. Candidate sites of action for microdosimetry associated with exposure to extremely-low-frequency magnetic fields, electric fields and contact currents. *Health Phys* 2002; 83: 387–394.
70. Sheppard AR, Kavet R, Renew DC. Exposure guidelines for low-frequency electric and magnetic fields: Report from the Brussels workshop. *Health Phys* 2002; 83: 324–332.
71. Kowalski T, Silny J, Buchner H. Current density threshold for the stimulation of neurons in the motor cortex area. *Bioelectromagnetics* 2002; 23: 421–428.
72. Swanson J, Renew DC. Power-frequency fields and people. *Eng Sci Ed J* 1994; 3: 71–79.
73. EPRI. Handbook of shielding principles for power system magnetic fields. Volume 1: Introduction and application. The Electric Power Research Institute (EPRI) (TR-103630-V1), Palo Alto, CA, 1994.

4 Bioeffects of Electric and Magnetic Fields

4.1 INTRODUCTION

A biological effect occurs when exposure to EMF causes some noticeable or detectable physiological change in a living system. Such an effect may sometimes, but not always, lead to an adverse health effect, which means a physiological change that exceeds normal range for a brief period of time. It occurs when the biological effect is outside the normal range for the body to compensate, and therefore leads to some detrimental health condition. Health effects are often the result of biological effects that accumulate over time and depend on exposure dose. Determining actual health risks from EMF exposure is complex. Not all investigators agree about the risk. In its EMF assessment, the National Institute of Environmental Health Sciences (NIEHS), based on the report of its expert Working Group [1,2], stated that biological effects are plausible at a tissue dose of 1 mV/m. According to Dawson et al. [3], contact current levels on the order of 10 μA or less, considerably below ICNIRP limits, can produce electric fields in some tissues that are well above the NIEHS's 1 mV benchmark [4]. In addition, a growing number of studies in the literature suggest that there may be health risks at such EMF levels, possibly depending on many variables including duration of field exposure, strength of the field, person's mass and age, general health, and probably genetic predisposition or vulnerability to cancer. Therefore, detailed knowledge of the biological effects is important to understand the generated health risks.

Public concern over human effects of exposure to EMF is largely based on a series of key epidemiological assessment studies. Such studies identify the association between diseases and particular environmental characteristics. It may indicate a cause-and-effect relationship, depending upon the strength of the observed association. Epidemiological studies correlate historical biological data for a large population of people. Any biological data are purely statistical in nature; however, people usually fit a particular category based on location or occupation. The results may only show an association with a stimulus, since there are many factors involved with each person.

In addition to epidemiological studies, this chapter reviews a significant number of studies that have been carried out to date to explore the relationship between exposure to EMF and illnesses including cancer. These studies describe various clinical and experimental investigations with humans, laboratory animals, tissue preparations, and cells. Detailed information and suggestions for future research on the bioeffects of EMF are also included.

4.2 EPIDEMIOLOGICAL STUDIES

The major objectives of most epidemiological studies are to determine whether a specific exposure or factor is likely to cause a given disease and to quantify the strength of the relationship. The epidemiological studies correlate EMF exposure and health effects on human populations to establish quantitative dose–response relations. At best, the epidemiological findings indicate a correlation between EMF exposure and a health effect, but not necessarily a causal relation. Two major types of studies are used to evaluate whether an exposure is linked with a given disease: the cohort and the case-control study designs. In a cohort study, exposed and unexposed populations are ascertained, then followed up to compare risks of developing particular disease outcomes. In an ideal case-control study, cases are those who have developed a particular disease in a specified population during the study period, and control subjects are a random sample of those in the population who have not developed disease [5,6]. Most epidemiological studies are limited by the use of surrogate indicators rather than direct measurements of exposure. An epidemiological association, if found, might not be related directly to exposure; rather, it may be due to chance, confounding factors, or some unrecognized factors related to the way the data have been collected.

Consideration of the extent to which epidemiological studies may be successful in assessing EMF risk is essential when reviewing the literature. Most epidemiological studies reported in the literature have been criticized as having significant limitations including failure to consider variability in exposure intensity, transients, intensity spikes, harmonics of the fundamental frequency, historical exposures, and concomitant exposures to other agents experienced in occupational settings.

Milham and Ossiander [7] investigated the history of electrification and its association to cancer. They hypothesized that electrification of homes during last century caused peak leukemia mortality among children 2–4 years of age. This occurred as domestic, urban, and rural reticulation of electric power was extended. This new age-related peak occurred in the United Kingdom in 1920s, the United States in the 1930s, and in other countries as they reticulated power. The same time delay concept was clear between the wealthier and poorer neighborhoods in the United States. The authors concluded that childhood acute lymphocytic leukemia (ALL) is attributable to residential electrification.

Health outcomes of particular interest in this section are childhood and adult cancer, as well as noncancer health effects, including reproductive effects, neurodegenerative diseases, suicide and depression, and cardiovascular diseases.

4.2.1 Public Environments

Public environments in which EMF exposures can occur include residences and schools, and transportation facilities. The primary sources of residential and school fields are power lines, distribution lines, substations, wiring, grounding systems, and various electrical appliances. Sources of fields in trains and cars are mainly from the power lines supplying energy to the trains.

Li et al. [8] investigated whether the age at cancer diagnosis was associated with residential exposure to magnetic fields. They compared average ages at diagnosis for cases of leukemia, brain tumor, or female breast cancer with elevated exposure (magnetic flux density 0.2 µT, or residential distance from major power lines 100 m) to average ages at diagnosis for cancer cases with same diagnoses but with a background exposure (<0.2 μT or >100 m from major power lines). They noted an association between magnetic field exposure and a greater mean age at diagnosis for brain tumors. The difference was greater for males than for females. No such phenomenon at a significant level was observed for leukemia, female breast cancer, or a random sample of general population. These phenomena suggest a delayed occurrence of brain tumors following a higher than background residential magnetic field exposure and they deserve further investigation.

Numerous studies have shown that most high-level fields measured in houses are a result of proximity to power lines. Residential studies address the exposure of children and adults to EM fields as either population-based or case-control cases. A number of studies summarized here address the issue of residential EMF exposure.

4.2.1.1   Childhood Cancer and Leukemia

Leukemia is the most common cancer to affect children, accounting for approximately a third of all childhood cancers. As with most other cancers, the mechanism by which leukemia arises is likely to involve gene–environment interactions. Accordingly, it is important to identify exposures that cause DNA damage and induce chromosome breaks, which are inadequately repaired, ultimately leading to initiation and disease progression [9]. Childhood exposure to EMF has been studied intensively for many decades. However, research into this area gained momentum in 1979, when one of the first epidemiological studies [10] showed an association between exposure to EMF and cancer among children living near power lines. This study was followed by other studies of childhood cancer [11–20]. Although some studies have supported the findings of Wertheimer and Leeper [10], more studies have failed to provide support for the hypothesis that EMF exposure increases the risk of childhood cancer. These studies include three collaborative population-based Nordic studies [13–15], a study in the United States [16], two Canadian studies [17,18], and a study in the UK [20]. One Canadian study [17] included 399 children with leukemia and 399 controls. The investigators found that EMF exposures actually provide a significant protective effect against cancer for fairly raised field levels but not significantly protective for still higher fields. Feychting et al. [21] observed that children of fathers with occupational magnetic field exposure had a higher incidence of leukemia than expected. No link was found for childhood leukemia and maternal occupational magnetic field exposure. For maternal exposure, assessments were done both for exposure before pregnancy and exposure during pregnancy. Exposure assessment was based on actual measurements made with people with the same job titles. However, Infante-Rivard and Deadman [22] reported that maternal occupational exposure to power-frequency fields during pregnancy was associated with an excess incidence of childhood leukemia. Exposure assessment was based on actual measurements made with people with similar jobs.

Henshaw and Reiter [23] proposed that the melatonin hypothesis, in which power frequency magnetic fields suppress the nocturnal production of melatonin in the pineal gland, accounts for the observed increased risk of childhood leukemia.

Such melatonin disruption has been shown in animals, especially with exposure to electric and rapid on/off magnetic fields. Support for the hypothesis is found in the body of studies showing magnetic field disruption of melatonin in related animal and human studies. Additional support comes from the observation that melatonin is highly protective of oxidative damage to the human hemopoietic system.

In children, a variety of distinct tumor types arise in the CNS but they are frequently considered by epidemiologists as a single entity. CNS tumors are the second most common childhood malignancy and occur more frequently in developed countries than developing nations. Approximately 50% of pediatric CNS tumors are gliomas, with astrocytomas of the piloctyic-type predominating. The causes of childhood CNS tumors are largely unknown; and although an estimated 5% or more may be explained by genetic predisposition, investigations of environmental etiology have not been fruitful. Exposure to ELF/EMF, at any level, has not been associated with childhood CNS tumors, but the current evidence base is inadequate for complete evaluation. The rarity of childhood CNS tumors necessitates careful attention being paid to the design of future etiological studies [24].

Overall, the association between EMF exposure and childhood cancer remains inadequate and inconclusive (Table 4.1). Some studies have suggested a link between EMF and cancer, although the risks tend to be small by epidemiological standards, and were unable to exclude other environmental influences. While the level of epidemiological evidence in support of this association is limited, further research in this area is needed to clarify this issue.

4.2.1.2 Breast Cancer

Breast cancer is the most commonly occurring malignancy among women; however, male breast cancer is rare. There are several established risk factors for breast cancer in females. The disease increases with age and is found most commonly among women of higher social class, women without children or with few children, and women who have their first child at an older age [25]. Of the first epidemiological studies that have addressed the risk of breast cancer and residential exposure to EMF is the study of Wertheimer and Leeper [26,27]. The authors found an association between high-current electric wiring configuration and breast cancer in a case-control study conducted in Colorado. The study compared residence in homes among 1179 cases of adult cancers with the residences of matched controls. McDowall [28] followed approximately 8000 people (3861 women) from 1971 through 1983 who were living within a 50 m radius of electrical transmission facilities at the time of the 1971 census in East Anglia, England. Among this cohort the overall mortality was lower than expected and there was no evidence of increased risk for breast cancer.

Researchers hypothesize that EMF may be linked to breast cancer through the hormone melatonin. Feychting et al. [29] conducted a case-control study based on people who had lived within 300 m of 220- or 400-kV power lines in Sweden between 1960 and 1985. For calculated magnetic field levels >0.2 µT closest in time before diagnosis, they estimated the risk ratio (RR) = 1.0 for women and 2.1 for men. Women younger than 50 years of age at diagnosis had a RR = 1.8. For women with estrogen receptor-positive breast cancer, RR = 1.6, using the magnetic exposure >0.1 µT. Among estrogen receptor-positive women younger than 50 years at diagnosis, RR increased to 7.4.

Gammon et al. [30] conducted a case-control study to investigate the effects of electric blanket use. There were 2199 case patients under age 55 years that had been newly diagnosed with breast cancer between 1990 and 1992. The 2009 controls were frequency-matched to cases by 5-year age group and geographic area. A nonsignificant increased risk was observed in women who had ever used electrical appliances, especially blankets, mattress pads, or heated waterbeds. Similar findings were observed by other investigators [31–38]. All the above studies provide evidence against a positive association between electric blanket or mattress cover use and breast cancer.

Erren [39] reviewed this topic in detail. The author concluded that no human health risk has been proven. At the same time, the data were inadequate to confirm that a kind of effect could not exist.

An association between residential EMF exposure including the use of appliances and breast cancer is far from being established. Nevertheless, interest in this subject will continue based on the melatonin hypothesis.

4.2.2 OCCUPATIONAL ENVIRONMENTS

Occupational exposure environments are studied in the context of specific industries and workplaces, particularly in the electric power-utility industry where high exposure to EMF is likely. Workers can be exposed to EMF from electrical systems in their building and the equipment they use. A variety of methods for exposure assessment are applied to studies in occupational environments. These methods range from job classification to modeling techniques based on personal exposure measurements and occupational history. Occupational history is a collection of data for a study subject, which may contain information on jobs that the subject held during their employment. Such information is obtained through many means such as interviews or through various employment records. The information contains industry title, company name, description, and duration of the job. Medical records may also be obtained from clinics or disease registries.

Electrical appliances, tools, and power supplies in buildings are the main sources of EMF exposure that most people receive at work. People who work near transformers, electrical closets, circuit boxes, or other high-current electrical equipment may have high-field exposures. In offices, magnetic field levels are often similar to those found at homes, typically 0.5–4.0 milligause (mG). However, these levels may increase dramatically near certain types of equipment. In general, the literature is rich with more occupational studies investigating exposure of workers to EMF at various places using different techniques of evaluation.

4.2.2.1 Adult Cancers

Occupational exposure was studied considering various health problems as well as adult cancers including brain tumors and leukemia [40–60], breast cancer among both men and women [61–66], lymphoma [49,56,67], lung cancer [48,49,54,66,67], and other cancers [49,67–69].

TABLE 4.1
Epidemiological Studies of EMF Exposure and Childhood Leukemia

Investigator	Type/Location/Size	Risk Measure	Outcome
Wertheimer and Leeper (1979) [10]	CC: USA (Denver, CO; <19 years) 155 cases/ 155 controls	OR WC: 2.98 (1.78–4.98)	Children had double or triple the chance of developing leukemia or tumors of the nervous system if they live near transmission lines as compared to those who do not.
Savitz et al. (1988) [11]	CC: USA (Denver, CO; <15 years); ≥0.25 µT spot 448 cases/466 controls	OR WC: 2.75 (0.94–8.04) MF: 1.93 (0.67–5.56)	Increased cases of childhood cancer and leukemia associated with magnetic field exposures above 0.25 µT.
London et al. (1991) [12]	CC: USA (Los Angeles; CA) <10 years; ≥0.125 µT; 373 cases/348 controls	OR WC: 2.15 (1.08–4.26) MF: 1.22 (0.52–2.82)	Largest study.
Feychting and Ahlbom (1993) [13]	PBCC: Sweden; <15 years; 38 cases/556 controls	RR WC: 3.8 (1.4–9.3)	39 leukemia and 33 CNS tumor cases. 3.8-fold increase of leukemia.
Olsen et al. (1993) [14]	PBCC: Denmark; <15 years; 833 cases/1666 controls	OR WC: 6 (0.8–44)	Increased risk of leukemia among children with exposure to magnetic fields from high-voltage lines of 0.1 µT or greater.
Verkasalo et al. (1993) [15]	PBCC: Finland; <17 years; 35 cases	OR WC: 1.6 (0.32–4.5)	1.6-fold increased risk of leukemia. Excess of brain tumor (OR = 2.3) was found in boys (not girls) exposed to magnetic fields ≥0.2 µT.
Linet et al. (1997) [16]	CC: USA (nine states); <19 years; ≥0.3 µT; 24-h measurements; 1026 cases/1017 controls	OR WC: 0.98 (0.72–1.33) MF: 1.24 (0.86–1.79)	No overall correlation between the level of field exposure and risk of ALL. There was a small increase in the risk of ALL for children whose residences measured in the very highest range of magnetic fields.

Reference	Study	OR	Conclusion
McBride et al. (1999) [17]	CC: Canada (five provinces); <15 years; ≥0.2 µT calculated; WC/48-h measurement; 596 cases/648 controls	OR WC: 0.77 (0.37–1.60) MF: 1.04 (0.69–1.57)	Elevated risk of ALL with high wiring configurations among residences of subjects 2 years before the diagnosis/reference date (OR = 1.72 compared with underground wiring (0.54–5.45)).
Schüz et al. (2001) [19]	CC: Germany; 24-h measurements; residential exposure to 16.7 (railway frequency); 489 cases/1240 controls	OR <0.1 µT: 1 0.1 – <0.2 µT: 0.31 (0.07–1.38) ≥0.2 µT: 1.91 (0.41–8.89)	A moderate but statistically non-significant association between magnetic field and childhood leukemia.
Skinner et al. (2002) [20]	PBCC: UK; >20 V m^{-1}; spot measurement; 273 cases/276 controls	O EF: 0.90 (0.59–1.35) for all malignancies	Residential electric fields and fields from power lines (66–400 kV) and electric blankets not associated with significant increase in risk of childhood cancer.
Infante-Rivard and Deadman (2003) [22]	PBCC: Canada (Quebec); >0.4 µT calculated; 491 cases/491 controls	OR MF: 2.5 (1.2–5.0)	The results are compatible with an increased risk of childhood leukemia among children whose mothers were exposed to the highest occupational levels of magnetic fields during pregnancy.

Note: CC: case-control; PBCC: population-based case-control; WC: wire code; MF: magnetic field measurement; EF: electric field measurement.

Sahl et al. [41] studied utility workers at Southern California Edison. Comparisons in the cohort study focused on electrical versus nonelectrical workers, and exposure was characterized on the basis of job history. The authors noticed no difference in risk for brain cancer among electrical workers compared with the reference group. However, small but significant increases in brain cancer risk were observed for electricians (RR = 1.6) and plant operators (RR = 1.6).

Researchers from Canada and France [42] conducted a study of 223,292 workers at three large utilities, two in Canada (Hydro Québec and Ontario Hydro) and a national utility in France (Électricité de France). The result shows that workers with acute myeloid leukemia (AML) were about three times more likely to be in the half of the workforce with higher cumulative exposure to magnetic fields. In the analysis of median cumulative magnetic field exposure, no significant elevated risks were found for most types of cancer studied.

Floderus et al. [47] at the Swedish National Institute of Working Life reported an association between cancer and magnetic field exposure in a broad range. The study included an assessment of EMF exposure at 1015 different workplaces in Sweden and involved over 1600 people in 169 different occupations. The researchers reported an association between estimated field exposure and increased risk for chronic lymphocytic leukemia (CLL). In addition, an increased risk of brain tumors was reported for men under the age of 40 years whose work involved an average magnetic field exposure of more than 2 mG.

Johansen and Olsen [51,52] conducted a study involving 32,006 men and women who had been employed at 99 electric utilities in Denmark with employment history dating back to 1909. Cancer incidence was obtained from the cancer registry over the same period. The authors predicted that utility workers would have a higher incidence of cancer compared with the general population. They reported that the workers had slightly more cancer than expected from general population statistics, but there was no excess of leukemia, brain cancer, or breast cancer.

Willett et al. [60] investigated whether the risk of acute leukemia among 764 adults was associated with occupational exposure to EM fields during 1991–1996. Risks were assessed using conditional logistic regression for a matched analysis. This large population-based case-control study found little evidence to support an association between occupational exposure to EM fields and acute leukemia. While an excess of acute lymphoblastic leukemia among women was observed, it is unlikely that occupational exposure to electromagnetic fields was responsible, given that increased risks remained during periods when exposure above background levels was improbable.

Most of the above studies concentrated on magnetic field exposures, assuming that they are the more biologically active components of the EMF and thus more likely to cause cellular damage. However, there are studies that indicate that electric field exposures may enhance cancer risk. Miller et al. [49] examined the cumulative effects of both magnetic and electric field exposures on the cancer incidence, and reported a marked increase in leukemia risk. At the highest level of exposure to both magnetic and electric fields, odds ratio (OR) increased from 3.51 to 11.2 when the researchers included the interaction of the combined effects of EMF. These investigators also reported an increase in the risk of all types of leukemia as well as some of the highest leukemia risks ever reported in a study of EMF and cancer. They also found evidence a dose–response relationship, with the risk of leukemia increasing with cumulative exposure to electric fields (an effect noticeably absent with exposure to magnetic fields alone, both in this and in previous studies).

An elevated risk of leukemia was also seen among senior workers who spent the most time in electric fields above certain thresholds, in the range of 10–40 V/m [56]. In a recent Canadian population-based control study, Villeneuve et al. [57] conducted a study among men in eight Canadian provinces, for 543 cases of brain cancer confirmed histologically (no benign tumors included). Astrocytoma and glioblastomas accounted for over 400 of these. Population-based controls (543) were selected to be of similar age. They reported a nonsignificant increased risk of brain cancer among men who had ever held a job with an average magnetic field exposure >0.6 µT relative to those with exposures <0.3 µT. A more pronounced risk was observed among men diagnosed with glioblastoma multiforme (the most malignant of neuroepithelial neoplasms) (OR = 5.36).

There are rather notable differences in adult cancer studies, with two kinds of results: (1) null association found in southern California Edison workers [41], study of Norwegian railway workers [44], study of electric utilities in Denmark [51,52], and (2) mixed but in general positive results from a few studies of power-frequency magnetic fields [42,45,50,54,58,66] and of electric field exposure [49,56,57,67]. The relative risks in the upper exposure categories were above 2.0 and for the more highly exposed groups between 1.1–1.3. Relative risks of this magnitude are below the level at which a causal association between EMF exposure and cancer can be assessed.

4.2.2.2 Cardiovascular Diseases

Savitz et al. [53] investigated risk of cardiovascular disease in a cohort of 139,000 male utility workers. Exposure was assessed according to the duration of employment in occupations with exposure to magnetic fields. Overall mortalities due to cardiovascular disease were low. Sahl et al. [70] found that men working longer in high-exposure occupations or working as electricians, linemen, or power plant operators had no increased risk of dying from either acute myocardial infarction (AMI) or chronic coronary heart disease (CCHD) compared with men who never worked in high-exposure occupations. Their study was based on cohort of 35,391 male workers at the Southern California Edison Company between 1960 and 1992. In addition, another study of electrical utility workers [71] found no evidence that exposure to power-frequency fields was associated with heart disease.

4.2.2.3 Neurodegenerative Diseases

There could be moderate support for an association between occupational exposure to elevated levels of EMF and Alzheimer's disease (AD) and amyotrophic lateral sclerosis (ALS). A very large and detailed study conducted by van Wijngaarden et al. [72] at the University of North Carolina has uncovered what appears to be a distinct association between exposure to EMF and suicide among electric utility workers. A group of 138,905 male U.S. electric utility workers from five companies were considered in the study. Electricians faced twice the expected risk of suicide. Linemen faced 1.5 times the expected risk. Meanwhile, suicides among power plant operators occurred at a rate slightly lower than expected. Baris et al. [73] found no association between the suicide and exposure to EMF.

Ahlbom [74] conducted a systematic review of the literature on neurodegenerative diseases and exposure to EMF. The author concluded, "For AD the combined data on an association with EMF are weaker than that for ALS. The association between suicide and EMF exposure was also weak. For depressive symptoms an assessment is more complex. For diseases such as Parkinson's, there is not enough information for an assessment."

Overall, currently available data suggest a weak association between EMF exposure and noncancer health effects. More research, particularly from large epidemiological studies, is needed.

4.2.2.4   Reproductive Toxic Effects

Wertheimer and Leeper [75] investigated the relationship between use of electrically heated waterbeds and electric blankets and pregnancy outcome, especially length of gestation, birth weight, congenital abnormalities, and fetal loss in Colorado. The study population consisted of 1806 (out of 4271) families in which a birth had occurred in two Denver-area hospitals in 1982. Seasonal patterns of occurrence of slow fetal development were observed among users of electric waterbeds and blankets, suggesting that use of such appliances at the time of conception might cause adverse health effects.

Dlugosz et al. [76] investigated a possible relationship between the use of electric bed heaters and birth defects. They asked mothers of children born with cleft palates or neural tube defects if they had used an electric bed heater during the 4 months around the estimated date of conception. A total of 663 case mothers were matched with a similar number of control women who had given birth to children without birth defects. The comparison showed that mothers of children with birth defects were no more likely to have used an electric bed heater than other mothers.

Blaasaas et al. [77] found little evidence that residence near power lines affected the risk of birth defects. The authors observed decreased risks of cardiac and respiratory defects and an increased risk of esophageal defects. They interpreted that to the number of endpoints, the imprecision in the calculations of the distance from the residence to the power line, and the limited information on pregnant women's change of residence. Blaasaas et al. [78] found that the total risk of birth defects was not associated with parental exposure to 50-Hz EMF. Feychting [79] summarized the evidence on adverse pregnancy outcomes in relation to ELF and RF exposures and briefly discussed other potential health effects, excluding cancer, following childhood exposures to these fields. The author concluded, "Most studies of ELF exposures have not demonstrated any consistent risk increases for adverse pregnancy outcomes, but limitations in the exposure assessment methods and very limited power to study high exposure levels prevents any conclusions. Different types of symptoms and effects on cognitive function in relation to both ELF and RF fields have been reported in adults, but scientific studies have not confirmed that these symptoms are caused by the EM fields. No information is available for children."

An exception to the lack of association of miscarriages and exposure to 50-Hz magnetic fields are three studies [80–82]. They reported that high peak power-frequency exposures were associated with an increased risk of miscarriages in humans. The first population-based prospective cohort study [80] was conducted among pregnant women within a large health maintenance organization. All women with a positive pregnancy test at less than 10 weeks of gestation and residing in the San Francisco area were contacted for participation in the study. All participants were also asked to wear a magnetic field-measuring meter for 24 h and to keep a diary of their activities. Pregnancy outcomes were obtained for all participants by searching the health maintenance organizations' databases, reviewing medical charts, and telephone follow-up. A total of 969 subjects were included in the final analysis. Miscarriage risk increased with an increasing level of maximum magnetic field exposure with a threshold around 16 mG. The risk associated with magnetic field exposure of 16 mG was 1.8. The risk remained elevated for levels of maximum magnetic field exposure of 16 mG. The association was stronger for early miscarriages (<10 weeks of gestation) (RR = 2.2) and among "susceptible" women with multiple prior fetal losses or subfertility (RR = 3.1). The findings provide strong prospective evidence that prenatal maximum magnetic field exposure above a certain level (possibly around 16 mG) may be associated with miscarriage risk.

The second case-control study [81] was conducted within a cohort of some 3400 pregnant women who were participating in a prospective reproductive health study. A sample was drawn of 531 women, of whom 219 allowed their exposures to be measured when they were or would have been 12 weeks pregnant, including 18 who miscarried. Of these women, 176 (10 with miscarriages) agreed to a second exposure measurement at 30 weeks pregnancy and they formed part of the study sample. The 328 women that were found to have miscarried (cases) and a random sample of 806 of those who had not miscarried was selected to provide controls. Of the five measures assumed to be associated with miscarriage, three were very weakly or not associated, while two were associated.

The third study [82] considered a cohort of 969 primiparous women who wore a meter for 24 h for not more than 15 weeks after they had become pregnant. They found significantly higher risk of miscarriage for women exposed to magnetic fields of 1.6 μT or greater (RR > 2.2). Their findings of increased miscarriages are consistent with the findings of Wertheimer and Leeper [75].

Following the publication of these two studies, Savitz [83] commented on the same issue: "Prior to this research, the evidence supporting an etiological (causal) relation between magnetic fields and miscarriage could have been summarized as 'extremely limited.' With publication of these reports, I believe the evidence in support of a causal association is raised only slightly. These two new studies provide fairly strong evidence against an association with time-weighted average (TWA) magnetic fields and moderately strong evidence for an association with other indices; both of these findings may be due to an artifact resulting from a laudable effort to integrate behavior and environment."

4.2.3 SUMMARY OF EPIDEMIOLOGICAL STUDIES

The consistency of the epidemiological studies is puzzling, especially when we consider that all the studies suffer from profound and diverse methodological limitations such as unknown and probable low accuracy of measurement, potential selection bias, potential confounding, or very small numbers of exposed cases. In addition, there are no accepted biophysical mechanisms that could explain how such low-level field exposures could be carcinogenic [84], although it has been suggested that children may be more sensitive to some or all parts of the EM spectrum. These problems have resulted in continued uncertainty as to the existence as well as size of the field effect. The potential impact of fields on overall childhood leukemia incidence is further clouded by the low prevalence of exposures associated with elevated risk. In most data, no association is visible among average field levels below 2 mG, where the vast majority of measurements lie, and an association is not consistently apparent until above 3 mG [85,86].

Though these epidemiologic outcomes are suggestive, the health impact of EMF is still uncertain. As has been the case with various environmental chemicals and physical agents, definitive conclusions as to the health risk of EMF are likely to require supporting evidence from whole animal studies along with a greater understanding of relevant biological mechanisms.

4.3 CELLULAR AND ANIMAL STUDIES

Laboratory studies provide another valuable source of information on the potential health risks of EMF. Laboratory studies on cells or on whole organisms play a key role in evaluating the response of different systems of the body. They lead to information about molecular mechanisms that can establish the scientific plausibility of effects under particular conditions. Laboratory studies are easier to control and provide the opportunity to check whether EMF exposure causes cancer or other illnesses, something that is not possible with human volunteers. However, laboratory studies entail complications of their own. For example, how should results obtained in only one animal be relevant or extrapolated to humans?

Cellular and animal experiments have enhanced our understanding of the health consequences of EMF exposure. They generally examine the effects of EMF exposure on cells and various systems of the body, in particular the immune, nervous, and endocrine systems. These systems are largely responsible for maintaining the internal environment of the body.

During the past 30 years, a number of experiments and major scientific reviews have been conducted to assess the biological effects of EMF. Considering the interaction mechanism of these fields with biological systems, the effect of magnetic fields has been the central point of research, focusing primarily on fields of the magnitude encountered in everyday life (below 100 μT).

4.3.1 MELATONIN HYPOTHESIS

One area attracting attention as a likely potential mechanism for EMF intervention in living organisms is consideration of a cancer-promoting effect of EMF by altered circadian rhythms of pineal activity and melatonin release. The "melatonin hypothesis," first proposed many years ago, explained how EMF exposure is related to certain kinds of hormone-dependent cancers, particularly breast cancer.

Kato et al. [87], Wilson et al. [88], and Huuskonen et al. [89] reported that exposure to magnetic fields between 1 and 130 µT caused a decrease in melatonin levels in rats and hamsters. However, other studies found no evidence of any effect on melatonin in baboons, rats, and mice at fields between 1 and 100 µT [90–97].

Karasek and Lerchl [98] reported the results of 60 independent assessments in animals of EMF exposure and nocturnal melatonin. Fifty-four percent reported no effect or inconsistent effects, 43% reported decreased melatonin, and 3% reported increased melatonin.

Juutilainen and Kumlin [99] reported that daytime occupational exposure to magnetic fields enhances the effects of nighttime light exposure on melatonin production. Juutilainen and Kumlin reanalyzed data from a previously published study on 6-hydroxy melatonin sulfate (6-OHMS) secretion in 60 women occupationally exposed to ELF magnetic fields.

Altogether, there is still not enough evidence to support the hypothesis that EMF exposure suppresses melatonin or causes an increase in cancer.

4.3.2 GENOTOXICITY AND CARCINOGENICITY

The weight of any positive association between EMF exposure and cancer depends on the ability of exposure to interact with genetic material to damage it, therefore causing mutations, which may lead to cancer. There have been many studies that show EMF may affect DNA or induce mutations. Lai and Singh [100] at the University of Washington, Seattle, observed an increase in double-strand DNA breaks in brain cells of rats being exposed to a 60-Hz magnetic field at flux densities of 0.25 and 0.5 mT. In 2004, the same authors found an increase in DNA single-strand breaks after 2 h of exposure to magnetic field at intensities of 0.1–0.5 mT [101]. Wu et al. [102] reported carcinogenic effects for both 50-Hz and 15.6-kHz magnetic fields on DNA damage/repair in the normal human amniotic fetal liver (FL) cell. Ivancsits et al. [103] reported that a 1-mT field caused DNA strand breaks if the exposure was intermittent, but not if the exposure was continuous. McNamee et al. [104] investigated the effect of an acute 2-h exposure of a 1-mT, 60-Hz magnetic fields on DNA damage in the brains of immature (10-day-old) mice. DNA damage was observed at 0, 2, 4, and 24 h after exposure. No supporting evidence of increased DNA damage was detected.

Other studies [105,106] suggested that environmental EMF exposures at 1–500 µT flux densities are unlikely to cause DNA damage. However, the second study [106] did report that 7 mT caused DNA strand breaks when a strong oxidant was present. Williams et al. [107] reported that 14.6-mT ELF magnetic field exposure does not cause DNA breaks in Salmonella test system.

A possible scenario for an effect of EMF on DNA is as follows: The two chains of DNA are held together by H-bonds joining the complementary bases of DNA. H-bonds are hydrogen (protons) that are bonded to both chains by electron pairs. They are relatively weak. If EMF forces displace electrons in H-bonds, this would lead to local charging and generate forces that overcome the H-bonds and initiate disaggregation of the chains [6].

Khalil and Qassem [108] reported chromosomal aberrations by exposing human lymphocyte cultures to a pulsing EM field (50 Hz, 1.05 mT) for various durations (24, 48, and 72 h). Suzuki et al. [109] reported chromosome damage in the bone marrow cells of mice after exposing them to a high-intensity magnetic field (3–4.7 T) for 24–72 h. However, other studies [105,110,111] were unable to induce chromosomal aberrations even under relatively strong magnetic field exposure.

Stronati et al. [112] found that a short exposure (2 h) to ELF magnetic fields at the intensity of 1 mT is not able to exert any genotoxic effect on human blood cells.

DNA damage and chromosome aberrations are closely related to carcinogenesis or "cancer-causing" effects. Operationally, the carcinogenic process is a multistep process involving genetic and epigenetic changes. The concern for possible carcinogenic effects of EMF exposure has been studied for some time. Environmental magnetic fields at 1–500 μT flux density were unlikely to induce carcinogenesis through a mechanism involving altered expression of the immediate early response genes [113].

It seems that the energy associated with EMF environmental exposure is not enough to cause direct damage to DNA; however, indirect effects are possible by changing cellular architecture and metabolic processes within cells that might lead to DNA damage. Together, there is negative evidence against DNA damage and chromosomal effects at the EMF environmental levels. Studies that do exhibit evidence for genotoxicity reported a mix of positive and negative results. In addition, there have been problems with replication of these findings.

4.3.3   CELL FUNCTIONS

The basic research studies on effects of EMF on cellular function have provided information about biological thresholds and mechanism that may be a basis for possible health impact. The literature has numerous reports on the effects of EMF exposure on ion transport, cell proliferation and differentiation, stress responses, and enzyme activity.

4.3.3.1   Intracellular Calcium

The phenomenon of Ca^{++} efflux (release of calcium ions from a sample into a surrounding solution) from cells due to EM exposure is well known, especially in brain and lymphatic cells. Investigation has shown that EMF exposures at high-flux densities influence the calcium efflux [114–121]. However, no change in calcium influx could be detected by other investigators [122,123]. Considerable attention has been given to explain the mechanisms for the effects of exposure to a time-varying magnetic field on the intracellular signaling pathway [122].

4.3.3.2   Cell Proliferation

Altered proliferation of cells *in vitro* due to EMF exposure has been observed in a number of studies [124–127]. However, Aldinucci et al. [121] investigated whether static fields at a flux density of 4.75 T, generated by an nuclear magnetic resonance (NMR) apparatus, could promote movements of Ca^{++}, cell proliferation, and the eventual production of proinflammatory cytokines in human peripheral blood mononuclear cells (PBMC) as well as in Jurkat cells, after exposure to the field for 1 h.

The results clearly demonstrate that static NMRF exposure has neither prolifera-
tive, nor activating, nor proinflammatory effects on either normal or PHA-activated
PBMC. Similar findings were observed by Supino et al. [128] but at lower magnetic
field densities (50 Hz; 20 or 500 µT) for different lengths of time (1–4 days).

4.3.3.3 Stress Response

Stress response is defined as a defense reaction of cells to damage that environmental forces inflict on macromolecules [129]. It has been shown that EMF stimulates
the cellular stress response, a reaction to potentially harmful stimuli in which cells
start to synthesize stress proteins [130]. Protein synthesis occurs only when the two
chains of DNA come apart and transfer the code for making a protein to mRNA. The
stress response shows that EMF must cause the DNA to come apart even in the weak
ELF range. These observations suggest that EMF stimuli could cause greater damage to DNA at more intense and longer exposures [6]. On the other hand, Shi et al. [131]
failed to detect any of a number of stress responses in human keratinocytes exposed
to 100 µT EMF from 20 min to 24 h.

4.3.3.4 Ornithine Decarboxylase (ODC)

ODC is an enzyme that plays an important role in regulating cell growth through
synthesis of polyamines necessary for protein and DNA synthesis. It is an enzyme
activated during carcinogenesis. Studies were carried out to investigate whether
there were effects on ODC due to EMF exposure. An *in vitro* study [132,133] found
increased ODC activity in three cell lines in response to a sinusoidal 60-Hz electric
field (10 mV/cm) for only 10 s duration. Stimulation in the activity of ODC in cultured cells by RFR with ELF modulation was also reported [134,135]. The results
depended upon the type of modulation employed. These effects were noted only
for certain modulations of the carrier wave, portraying the window effect (an effect
that appears at certain frequency but not at higher or lower frequencies). In addition,
changes in ODC have also been reported from EMF exposure *in vivo* [136]. It is clear
from the literature that a variety of *in vitro* studies have demonstrated that EMF
exposure affects ODC activity and cellular proliferation, while exposure to fields
below 0.1 mT have not been convincingly associated with adverse health effects.

4.3.3.5 Immune System

In most studies, EMF exposure appears to have no effect on the immune system.
House et al. [137] exposed mice and rats to 2, 200, and 1000 µT (60 Hz) continuously. No significant change in the distribution of lymphocyte subsets in the spleens
of exposed mice was observed when compared with controls. They concluded that
exposure of mice to linearly polarized, sinusoidal 60-Hz magnetic fields at strengths
up to 1000 µT for up to 3 months did not significantly affect a broad range of immune
effect or functions. In a study of human white blood cells, Aldinucci et al. [120]
found no effect of a 4275-mT field on the inflammatory response of normal or leukemic cells. Onodera et al. [138] reported that exposure of immune system cells to 1-T
field caused the loss of some cell types if the cells had been stimulated to divide, but

no effect if the cells had not been stimulated into division. Ikeda et al. [139] reported that exposure of human immune system cells to 2–500 µT fields (50 and 60 Hz linearly, elliptically, and circularly polarized) could not find any effects on the cytotoxic activities and the cytokines production of human PBMCs. However, Tremblay et al. [140] found that 60-Hz linearly polarized, sinusoidal, continuous-wave magnetic fields (2, 20, 200, and 2000 mT) can induce immunological perturbations on cells of both natural and adaptive immunity in a dose-dependent fashion.

4.3.4   ANIMAL CANCER STUDIES

There has been no absolute evidence in any study that low-level EMF alone can cause cancer in animals. This is supported by the findings of many studies [141–148]. Meanwhile, a few other studies show influence; for example, Vallejo et al. [149] reported that exposure of mice for 15 or 52 weeks to a 50-Hz field at 15 µT resulted in a significant increase in leukemia.

Animal studies presented mixed results but no direct carcinogenic effects have been observed. Future research may focus on the role of EMF as a tumor promoter or copromoter. Only a limited number of *in vivo* studies suggest a positive relationship between breast cancer in animals treated with carcinogens and magnetic-field exposure at approximately 0.02–0.1 mT. According to Löscher [150], one area with some positive laboratory evidence of cancer incidence could involve animals treated with carcinogens during an extended period of tumor development.

4.3.5   NONCANCER ANIMAL STUDIES

A number of noncancer studies were investigated for possible adverse effects of EMF exposure.

4.3.5.1   Behavioral Effects

There is insufficient evidence that EMF exposure at environmental levels causes behavioral changes of animals. Coelho et al. [151] reported that exposure to electric fields at 30 kV/m (60 Hz) increased the occurrence of three out of ten categories of social behavior of baboons during a 6-week exposure, compared with equivalent rates observed in 6-week pre- and post-exposure periods. Trzeciak et al. [152] noted that exposure to magnetic fields (50 Hz, 18 mT) had no effect on open-field behavior of 10–12 adult male and female Wistar rats. But the investigators recommended the need for further studies to fully determine conditions under which an effect can be observed. Meanwhile, Sienkiewicz et al. [153] reported that short-term, repeated exposure to intense magnetic fields might affect the behavior of mice. Mice were exposed each day to a 50-Hz magnetic field before being tested in a radial arm maze, a standard behavioral test of the ability of mice to learn a procedure for seeking food. Recently, Houpt et al. [154] reported that exposure of rats to high-strength magnetic fields (7000 or 14,000 mT) caused behavioral changes within 5 min. Similar behavioral effects were observed by Lockwood et al. [155] when mice were exposed to a 14.1 T field for 30 min. These effects, similar to the effects in rats [154], may be the result of a vestibular disturbance caused by the magnetic field, Lockwood et al. said.

4.3.5.2 Blood–Brain Barrier

The BBB is a physiologically complex system. It separates the brain and cerebral spinal fluid of the CNS from the blood. It primarily consists of an essentially continuous layer of cells lining the blood vessels of the brain. It protects sensitive brain tissues from ordinary variations in the composition of blood while allowing transport of nutrients into the brain. But the BBB is not an absolute barrier between the blood and the brain; rather it retards the rate at which substances cross between the blood stream and the brain. Any disruption to the BBB has serious consequences for health. The BBB may break down following brain trauma or brain heating. The BBB breakdown is risky if it allows enough concentrations of blood-borne neurotoxins (such as urea) to enter the brain.

Several investigations have indicated that ELF exposure has influence on the BBB permeability [156–158]. However, Öztas et al. [159] suggested that magnetic field has no effect on the BBB permeability.

4.3.5.3 Reproductive and Development

There is no strong evidence of reproductive or developmental effects of exposure to magnetic fields in experimental animals. Studies using mice and rats have shown that exposure to magnetic fields results skeletal malformations [160,161], increase in placental resorptions [162], and fertility [163]. However, Ryan et al. [164] studied the effect of magnetic field (2, 200, and 1000 µT continuous exposure and 1000 µT intermittent exposure) on fetal development and reproductive toxicity in the rodent. There was no evidence of any maternal or fetal toxicity or malformation. Elbetieha et al. [165] found that exposure of male and female mice to 50-Hz sinusoidal magnetic field (25 µT) for 90 days before they were mated with unexposed counterparts had no adverse effects on fertility and reproduction in mice. Other studies also have reported no major effects on reproduction and development in mice [166–171].

Brent [172] reviewed *in vivo* animal studies and *in vitro* tests, as well as the biological plausibility of the allegations of reproductive risks and concluded, "The studies involving nonhuman mammalian organisms dealing with fetal growth, congenital malformations, embryonic loss, and neurobehavioral development were predominantly negative and are therefore not supportive of the hypothesis that low-frequency EMF exposures result in reproductive toxicity."

Juutilainen [173] reviewed experimental studies on the effects of RF, ELF, and intermediate frequency (IF) EM fields on animal development. The author concluded, "ELF electric fields up to 150 kV/m have been evaluated in several mammalian species. The results are rather consistent and do not suggest adverse developmental effects. The results of studies on ELF magnetic fields suggest effects on bird embryo development, but not consistently in all studies. Results from experiments with other nonmammalian experimental models have also suggested subtle effects on developmental stability. In mammals, most studies have shown no effects of prenatal exposure to ELF or IF magnetic on gross external, visceral, or skeletal malformations. The only finding that shows some consistency is increase of minor skeleton alterations in several experiments. Taken as a whole, the results do not show robust adverse effects of ELF and IF fields on development."

4.4 CLINICAL STUDIES

Clinical studies carefully utilize screened volunteers who participate in double-blind studies, where appropriate, performed in a certified exposure facility. These studies investigate effects of EMF exposure on various senses, hormones, and organs, such as hearing, the brain, the cardiovascular system, the immune system, melatonin, and the eyes. EMF effects might be studied safely and effectively in the laboratory with human volunteers in spite of limitations to the duration of exposure and types of tests that are performed. The focus in human studies is usually on the effects that occur within a time frame of minutes, hours, days, or perhaps weeks. Longer-term studies with controlled exposure are difficult, if not impossible, to carry out with human volunteers in laboratory settings. The selection of physiological mechanisms for study is also limited to those that can be measured by noninvasive or minimally invasive procedures.

Various health effects are claimed by people due to EMF exposure, including headache, cardiovascular changes, behavioral changes, confusion, depression, difficulty in concentrating, sleep disturbances, decreased libido, and poor digestion. The main sources of information in this field are surveys of people and workers living close to potential sources of EMF, laboratory tests, and epidemiological data.

4.4.1 PERCEPTION AND SENSITIVITY

Exposure to electric fields, especially at low frequency (up to 300 Hz), can result in field perception as a result of alternating electric charge induced on the surface, causing body hair to vibrate. Electrically excitable cells in the retina can be affected by current densities of 10 mA/m^2 or more, induced by low-frequency magnetic fields or directly applied electric currents but with no adverse health effects [174]. Most people can perceive electric fields greater than 20 kV/m, and a small percentage of people perceive field strengths below 5 kV/m [175].

Humans experience flickering visual sensations caused by nonphotic stimulation such as pressure on the eyes and mechanical shocks. They are caused by induced currents in the retina, where the threshold at 20 Hz (maximum sensitivity occurs between 20 and 30 Hz) is about 20 mA/m^2. This is a level much higher than endogenous current densities in electrically excitable living tissues [176]. The effect observed in humans at the lowest magnetic field is a kind of visual sensation called a "magnetophosphene," where a flickering sensation is produced in surrounding vision by 50/60-Hz magnetic fields above about 10 mT. The effect is also connected to biomagnetic particles, which have been reported in the human brain [177].

A syndrome called "electrosensitivity" or electromagnetic hypersensitivity (EHS) initially appeared in Norway in the early 1980s among users of VDTs [178]. The syndrome has included various nonspecific health symptoms such as skin reaction, electrophysiological changes in the CNS, respiratory, cardiovascular, and digestive effects. Mueller et al. [179] reported that some people appear able to detect weak (100 V/m and 6 µT) EMF, but the ability to detect the fields is unrelated to whether the person is electrosensitive.

Leitgeb and Schröttner [180] considered an extended sample of the general population of 708 adults, including 349 men and 359 women aged between 17 and

60 years. Electrosensibility was investigated and characterized by perception threshold and its standard deviation (SD). By analyzing the probability distributions of the perception threshold of electric 50 Hz currents, evidence could be found for the existence of a subgroup of people with significantly increased hypersensibility who as a group could be differentiated from the general population. The presented data show that the variation of the electrosensibility among the general population is significantly larger than has yet been estimated by nonionizing radiation protection bodies, but much smaller than claimed by hypersensitivity self-aid groups.

4.4.2 Brain and Behavior

The CNS is a potential site of interaction with EMF because of the electrical sensitivity of the tissues. Lyskov et al. [181,182] performed spectral analysis of EEG recorded from volunteers exposed to a 45-Hz, 1.26-mT magnetic field. Significant increases in the mean frequency and spectral power were observed in the α and β bands of the spectrum.

Studies conducted at 50 Hz on visual evoked potentials exhibited no effect on visual evoked potentials while using combined 60-Hz EMF up to 12 kV/m and 0.03 mT [183]. However, Crasson et al. [184] indicated that a 50-Hz at 0.1-mT magnetic fields may have a slight influence on event-related potentials and reaction time under specific circumstances of sustained attention.

Magnetic or electric fields in the occupational environment (up to 5 mT or 20 kV/m) are generally reported to have no or minimal effects on neurophysiologic (EEG rhythms and evoked potentials) or cognitive responses of human subjects [184,185]. Preece et al. [186] reported small reductions in attention and mnemonic aspects of task performance when volunteers were exposed to a 50-Hz, 0.6-mT magnetic field. An insignificant effect on memory function has also been reported at a magnetic flux density of 1 mT [187]. Podd et al. [188] failed to find any effects of the field on reaction time and accuracy in the visual discrimination task when using a 50-Hz, 100-μT magnetic fields. Recently, Legros and Beuter [189] suggested that magnetic field could have a subtle delayed effect on human behavior, which is clearly not pathological. The aim of the above study was to determine the effect of a 50-Hz, 1000-μT magnetic field centered at the level of the head on human index finger microdisplacements.

Cook et al. [190] reviewed the behavioral and physiological effects of EMF on humans and concluded, "The variability in results makes it extremely difficult to draw any conclusions with regard to functional relevance for possible health risks or therapeutic benefits." For more details, please see a review on the recent studies (2001–2005) [191]. In their concluding remarks, the authors discussed a number of variables that are not often considered in human bioelectromagnetics studies, such as personality, individual differences, and the specific laterality of ELF magnetic field and mobile phone exposure over the brain. They also considered the sensitivity of various physiological assays and performance measures in the study of biological effects of EM fields.

Although the evidence for an association between EMF exposure at levels lower than MPE values and brain activity is inconclusive, research on brain functions due to prolonged exposure should be investigated in future research.

4.4.3 Cardiovascular System

Heart rate, blood pressure, and the performance of electrocardiogram (ECG) are commonly used to assess cardiovascular functions. Current densities of about 0.1 A/m^2 can stimulate excitable tissues, while current densities above about 1 A/m^2 interfere with the action of the heart by causing ventricular fibrillation, as well as producing heat. Korpinen et al. [192] found no field-related changes in mean heart rate as a result of exposure to 50-Hz fields directly under power lines ranging from 110 to 400 kV. However, Sastre et al. [193] and Sait et al. [194] reported that exposure of human volunteers to 60-Hz magnetic fields (15 and 20 µT, respectively) caused changes in heart rate. Kurokawa et al. [195] reported the absence of effects on heart rate in human volunteers exposed to 50- to 1000-Hz magnetic fields at 20–100 mT for 2 min to 12 h.

According to a review by Stuchly [196], exposure of healthy male volunteers to 20-µT EMF at 60 Hz has been linked to a statistically significant slowing of the heart rate and to changes in a small fraction of the tested behavioral indicators. In another review, Jauchem [197] concludes that no obvious acute or long-term cardiovascular-related hazards have been demonstrated at levels below current exposure limits for EMF.

In a recent review of the literature involving the effects of magnetic fields on microcirculation and microvasculature, McKay et al. [198] indicates that nearly half of the cited experiments (10 of 27 studies) report either a vasodilatory effect due to magnetic field exposure, increased blood flow, or increased blood pressure. Conversely, three of the 27 studies report a decrease in blood perfusion/pressure. Four studies report no effect. The remaining 10 studies found that magnetic field exposure could trigger either vasodilation or vasoconstriction depending on the initial tone of the vessel.

4.4.4 Melatonin in Humans

Several studies examining the suppression of human melatonin due to exposure to EMF from VDTs [199] and electric utilities [34,200–203] have been reported. Many studies found no effect on melatonin levels among healthy volunteers exposed to fields at 1–200 µT [204–210].

Wood et al. [211] reported that the nighttime melatonin peak was delayed by exposure to a 20-µT magnetic field, but that overall melatonin levels were not affected. Juutilainen et al. [212] showed some ambiguous evidence for a decrease in nighttime melatonin production among female Finnish garment workers (who are exposed to power-frequency fields from sewing machines). Griefahn et al. [207] reported that the effect of magnetic fields on melatonin secretion will most likely occur after repetitive exposures to intermittent fields. This conclusion was obtained after conducting a study on seven healthy young men aged between 16 and 22 years.

Liburdy et al. [213] indicated that melatonin reduces the growth rate of human breast cancer cells in culture, but a 1.2-µT (60 Hz) magnetic field can block the ability of melatonin to inhibit breast cancer cell growth. Recently, Juutilainen and Kumlin [99] noted that daytime occupational exposure to magnetic fields enhances the effects of nighttime light exposure on melatonin production in middle-aged women. However, the results were not conclusive because of several limitations of the data, such as imprecise light measurements and low number of subjects who were exposed to magnetic fields. According to the authors, the value of the findings supports evidences from other studies and indicates that possible interaction with light should be considered in any further studies of magnetic fields and melatonin.

In a review, Karasek and Lerchl [98] concluded, "At present there are no convincing data showing a distinct effect of magnetic fields on melatonin secretion in (human) adults." It is also not clear whether the decreases in melatonin reported in the positive papers are related to the presence of EMF exposure or to other factors.

4.5 CONCLUDING REMARKS AND FUTURE RESEARCH

Since 1979, there has been a flurry of scientific activity to evaluate the possibility that exposure to EMF from power lines and other sources may cause cancer. Overall, the currently available epidemiological and toxicological data do not provide clear evidence that EMF is associated with an increased risk of cancer, although there is some epidemiological evidence of linkages between EMF and childhood leukemia. There is also no convincing evidence from cellular and animal studies that EMF can directly damage DNA or promote tumor growth.

Current evidence from laboratory and epidemiological studies on the association between EMF exposure and cancer or other harmful health outcomes is inconsistent and inconclusive. Whereas early studies focusing on residents living near high-voltage transmission lines provided some evidence of a link between the risk of leukemia and EMF as characterized by Wertheimer and Leeper [10], most of the subsequent studies using actual field measurements failed to confirm the initial findings.

Investigations of weak EM field (including ELF associated with cellular phones) effects on human physiology have yielded some evidence of effects in a number of different areas such as heart-rate variability, sleep disturbance, and melatonin suppression [2,190,205]. The lack of consistent positive findings in experimental studies weakens the argument that this association is actually due to EMF exposure only. Although experimental studies cannot be used to rule out the possibility of small risks, they can provide evidence of a positive association under certain exposure conditions. In order to achieve possible proof, there is a need for better EMF exposure assessments (including transients), increased cellular and animal studies that better simulate the effect on humans, and increased human population studies that evaluate exposures with adverse health outcomes.

Most studies of adult cancers, particularly brain cancer, have been based on occupational groups, especially electrical workers with possibly high exposure. The few studies examining brain cancer and residential exposures found little or no evidence of association.

Studies examining health outcomes other than cancer do not provide sufficient evidence to support an association between EMF exposure and pregnancy outcomes, heart diseases, Alzheimer's disease, depression, or symptoms attributed by some to sensitivity. However, a number of epidemiological and experimental studies suggest that relatively strong EMF can alter cardiac rhythm, which is not surprising in view of the electrical nature of the mechanisms controlling heart rate.

In evaluation of all epidemiological studies, researchers were particularly concerned with the methodological challenges, especially with respect to exposure control and assessment. The challenges include better knowledge about exposure metrics, periods of exposure, characterization of exposure sources, availability of population registry databases, and residential area measurements.

Laboratory research has given no consistent evidence that EMF at environmental levels for a substantial period can affect biological processes or cause cancer. It is generally considered that EMF exposure does not possess enough energy to damage DNA directly, but there have been some reports in the literature of damage to DNA after exposure to EMF, and some of these reports are presented and discussed. Recent studies of disturbances in melatonin release in both animals and humans have been inconsistent. The NIEHS concluded that there was inadequate evidence for carcinogenicity in animals exposed to EMF exposure.

4.5.1 Review Studies

Several major large-scale national and international programs and reviews have been undertaken recently [39,74,198,214–223]. In 1991, the National Research Council (NRC) convened an expert committee to review and evaluate the existing scientific information on the possible effects of EMF exposure on the incidence of cancer, on reproduction and developmental abnormalities, and on neurobiological response, as reflected in learning and behavior. The committee concluded in its 1997 report that the evidence does not support the notion that EMF exposure is a human health hazard.

In the United States, the mandate of the NRC committee was restricted in its scope; however, the National Institute of Environmental Health Sciences (NIEHS) [1,2] was charged to prepare and submit a wider evaluation of the potential human health effects from EMF exposure. In addition, the World Health Organization (WHO) has completed extensive reviews of related studies. Details of the above reviews are summarized in reports, scientific journals, and conferences.

Evidence linking EMF to most cancers (except childhood and CLL, where the evidence has been characterized as suggestive or as "possibly carcinogenic" to humans) was deemed inadequate by NIEHS. WHO's International EMF Project reached similar conclusions [175]. The National Academy of Science concluded that there was no consistent evidence linking EMF and cancer [214]. Each of these reports noted a lack of studies properly designed to investigate this issue.

Childhood leukemia is the only cancer for which there is statistically consistent evidence of an association with exposure to EMF above 0.4 µT. The evidence for a causal relationship is still inconclusive. The NIEHS concluded that there was limited evidence for an association with EMF exposure. Specifically, investigators found some evidence of an increased risk of leukemia associated with increased EMF exposure [2]. Similar conclusions were made by the NRPB [215], the ICNIRP [174], the International Agency for Research on Cancer (IARC) [218], and the California EMF Program [219]. The IARC has concluded that EMF exposures are possibly carcinogenic to humans, based on a consistent statistical association of high-level residential magnetic fields with an increased risk of childhood leukemia, by approximately a factor of 2.

In most cases, the NIEHS concluded that there was no solid evidence to suggest that EMF in the environmental levels affect cells or systems. Two exceptions involved reports of weak evidence that EMF exposures contribute to behavioral, pharmacological, physiological, and biochemical changes in the nervous system and alter melatonin levels. EMF exposure, however, has been reported to enhance healing of damaged bones and is currently used in clinics for therapeutic purposes.

On behalf of the California Public Utilities Commission, three scientists who work for the California Department of Health Services (DHS) reviewed the studies about possible health risks from EMF exposure [219]. The reviewers are inclined to believe that EMF exposure can cause some degree of increased risk of childhood leukemia, adult brain cancer, and miscarriage. They believe that exposure to EMF is not a universal carcinogen and does not increase the risk of birth defects, low birth weight, depression, or heart disease.

4.5.2   FUTURE RESEARCH

Looking to the future, further studies are required to address the following issues: (1) elucidation of the biophysical interaction mechanisms that may explain how the signal from a low-energy source could affect biological systems; (2) improved dosimetry to reduce uncertainties in exposure assessment; (3) *in vitro* and *in vivo* studies on genetic effects, melatonin secretion, and tumorigenesis (with particular emphasis on characterization of dose–response relationships under a range of exposure conditions); (4) understanding the neurophysiologic implications of EMF; and (5) epidemiological studies to clarify the relationship between EMF and cancer in children, particularly leukemia.

A comprehensive research program that addresses these topics will require a transdisciplinary approach, involving specialists in EMF dosimetry, epidemiology, toxicology, and clinical research. This information will provide a firmer basis for assessing the potential health risks of EMF, and for both the updating and harmonization of current protection guidelines. In addition, work is also needed to better understand public perception of EMF risks, which can inform the design of risk communication strategies related to the management of EMF health risks.

REFERENCES

1. NIEHS. Assessment of health effects from exposure to power-line frequency electric and magnetic fields: working group report. National Institute of Environmental Health Sciences. NIH Publication No. 98-3981. Research Triangle Park, NC, USA, 1998.
2. NIEHS. Health effects from exposure to power-line frequency electric and magnetic fields. National Institute of Environmental Health Sciences. NIH Publication No. 99-4493. Research Triangle Park, NC, USA, 1999.
3. Dawson TW, Caputa K, Stuchly MA, Kavet R. Electric fields in the human body resulting from 60-Hz contact currents. *IEEE Trans Biomed Eng* 2001; 48: 1020–1026.
4. Niple JC, Daigle JP, Zaffanella LE, Sullivan T, Kavet R. A portable meter for measuring low frequency currents in the human body. *Bioelectromagnetics* 2004; 25: 369–373.
5. Linet MS, Wacholder S, Zahm SH. Interpreting epidemiologic research: lessons from studies of childhood cancer. *Pediatrics* 2003; 112: 218–232.

6. Blank M. The precautionary principle must be guided by EMF research. *Electromag Biol Med* 2006; 25: 203–208.

7. Milham S, Ossiander EM. Historical evidence that residential electrification caused the emergence of the childhood leukemia peak. *Med Hypotheses* 2001; 56: 290–295.

8. Li C-Y, Lin RS, Sung F-C. Elevated residential exposure to power frequency magnetic field associated with greater average age at diagnosis for patients with brain tumors. *Bioelectromagnetics* 2003; 24: 218–221.

9. Lightfoot L. Aetiology of childhood leukemia. *Bioelectromagnetics* 2005; 26: S5–S11.

10. Wertheimer N, Leeper E. Electric wire configurations and childhood cancer. *Am J Epidemiol* 1979; 109: 273–284.

11. Savitz DA, Wachtel H, Barnes FA, John EM, Tvrdik JG. Case-control study of childhood cancer and exposure to 60 Hz magnetic fields. *Am J Epidemiol* 1988; 128: 21–38.

12. London SJ, Thomas DC, Bowman JD, Sobel E, Chen TS, Peters JM. Exposure to residential electric and magnetic fields and risk of childhood leukemia. *Am J Epidemiol* 1991; 134: 923–937.

13. Feychting M, Ahlbom A. Magnetic fields and cancer in children residing near Swedish high-voltage power lines. *Am J Epidemiol* 1993; 138: 467–481.

14. Olsen JH, Nielsen A, Schulgen G. Residence near high-voltage facilities and the risk of cancer in children. *Br Med J* 1993; 307: 891–895.

15. Verkasalo PK, Pukkala E, Hongisto MY, Vajus JE, Jarvinen PJ, Heikkila KV, Koskenvuo M. Risk of cancer in Finnish children living close to power lines. *Br Med J* 1993; 307: 895–899.

16. Linet MS, Hatch EE, Kleinerman RA, Robison LL, Kaune WT, Friedman DR, Severson RK, Haines CM, Hartsock CT, Niwa S, Wacholder S, Tarone RE. Residential exposure to magnetic fields and acute lymphoblastic leukemia in children. *N Engl J Med* 1997; 337: 1–7.

17. McBride ML, Gallagher RP, Theriault G, Armstrong BG, Tamaro S, Spinelli JJ, Deadman JE, Finchman S, Robson D, Choi W. Power-frequency electric and magnetic fields and risk of childhood of leukemia in Canada. *Am J Epidemiol* 1999; 149: 831–842.

18. Green LM, Miller AB, Agnew DA, Greenberg ML, Li J, Villeneuve PJ, Tibshirani R. Childhood leukemia and personal monitoring of residential exposures to electric and magnetic fields in Ontario, Canada. *Cancer Cause Control* 1999; 10: 233–243.

19. Schüz J, Grigat JP, Brinkmann K, Michaelis J. Leukaemia and residential 16.7 Hz magnetic fields in Germany. *Br J Cancer* 2001; 84: 697–699.

20. Skinner J, Mee TJ, Blackwell RP, Maslanyj MP, Simpson J, Allen SG. Exposure to power frequency electric fields and the risk of childhood cancer in the UK. *Br J Cancer* 2002; 87: 1257–1266.

21. Feychting M, Floderus B, Ahlbom A. Parental occupational exposure to magnetic fields and childhood cancer (Sweden). *Cancer Causes Control* 2000; 11: 151–156.

22. Infante-Rivard C, Deadman JE. Maternal occupational exposure to extremely low frequency magnetic fields during pregnancy and childhood leukemia. *Epidemiology* 2003; 14: 437–441.

23. Henshaw DL, Reiter RJ. Do magnetic fields cause increased risk of childhood leukemia via melatonin disruption? *Bioelectromagnetics* 2005; 26: 68–97.

24. McKinney PA. Central nervous system tumours in children: epidemiology and risk factors. *Bioelectromagnetics* 2005; 26: S60–S68.

25. Kheifets L, Matkin CC. Industrialization, electromagnetic fields, and breast cancer risk. *Environ Health Perspec* 1999; 107: S145–S154.

26. Wertheimer N, Leeper E. Adult cancer related to electrical wires near the home. *Int J Epidemiol* 1982; 11: 345–355.

27. Wertheimer N, Leeper E. Magnetic field exposure related to cancer subtypes. *Ann NY Acad Sci* 1987; 502: 43–53.

28. McDowall ME. Mortality of persons resident in the vicinity of electricity transmission facilities. *Br J Cancer* 1986; 53: 271–279.
29. Feychting M, Forssén U, Rutqvist LE, Ahlbom A. Magnetic fields and breast cancer in Swedish adults residing near high-voltage power lines. *Epidemiology* 1998; 9: 392–397.
30. Gammon MD, Schoenberg JB, Britton JA, Kelsey JL, Stanford JL, Malone KE, Coates RJ, Brogan DJ, Potischman N, Swanson CA, Brinton LA. Electric blanket use and breast cancer risk among younger women. *Am J Epidemiol* 1998; 148: 556–563.
31. Verkasalo PK, Pukkala E, Kaprio J, Heikkilä KV, Koskenvuo M. Magnetic fields of high voltage power lines and risk of cancer in Finnish adults: nationwide cohort studies. *Br Med J* 1996; 313: 1047–1051.
32. Zheng T, Holford TR, Mayne ST, Owens PH, Zhang B, Boyle P. Exposure to electromagnetic fields from use of electric blankets and other in-home electrical appliances and breast cancer risk. *Am J Epidemiol* 2000; 151: 1103–1111.
33. McElroy JA, Newcomb PA, Remington PL, Egan KM, Titus-Ernstoff L, Trentham-Dietz A, Hampton JM, Baron JA, Stampfer MJ, Willett WC. Electric blanket or mattress cover use and breast cancer incidence in women 50–79 years of age. *Epidemiology* 2001; 12: 613–617.
34. Davis S, Kaune WT, Mirick DK, Chen C, Stevens RG. Residential magnetic fields, light-at-night, and nocturnal urinary 6-sulfatoxymelatonin concentration in women. *Am J Epidemiol* 2001; 154: 591–600.
35. Davis S, Mirick DK, Stevens RG. Residential magnetic fields and the risk of breast cancer. *Am J Epidemiol* 2002; 155: 446–454.
36. Li D–K, Odouli R, Wi S, Janevic T, Golditch I, Bracken TD, Senior R, Rankin R, Iriye R. A population-based prospective cohort study of personal exposure to magnetic fields during pregnancy and the risk of miscarriage. *Epidemiology* 2002; 13: 9–20.
37. Schoenfeld ER, O'Leary ES, Henderson K, Grimson R, Kabat GC, Ahnn S. Electromagnetic fields and breast cancer on Long Island: a case-control study. *Am J Epidemiol* 2003; 158: 47–58.
38. Kabat GC, O'Leary ES, Schoenfeld ER, Green JM, Grimson R. Electric blanket use and breast cancer on Long Island. *Epidemiology* 2003; 14: 514–520.
39. Erren TC. A meta-analysis of epidemiologic studies of electric and magnetic fields and breast cancer in women and men. *Bioelectromagnetics* 2001; S5: S105–S119.
40. Lin RS, Dischinger PC, Conde J, Farrell KP. Occupational exposure to electromagnetic fields and the occurrence of brain tumors. *J Occup Med* 1985; 27: 413–419.
41. Sahl JD, Kelsh MA, Greenland S. Cohort and nested case-control studies of hematopoietic cancers and brain cancer among electric utility workers. *Epidemiology* 1993; 4: 104–114.
42. Theriault G, Goldberg M, Miller AB, Armstrong B, Guenel P, Deadman J, Imbernon E, To T, Chevalier A, Cyr D, Wall C. Cancer risks associated with occupational exposure to magnetic fields among electric utility workers in Ontario and Quebec, Canada, and France: 1970–1989. *Am J Epidemiol* 1994; 139: 550–572.
43. London SJ, Bowman JD, Sobel E, Thomas DC, Garabrant DH, Pearce N, Bernstein L, Peters JM. Exposure to magnetic fields among electrical workers in relation to leukemia risk in Los Angeles County. *Am J Ind Med* 1994; 26: 47–60.
44. Tynes T, Jynge H, Vistnes Al. Leukemia and brain tumors in Norwegian railway workers, a nested case-control study. *Am J Epidemiol* 1994; 139: 643–653.
45. Savitz DA, Loomis DP. Magnetic field exposure in relation to leukemia and brain cancer mortality among electric utility workers. *Am J Epidemiol* 1995; 141: 123–134.
46. Coogan PF, Clapp RW, Newcomb PA, Wenzle TB, Bogdan G, Mittendorf R, Baron JA, Longnecker MP. Occupational exposure to 60-hertz magnetic fields and risk of breast cancer in women. *Epidemiology* 1996; 7: 459–464.

47. Floderus B, Persson T, Stenlund C. Magnetic field exposure in the workplace: reference distributions and exposures in occupational groups. *Int J Occup Environ Health* 1996; 2: 226–238.
48. Fear NT, Roman E. Cancer in electrical workers: an analysis of cancer registrations in England, 1981–1987. *Br J Cancer* 1996; 73: 935–939.
49. Miller AB, To T, Agnew DA, Wall C, Green LM. Leukemia following occupational exposure to 60 Hz electric and magnetic fields among Ontario electricity utility workers. *Am J Epidemiol* 1996; 144: 150–160.
50. Feychting M, Forssen U, Floderus B. Occupational and residential magnetic field exposure and leukemia and central nervous system tumors. *Epidemiology* 1997; 8: 384–389.
51. Johansen C, Olsen J. Mortality from amyotrophic lateral sclerosis, other chronic disorders, and electric shocks among utility workers. *Am J Epidemiol* 1998a; 148: 362–368.
52. Johansen C, Olsen J. Risk of cancer among Danish utility workers—a nationwide cohort study. *Am J Epidemiol* 1998b; 147: 548–555.
53. Savitz DA, Liao D, Sastre A, Kleckner RC. Magnetic field exposure and cardiovascular disease mortality among electric utility workers. *Am J Epidemiol* 1999; 149: 135–142.
54. Floderus B, Stenlund C, Persson T. Occupational magnetic field exposure and site-specific cancer incidence: a Swedish cohort study. *Cancer Causes Control* 1999; 10: 323–332.
55. Carozza SE, Wrensch M, Miike R, Newman B, Olshan AF, Savitz DA, Yost M, Lee M. Occupation and adult gliomas. *Am J Epidemiol* 2000; 152: 838–846.
56. Villeneuve PJ, Agnew DA, Johonson KC, Mao Y. Brain cancer and occupational exposure to magnetic fields among men: results from a Canadian population-based case-control study. *Int J Epidemiol* 2002; 31: 210–217.
57. Villeneuve PJ, Agnew DA, Miller AB, Corey PN, Purdham JT. Leukemia in electric utility workers: the evaluation of alternative indices of exposure to 60 Hz electric and magnetic fields. *Am J Ind Med* 2000; 37: 607–617.
58. Minder CE, Pfluger DH. Leukemia, brain tumors, and exposure to extremely low frequency electromagnetic fields in Swiss railway employees. *Am J Epidemiol* 2001; 153: 825–835.
59. Navas-Acién A, Pollán M, Gustavsson P, Floderus B, Plato N, Dosemeci M. Interactive effect of chemical substances and occupational electromagnetic field exposure on the risk of gliomas and meningiomas in Swedish men. *Cancer Epidemiol Biomarkers Prev* 2002; 11: 1678–1683.
60. Willett EV, Mckinney PA, Fear NT, Cartwright RA, Roman E. Occupational exposure to electromagnetic fields and acute leukaemia: analysis of a case-control study. *Occup Environ Med* 2003; 60: 577–583.
61. Demers PA, Thomas DB, Rosenblatt KA, Jiminez LM, McTiernan A, Stalsberg H, Stemhagen A, Thompson WD, Curnen M, Satariano A, Austin DF, Isacson P, Greenberg RS, Key C, Kolonel L, West D. Occupational exposure to electromagnetic radiation and breast cancer in males. *Am J Epidemiol* 1991; 134: 340–347.
62. Tynes T, Andersen A, Langmark B. Incidence of cancer in Norwegian workers potentially exposed to electromagnetic fields. *Am J Epidemiol* 1992; 136: 81–86.
63. Stenlund C, Floderus, B. Occupational exposure to magnetic fields in relation to male breast cancer and testicular cancer: a Swedish case-control study. *Cancer Causes Control* 1997; 8: 184–191.
64. Petralia SA, Vena JE, Freudenheim JL, Dosemeci M, Michalek A. Occupational risk factors for breast cancer among women in Shanghai. *Am J Ind Med* 1998; 34: 477–483.
65. Cocco P, Figgs L, Dosemeci M, Hayes R, Linet MS, Hsing AW. Case-control study of occupational exposures and male breast cancer. *Occup Environ Med* 1998; 55: 599–604.

66. Håkansson N, Floderus B, Gustavsson P, Johansen C, Olsen JH. Cancer incidence and magnetic field exposure in industries using resistance welding in Sweden. *Occup Environ Med* 2002; 59: 481–486.

67. Guenel P, Nicolau J, Imbernon E, Chevalier A, Goldberg M. Exposure to 50-Hz electric field and the incidence of leukemia, brain tumors, and other cancers among French electric utility workers. *Am J Epidemiol* 1996; 144: 1107–1121.

68. Firth HM, Cooke KR, Herbison GP. Male cancer incidence by occupation: New Zealand, 1972–1984. *Int J Epidemiol* 1996; 25: 14–21.

69. Charles LE, Loomis D, Shy CM, Newman B, Millikan R, Nylander-French LA, Couper D. Electromagnetic fields, polychlorinated biphenyls, and prostate cancer mortality in electric utility workers. *Am J Epidemiol* 2003; 157: 683–691.

70. Sahl J, Mezel G, Kavet R, McMillan A, Silvers A, Sastre A, Kheifets L. Occupational magnetic field exposure and cardiovascular mortality in a cohort of electric utility workers. *Am J Epidemiol* 2002; 156: 913–918.

71. Johansen C, Feychting M, Moller M, Arnsbo P, Ahlbom A, Olsen JH. Risk of severe cardiac arrhythmia in male utility workers: a nationwide Danish cohort study. *Am J Epidemiol* 2002; 156: 857–861.

72. van Wijngaarden E, Savitz DA, Kleckner RTC, Cai J, Loomis D. Exposure to electromagnetic fields and suicide among electric utility workers: a nest case-control study. *Occup Environ Med* 2000; 57: 258–263.

73. Baris D, Armstrong BG, Deadman J, Theriault G. A case cohort study of suicide in relation to exposure to electric and magnetic fields among electrical utility workers. *Occup Environ Med* 1996; 53: 17–24.

74. Ahlbom, A. Neurodegenerative diseases, suicide and depressive symptoms in relation to EMF. *Bioelectromagnetics* 2001; S5: S132–S143.

75. Wertheimer N, Leeper E. Possible effects of electric blankets and heated waterbeds on fetal development. *Bioelectromagnetics* 1986; 7: 13–22.

76. Dlugosz L, Vena J, Byers T, Sever L, Bracken M, Marshall E. Congenital defects and electric bed heating in New York State: a register-based case-control study. *Am J Epidemiol* 1992; 135: 1000–1011.

77. Blaasaas KG, Tynes T, Rolv TL. Residence near power lines and the risk of birth defects. *Epidemiology* 2003; 14: 95–98.

78. Blaasaas KG, Tynes T, Irgens Å, Lie RT. Risk of birth defects by parental occupational exposure to 50 Hz electromagnetic fields: a population based study. *Occup Environ Med* 2002; 59: 92–97.

79. Feychting M. Non-cancer EMF effects related to children. *Bioelectromagnetics* 2005; 26: S69–S74.

80. Li D-K, Odouli R, Wi S, Janevic T, Golditch I, Bracken TD, Senior R, Rankin R, Iriye R. A population-based prospective cohort study of personal exposure to magnetic fields during pregnancy and the risk of miscarriage. *Epidemiology* 2002; 13: 9–20.

81. Lee GM, Neutra RR, Hristova L, Yost M, Hiatt RA. A nested case-control study of residential and personal magnetic field measures and miscarriages. *Epidemiology* 2002; 13: 21–31.

82. Li D-K, Neutra RR. Magnetic fields and miscarriage. *Epidemiology* 2002; 13: 237–238.

83. Savitz DA. Magnetic fields and miscarriage. *Epidemiology* 2002; 13: 1–3.

84. Greenland S, Kheifets L. Leukemia attributable to residential magnetic fields: results from analyses allowing for study biases. *Risk Analysis* 2006; 26: 471–482.

85. Greenland S, Sheppard AR, Kaune WT, Poole C, Kelsh MA. A pooled analysis of magnetic fields, wire coodes, and childhood leukemia. *Epidemiology* 2000; 11: 624–664.

86. Kheifets L, Repacholi M, Saunders R, van Deventer E. Sensitivity of children to EMF. *Pediatrics* 2005; 115: e303–e313.

87. Kato M, Honma K, Shigemitsu T, Shiga Y. Effects of exposure to a circularly polarized 50-Hz magnetic field on plasma and pineal melatonin levels in rats. *Bioelectromagnetics* 1993; 14: 97–106.

88. Wilson BW, Matt KS, Morris JE, Sasser LB, Miller DL, Anderson LE. Effects of 60 Hz magnetic field exposure on the pineal and hypothalamic-pituitary-gonadal axis in Siberian hamster (*Phodopus sungorus*). *Bioelectromagnetics* 1999; 20: 224–232.

89. Huuskonen H, Saastamoinen V, Komulainen H, Laitinen J, Juutilainen J. Effects of low-frequency magnetic fields on implantation in rats. *Reprod Toxicol* 2001; 15: 49–59.

90. Rogers WR, Reiter RJ, Barlow-Walden L, Smith HD, Orr JL. Regularly scheduled, daytime, slow-onset 60 Hz electric and magnetic field exposure does not depress serum melatonin concentration in nonhuman primates. *Bioelectromagnetics* 1995a; 3: 111–118.

91. Rogers WR, Reiter RJ, Smith HD, Barlow-Walden L. Rapid-onset/offset, variably scheduled 60 Hz electric and magnetic field exposure reduces nocturnal serum melatonin concentration in nonhuman primates. *Bioelectromagnetics* 1995b; 3: 119–122.

92. Mevissen M, Lerchl A, Szamel M, Löscher W. Exposure of DMBA-treated female rats in a 50-Hz, 50 milliT magnetic field: effects on mammary tumor growth, melatonin levels, and T lymphocyte activation. *Carcinogenesis* 1996; 17: 903–910.

93. Löscher W, Mevissen M, Lerchl A. Exposure of female rats to a 100 microT 50 Hz magnetic field does not induced consistent changes in nocturnal levels of melatonin. *Radiat Res* 1998; 150: 557–567.

94. Selmaoui B, Touitou Y. Age-related differences in serum melatonin and pineal NAT activity and in the response of rat pineal to a 50-Hz magnetic field. *Life Sci* 1999; 64: 2291–2297.

95. Fedrowitz M, Westermann J, Löscher W. Magnetic field exposure increases cell proliferation but does not affect melatonin levels in the mammary gland of female Sprague–Dawley rats. *Cancer Res* 2002; 62: 1356–1363.

96. Bakos J, Nagy N, Thuróczy G, Szabó LD. One week of exposure to 50 Hz, vertical magnetic field does not reduce urinary 6-sulphatoxymelatonin excretion of male Wistar rats. *Bioelectromagnetics* 2002; 23: 245–248.

97. Tripp HM, Warman GR, Arendt J. Circularly polarised MF (500 T 50 Hz) does not acutely suppress melatonin secretion from cultured Wistar rat pineal glands. *Bioelectromagnetics* 2003; 24: 118–124.

98. Karasek M, Lerchl A. Melatonin and magnetic fields. *Neuroendocrin Lett* 2002; 23: 84–87.

99. Juutilainen J, Kumlin T. Occupational magnetic field exposure and melatonin: interaction with light-at-night. *Bioelectromagnetics* 2006; 27: 423–426.

100. Lai H, Singh NP. Acute exposure to a 60 Hz magnetic field increases DNA strand breaks in rat brain cells. *Bioelectromagnetics* 1997; 18: 156–165.

101. Lai H. Singh NP. Magnetic-field-induced DNA strand breaks in brain cells of the rat. *Environ Health Perspec* 2004; 112: 687–694.

102. Wu RW, Yang H, Chiang H, Shao BJ, Bao JL. The effects of low-frequency magnetic fields on DNA unscheduled synthesis induced by methylnitro-nitrosoguanidine. In vitro. *Electro- Magnetobiol* 1998; 17: 57–65.

103. Ivancsits S, Diem E, Pilger A, Rudiger HW, Jahn O. Induction of DNA strand breaks by intermittent exposure to extremely-low-frequency electromagnetic fields in human diploid fibroblasts. *Mutat Res* 2002; 519: 1–13.

104. McNamee JP, Bellier PV, McLeen JR, Marro L, Gajda GB, Thansandote A. DNA damage and apoptosis in the immature mouse cerebellum after acute exposure to a 1 mT, 60 Hz magnetic field. *Mutat Res* 2002; 513: 121–133.

105. Maes A, Collier M, Vandoninck S, Scarpa P, Verschaeve L. Cytogenetic effects of 50 Hz magnetic fields of different magnetic flux densities. *Bioelectromagnetics* 2000. 21: 589–596.

106. Zmyslony M, Palus J, Jajte J, Dziubaltowska E, Rajkowska E. DNA damage in rat lymphocytes treated in vitro with iron cations and exposed to 7 mT magnetic fields (static or 50 Hz). *Mutat Res* 2000; 453: 89–96.

107. Williams Pa, Ingebretsen RJ, Dawson RJ. 14.6 mT ELF magnetic field exposure yields no DNA breaks in model system Salmonella, but provides evidence of heat stress protection. *Bioelectromagnetics* 2006; 27: 445–450.

108. Khalil AM, Qassem W. Cytogenetic effects of pulsing electromagnetic field on human lymphocytes in vitro: chromosome aberrations, sister chromatid exchanges and cell kinetics. *Mutat Res* 1991; 247: 141–146.

109. Suzuki Y, Ikehata M, Nakamura K, Nishioka M, Asanuma K, Koana T, Shimizu H. Induction of micronuclei in mice exposed to static magnetic fields. *Mutagenesis* 2001; 16: 499–501.

110. Scarfi MR, Lioi MB, Zeni O, Franceschetti G, Franceschi C, Bersani F. Lack of chromosomal aberration and micronucleus induction in human lymphocytes exposed to pulsed magnetic fields. *Mutat Res* 1994; 306: 129–133.

111. Nakahara T, Yaguchi H, Yoshida M, Miyakoshi J. Effects of exposure of CHO–K1 cells to a 10-T static magnetic field. *Radiology* 2002; 224: 817–822.

112. Stronati L, Testa A, Villani P, Marino C, Lovisolo GA, Conti D, Russo F, Fresegna AM, Cordelli E. Absence of genotoxicity in human blood cells exposed to 50 Hz magnetic fields as assessed by comet assay, chromosome aberration, micronucleus, and sister chromatid exchange analyses. *Bioelectromagnetics* 2004; 25: 41–48.

113. Yomori H, Yasunaga K, Takahashi C, Tanaka A, Takashima S, Sekijima M. Elliptically polarized magnetic fields do not alter immediate early response genes expression levels in human glioblastoma cells. *Bioelectromagnetics* 2002; 23: 89–96.

114. Blackman CF, Benane SG, Kinney LS, Joines WT, House DE. Effects of ELF fields on calcium-ion efflux from brain tissue in vitro. *Radiat Res* 1982; 92: 510–520.

115. Blackman CF, Benane SG, House DE, Joines WT. Effects of ELF (1–120 Hz) and modulated (50 Hz) RF fields on the efflux of calcium ions from brain tissue in vitro. *Bioelectromagnetics* 1985; 6: 1–11.

116. Ikehara T, Park KH, Houchi H, Yamaguchi H, Hosokawa K, Shono M, Minakuchi K, Tamaki T, Kinouchi Y, Yoshizaki K, Miyamoto H. Effects of a time-varying strong magnetic field on transient increase in cytosolic free Ca^{2+} induced by bradykinin in cultured bovine adrenal chromaffin cells. *FEBS Lett* 1998; 435: 229–232.

117. Galvanovskis J, Sandblom J, Bergqvist B, Galt S, Hamnerius Y. Cytoplasmic Ca^{2+} oscillations in human leukemia T-cells are reduced by 50 Hz magnetic fields. *Bioelectromagnetics* 1999; 20: 269–276.

118. Pessina GP, Aldimucci C, Palmi M, Sgaragli G, Benocci A, Meini A, Pessina F. Pulsed electromagnetic fields affect the intracellular calcium concentrations in human astrocytoma cells. *Bioelectromagnetics* 2001; 22: 503–510.

119. Spadaro JA, Bergstrom WH. In vivo and in vitro effects of a pulsed electromagnetic field on net calcium flux in rat calvarial bone. *Clacif Tissue Int* 2002; 70: 496–502.

120. Aldinucci C, Garcia JB, Palmi M, Sgaragli G, Benocci A, Meini A, Pessina F, Rossi C, Bonechi C, Pessina GP. The effect of strong static magnetic field on lymphocytes. *Bioelectromagnetics* 2003a; 24: 109–117.

121. Aldinucci C, Blanco GJ, Palmi M, Sgaragli G, Benocci A, Meini A, Pessina F, Rossi C, Bonechi C, Pessina GP. The effect of exposure to high flux density static and pulsed magnetic fields on lymphocyte function. *Bioelectromagnetics* 2003b; 24: 373–379.

122. Ikehara T, Park KH, Yamaguchi H, Hosokawa K, Houchi H, Azuma M, Minakuchi K, Kashimoto H, Kitamura M, Kinouchi Y, Yoshizaki K, Miyamoto H. Effects of a time varying strong magnetic field on release of cytosolic free Ca^{2+} from intracellular stores in cultured bovine adrenal chromaffin cells. *Bioelectromagnetics* 2002; 23: 505–515.

123. Obo M, Konishi S, Otaka Y, Kitamura S. Effect of magnetic field exposure on calcium channel currents using patch clamp technique. *Bioelectromagnetics* 2002; 23: 306–314.

124. Antonopoulos A, Yang B, Stamm A, Heller W-D, Obe G. Cytological effects of 50 Hz electromagnetic fields on human lymphocytes in vitro. *Mutation Res* 1995; 346: 151–157.

125. Katsir G, Baram S, Parola A. Effect of sinusoidally varying magnetic fields on cell proliferation and adenosine deaminase specific activity. *Bioelectromagnetics* 1998; 19: 46–52.

126. Chen G, Upham BL, Sun W, Change C-C, Rothwell EJ, Chen K-M, Yamasaki H, Trosko JE. Effect of electromagnetic field exposure on chemically induced differentiation of friend erythroleukemia cells. *Environ Health Perspec* 2000; 108: 967–972.

127. Pirozzoli MC, Marino C, Lovisolo GA, Laconi C, Mosiello L, Negroni A. Effects of 50 Hz electromagnetic field exposure on apoptosis and differentiation in a neuroblastoma cell line. *Bioelectromagnetics* 2003; 24: 510–516.

128. Supino R, Bottone MG, Pellicciari C, Caserini C, Bottiroli G, Beller M, Veicsteinas A. Sinusoidal 50 Hz magnetic fields do not affect structural morphology and proliferation of human cells in vitro. *Histol Histopathol* 2001; 16: 719–726.

129. Kultz D. Molecular and evolutionary basis of the cellular stress response. *Ann Rev Physiol* 2005; 67: 225–227.

130. Goodman R, Blank M. Magnetic field stress induces expression of hsp70. *Cell Stress Chaperones* 1998; 3: 79–88.

131. Shi B, Farboud B, Nuccitelli R, Isseroff RR. Power-line frequency electromagnetic fields do not induce changes in phosphorylation, localization, or expression of the 27-kilodalton heat shock protein in human keratinocytes. *Environ Health Perspec* 2003; 111: 281–287.

132. Litovitz TA, Krause D, Mullins JM. Effect of coherence time of the applied magnetic field on ornithine decarboxylase activity. *Biochem Biophys Res Comm* 1991; 178: 862–865.

133. Litovitz TA, Krause D, Penafiel M, Elson EC, Mullins JM. The role of coherence time in the effect of microwaves on ornithine decarboxylase activity. *Bioelectromagnetics* 1993; 14: 395–403.

134. Byus CV, Kartun K, Pieper S, Adey WR. Increased ornithine decarboxylase activity in cultured cells exposed to low energy modulated microwave fields and phorbol ester tumor promoters. *Cancer Res* 1988; 48: 4222–4226.

135. Penafiel M, Litovitz T, Krause D, Desta A, Mullins JM. Role of modulation on the effect of microwaves on ornithine decarboxylase activity in L929 cells. *Bioelectromagnetics* 1997; 18: 132–141.

136. Mevissen M, Keitzmann M, Lösher W. In vivo exposure of rats to weak alternating magnetic field increases ornithine decarboxylase activity in the mammary gland by a similar extent as the carcinogen DMBA. *Cancer Lett* 1995; 90: 207–214.

137. House RV, Ratajczak HV, Gauger JR, Johnson TR, Thomas PT, McCormick DL. Immune function and host defense in rodents exposed to 60 Hz magnetic fields. *Fund Appl Toxicol* 1996; 34: 228–239.

138. Onodera H, Jin Z, Chida S, Suzuki Y, Tago H, Itoyama Y. Effects of 10-T static magnetic field on human peripheral blood immune cells. *Radiat Res* 2003; 159: 775–779.

139. Ikeda K, Shinmura Y, Mizoe H, Yoshizawa H, Yoshida A, Kanao S, Sumitani H, Hasebe S, Motomura T, Yamakawa T, Mizuno F, Otaka Y, Hirose H. No effects of extremely low frequency magnetic fields found on cytotoxic activities and cytokine production of human peripheral blood mononuclear cells in vitro. *Bioelectromagnetics* 2003; 24: 21–31.

140. Tremblay L, Houde M, Mercier G, Gagnon J, Mandeville R. Differential modulation of natural and adaptive immunity in Fischer rats exposed for 6 weeks to 60 Hz linear sinusoidal continuous-wave magnetic fields. *Bioelectromagnetics* 1996; 17: 373–383.

141. Sasser LB, Morris JE, Miller DL, Rafferty CN, Ebi KL, Anderson LE. Exposure to 60 Hz magnetic fields does not alter clinical progression of LGL leukemia in Fischer rats. *Carcinogenesis* 1996; 17: 2681–2687.

142. Sasser LB, Morris JE, Miller DL, Rafferty CN, Ebi KL, Anderson LE. Lack of a co-promoting effect of a 60 Hz magnetic field on skin tumorigenesis in SENCAR mice. *Carcinogenesis* 1998; 19: 1617–1621.

143. Harris AW, Basten A, Gebski V, Noonan D, Finnie J, Bath ML, Bangay MI, Repacholi MH. A test of lymphoma induction by long-term exposure of Eu-Pim1 transgenic mice to 50 Hz magnetic fields. *Radiat Res* 1998; 149: 300–330.

144. Morris JE, Sasser LB, Miller DL, Dagle GE, Rafferty CN, Ebi KL, Anderson LE. Clinical progression of transplanted large granular lymphocytic leukemia in Fischer 344 rats exposed to 60 Hz magnetic fields. *Bioelectromagnetics* 1999; 20: 48–56.

145. Boorman GA, McCormick DL, Findlay JC, Hailey JR, Gauger JR, Johnson TR, Kovatch RM, Sills RC, Haseman JK. Chronic toxicity/oncogenicity evaluation of 60 Hz (power frequency) magnetic fields in F344/N rats. *Toxicologic Pathology* 1999; 27: 267–278.

146. Galloni P, Marino C. Effects of 50 Hz magnetic field exposure on tumor experimental models. *Bioelectromagnetics* 2000; 21: 608–614.

147. Anderson LE, Morris JE, Miller DL, Rafferty CN, Ebi KL, Sasser LB. Large granular lymphocytic (LGL) leukemia in rats exposed to intermittent 60 Hz magnetic fields. *Bioelectromagnetics* 2001; 22: 185–193.

148. McLean JR, Thansandote A, McNamee JP, Tryphonas L, Lecuyer D, Gajda G. A 60 Hz magnetic field does not affect the incidence of squamous cell carcinomas in SENCAR mice. *Bioelectromagnetics* 2003; 24: 75–81.

149. Vallejo D, Sanz P. A hematological study in mice for evaluation of leukemogenesis by extremely low frequency magnetic fields. *Electro- Magnetobiol* 2001; 20: 281–298.

150. Löscher W. Do carcinogenic effects of ELF electromagnetic fields require repeated long-term interaction with carcinogens? Characteristics of positive studies using the DMBA breast cancer model in rats. *Bioelectromagnetics* 2001; 22: 603–614.

151. Coelho AM Jr, Easley SP, Rogers WR. Effects of exposure to 30 kV/m, 60 Hz electric fields on the social behavior of baboons. *Bioelectromagnetics* 1991; 12: 117–135.

152. Trzeciak HI, Grzesik J, Bortel M, Kuska R, Duda D, Michnik J, Maecki A. Behavioral effects of long-term exposure to magnetic fields in rats. *Bioelectromagnetics* 1993; 14: 287–297.

153. Sienkiewicz ZJ, Haylock RGE, Saunders RD. Deficits in spatial learning after exposure of mice to a 50 Hz magnetic field. *Bioelectromagnetics* 1998; 19: 79–85.

154. Houpt TA, Pittman DW, Barranco JM, Brooks EH, Smith JC. Behavioral effects of high-strength static magnetic fields on rats. *J Neurosci.* 2003; 23: 1498–1505.

155. Lockwood DR, Kwon B, Smith JC, Houpt TA. Behavioral effects of static high magnetic fields on unrestrained and restrained mice. *Physiol Behav* 2003; 78: 635–640.

156. Salford LG, Brun A, Sturesson K, Eberhardt JL, Persson BR. Permeability of the blood–brain barrier induced by 915 MHz electromagnetic radiation, continuous wave and modulated at 8, 16, 50, and 200 Hz. *Bioelectromagnetics* 1994; 27: 535–542.

157. Lapin GD. The EMP to BBB connection. Studying the effect of electromagnetic energy on the blood brain barrier. *IEEE Eng Med Biol* 1996; 15: 57–60.

158. Schirmacher A, Winters S, Fischer S, Goeke J, Galla HJ, Kullnick U, Ringelstein EB, Stogbauer F. Electromagnetic fields (1.8 GHz) increase the permeability to sucrose of the blood–brain barrier in vitro. *Bioelectromagnetics* 2000; 21: 338–345.

159. Öztas B, Kalkan T, Tuncel H. Influence of 50 Hz frequency sinusoidal magnetic field on the blood–brain barrier permeability of diabetic rats. *Bioelectromagnetics* 2004; 25: 400–402.

160. Huuskonen H, Juutilainen J, Komulainen H. Effects of low-frequency magnetic fields on fetal development in rats. *Bioelectromagnetics* 1993; 14: 205–213.

161. Mevissen M, Buntrnkotter S, Loscher W. Effect of static and time-varying (50 Hz) magnetic fields on reproduction and fetal development in rats. *Teratology* 1994; 50: 229–237.

162. Juutilainin J, Huuskonen H, Komulainen H. Increased resportions in CBA mice exposed to low-frequency magnetic fields: an attempt to replicate earlier observations. *Bioelectromagnetics* 1997; 18: 410–417.

163. Al-Akhras MA, Elbetieha A, Hasan MK, Al-Omari I, Darmani H, Albiss B. Effects of low-frequency magnetic field on fertility of adult male and female rats. *Bioelectromagnetics* 2001; 22: 340–344.

164. Ryan BM, Symanski RR, Pomeranz LE, Johnson TR, Gauger JR, McCormick DL. Multi-generation reproductive toxicity assessment of 60 Hz magnetic fields using a continuous breeding protocol in rats. *Teratology* 1999; 56: 159–162.

165. Elbetieha A, Al-Akhras A-A, Darmani H. Long-term exposure of male and female mice to 50 Hz magnetic field: effect on fertility. *Bioelectromagnetics* 2002; 23: 168–172.

166. Wiley MJ, Corey P, Kavet R, Charry J, Harvey S, Agnew D, Walsh M. The effects of continuous exposure to 20 kHz sawtooth magnetic fields on the litters of CD-1 mice. *Teratology* 1992; 46: 391–398.

167. Kowalczuk CI, Robbins L, Thomas JM, Butlnd BK, Saunders RD. Effects of prenatal exposure to 50 Hz magnetic fields development in mice. I. Implementation rate and fetal development. *Bioelectromagnetics* 1994; 15: 349–361.

168. Ryan BM, Mallett E, Johnson TR, Gauger JR, McCormick DL. Developmental toxicity study of 60 Hz (power frequency) magnetic fields in rats. *Teratology* 1996; 54: 73–83.

169. Okazaki R, Ootsuyama A, Uchida S, Norimura T. Effects of a 4.7 T static magnetic field on fetal development in ICR mice. *J Radiat Res* 2001; 42: 273–283.

170. Ohnishi Y, Mizuno F, Sato T, Yasui M, Kikuchi T, Ogawa M. Effects of power frequency alternating magnetic fields on reproduction and pre-natal development of mice. *J Toxicol Sci* 2002; 27: 131–138.

171. Chung M-K, Kim J-C, Myung S-H, Lee D-I. Developmental toxicity evaluation of ELF magnetic fields in Sprague–Dawley rats. *Bioelectromagnetics* 2003; 24: 231–240.

172. Brent RL. Reproductive and teratologic effects of low-frequency electromagnetic fields: a review of in vivo and in vitro studies using animal models. *Teratology* 1999; 59: 261–286.

173. Juutilainen J. Developmental effects of electromagnetic fields. *Bioelectromagnetics* 2005; 26: S107–S115.

174. ICNIRP. Guidelines for limiting exposure to time-varying electric, magnetic and electromagnetic fields (up to 300 GHz). *Health Phys* 1998; 74: 494–522.

175. Repacholi MH, Greenbaum B. Interaction of static and extremely low frequency electric and magnetic fields with living systems: health effects and research needs. *Bioelectromagnetics* 1999; 20: 133–160.

176. Foster KR. Electromagnetic field effects and mechanisms. *IEEE Eng Med Biol* 1996; 15: 50–56.

177. Adair AK. Effects of ELF magnetic fields on biological magnetite. *Bioelectromagnetics* 1993; 14: 1–4.

178. Ziskin MC. Electromagnetic hypersensitivity. *IEEE Eng Med Biol* 2002; 21: 173–175.

179. Mueller CH, Krueger H, Schierz C. Project NEMESIS: perception of a 50 Hz electric and magnetic field at low intensities (laboratory experiment). *Bioelectromagnetics* 2002; 23: 26–36.

180. Leitgeb N, Schröttner J. Electrosensibility and electromagnetic hypersensitivity. *Bioelectromagnetics* 2003; 24: 387–394.

181. Lyskov EB, Juulitainen J, Jousmaki V, Partanen J, Medvedev S, Hanninen O. Effects of 45-Hz magnetic fields on the functional state of the human brain. *Bioelectromagnetics* 1993a; 14: 87–95.
182. Lyskov EB, Juulitainen J, Jousmaki V, Hanninen O, Partanen J, Medvedev S, Hanninen O. Influence of short-term exposure of magnetic field on the bioelectrical processes of the brain and performance. *Int J Psychophysiol* 1993b; 14: 227–231.
183. Graham C, Cook MR, Cohen HD, Gerkovich MM. Dose response study of human exposure to 60 Hz electric and magnetic fields. *Bioelectromagnetics* 1994; 15: 447–463.
184. Crasson M, Legros JJ, Scarpa P. 50 Hz magnetic field exposure influence on human performance and psychophysiological parameters: two double-blind experimental studies. *Bioelectromagnetics* 1999; 20: 8: 474–486.
185. Graham C, Cook MR, Cohen HD. Human exposure to 60-Hz magnetic fields: neurophysiological effects. *Int J Psychophysiol* 1999; 33: 169–175.
186. Preece AW, Wesnes KA, Iwi GR. The effect of a 50 Hz magnetic field on cognitive function in humans. *Int J Radiat Biol* 1998; 74: 463–470.
187. Trimmel M, Schweiger E. Effects of an ELF (50 Hz, 1 mT) electromagnetic field (EMF) on concentration in visual attention, perception and memory including effects of EMF sensitivity. *Toxicol Lett* 1998; 96/97: 377–382.
188. Podd J, Abbott J, Kazantzis N, Rowland A. Brief exposure to a 50 Hz, 100 T magnetic field: effects on reaction time, accuracy, and recognition memory. *Bioelectromagnetics* 2002; 23: 189–195.
189. Legros A, Beuter A. Effect of a low intensity magnetic field on human motor behavior. *Bioelectromagnetics* 2005; 26: 657–669.
190. Cook CM, Thomas AW, Prato FS. Human electrophysiological and cognitive effects of exposure to ELF magnetic and ELF modulated RF and microwave fields: a review of recent studies. *Bioelectromagnetics* 2002; 23: 144–157.
191. Cook CM, Saucier DM, Thomas AW, Prato FS. Exposure to ELF magnetic and ELF-modulated radiofrequency fields: the time course of physiological and cognitive effects observed in recent studies (2001–2005). *Bioelectromagnetics* 2006; 27: 613–627.
192. Korpinen L, Partanen J, Uusitalo A. Influence of 50 Hz electric and magnetic fields on the human heart. *Bioelectromagnetics* 1993; 14: 329–340.
193. Sastre A, Coor MR, Graham C. Nocturnal exposure to intermittent 60 Hz magnetic fields alters human cardiac rhythm. *Bioelectromagnetics* 1998; 19: 98–106.
194. Sait ML, Wood AW, Sadafi HA. Human heart rate changes in response to 50 Hz sinusoidal and square waveform magnetic fields: a follow up study. In: Bersani F, Editor. *Electricity and Magnetism in Medicine and Biology.* Kluwer Academic/Plenum Publishers, New York, pp. 517–520, 1999.
195. Kurokawa Y, Nitta H, Imai H, Kabuto M. Can extremely low frequency alternating magnetic fields modulate heart rate or its variability in humans? *Auton Neurosci Basic Clin* 2003a; 105: 53–61.
196. Stuchly MA. Human exposure to static and time-varying magnetic fields. *Health Phys* 1986; 51: 215–225.
197. Jauchem JR. Exposure to extremely-low-frequency electromagnetic fields and radio frequency radiation: cardiovascular effects in humans. *Int Arch Occup Environ Health* 1997; 70: 9–21.
198. McKay JC, Prato FS, Thomas AW. A literature review: the effects of magnetic field exposure on blood flow and blood vessels in the microvasculature. *Bioelectromagnetics* 2007; 28: 81–98.
199. Arnetz BB, Berg M. Melatonin and adrenocorticotropic hormone levels in video display unit workers during work and leisure. *J Occup Environ Med* 1996; 38: 1108–1110.

200. Pfluger DH, Minder CE. Effects of exposure to 16.7 Hz magnetic fields on urinary 6-hydroxymelatonin sulfate excretion on Swiss railway workers. *J Pineal Res* 1996; 21: 91–100.
201. Burch JB, Reif JS, Yost MG, Keefe TJ, Pitrat CA. Nocturnal excretion of a urinary melatonin metabolite in electric utility workers. *Scand J Work Environ Health* 1998; 24: 183–189.
202. Burch JB, Reif JS, Yost MG, Keefe TJ, Pitrat CA. Reduced excretion of melatonin metabolite in electric utility workers. *Am J Epidemiol* 1999; 150: 2736.
203. Burch JB, Reif JS, Noonan CW, Yost MG. Melatonin metabolite levels in workers exposed to 60-Hz magnetic fields: work in substations and with 3-phase conductors. *J Occup Environ Med* 2000; 42: 136–142.
204. Graham C, Cook MR, Riffle DW, Gerkovich MM, Cohen HD. Nocturnal melatonin levels in human volunteers exposed to intermittent 60 Hz magnetic fields. *Bioelectromagnetics* 1996; 17: 263–273.
205. Graham C, Sastre A, Cook MR, Gerkovich MM. Nocturnal magnetic field exposure: gender-specific effects on heart rate variability and sleep. *Clin Neurophysiol* 2000; 111: 1936–1941.
206. Crasson M, Beckers V, Pequeux CH, Claustrat B, Legros JJ. Daytime 50 Hz magnetic field exposure and plasma melatonin and urinary 6-sulfatoxymelatonin concentration profiles in humans. *J Pineal Res* 2001; 31: 234–241.
207. Griefahn B, Künemund C, Blaszkewicz M, Golka K, Mehnert P, Degen G. Experiments on the effects of a continuous 16.7 Hz magnetic field on melatonin secretion, core body temperature, and heart rates in humans. *Bioelectromagnetics* 2001; 22: 581–588.
208. Levallois P, Dumont M, Touitou Y, Gingras S, Mâsse B, Gauvin D, Kröger E, Bourdages M, Douville P. Effects of electric and magnetic fields from high-power lines on female urinary excretion of 6-sulfatoxymelatonin. *Am J Epidemiol* 2001; 154: 601–609.
209. Youngstedt SD, Kripke DF, Elliott JA, Assmus JD. No association of 6-sulfatoxymelatonin with in-bed 60-Hz magnetic field exposure or illumination level among older adults. *Environ Res* 2002; A89: 201–209.
210. Kurokawa Y, Nitta H, Imai H, Kabuto M. Acute exposure to 50 Hz magnetic fields with harmonics and transient components: lack of effects on nighttime hormonal secretion in men. *Bioelectromagnetics* 2003b; 24: 12–20.
211. Wood AW, Armstrong SM, Sait ML, Devine L, Martin MJ. Changes in human plasma melatonin profiles in response to 50 Hz magnetic field exposure. *J Pineal Res* 1998; 25: 116–127.
212. Juutilainen J, Stevens RG, Anderson LE, Hansen NH, Kilpeläinen M, Kumlin T, Laitinen JT, Sobel EM, Wilson BW. Nocturnal 6-hydroxymelatonin sulfate excretion in female workers exposed to magnetic fields. *J Pineal Res* 2000; 28: 97–104.
213. Liburdy RP, Sloma TR, Sokolic R, Yaswen P. ELF magnetic fields, breast cancer and melatonin: 60 Hz fields block melatonin's oncostatic action on ER⁺ breast cancer cell proliferation. *J Pineal Res* 1993; 14: 89–97.
214. NRC. *Possible Health Effects of Exposure to Residential Electric and Magnetic Fields.* National Research Council. Washington, DC: National Academy Press, 1997.
215. NRPB. ELF electromagnetic fields and risk of cancer. Report of an Advisory Group on Non-Ionising Radiation of the National Radiological Protection Board 2001; 12(1): 1–179.
216. Shaw GM. Adverse human reproductive outcomes and electromagnetic fields: a brief summary of the epidemiologic literature. *Bioelectromagnetics* 2001; 5(Suppl): S5–S18.
217. Kheifets LI. Electric and magnetic field exposure and brain cancer: a review. *Bioelectromagnetics* 2001; 5(Suppl): S120–S131.

218. IARC. Non-ionizing radiation, Part 1: Static and extremely low-frequency (ELF) electric and magnetic fields. International Agency for Research on Cancer (IARC) Monographs on the Evaluation of Carcinogenic Risks to Humans, Report No. 80, Lyon, France, 2002.
219. Neutra R, DelPizzo V, Lee GM. An evaluation of the possible risks from electric and magnetic fields (EMF) from power lines, internal wiring, electrical occupations, and appliances. *California EMF Program*, Oakland, 2002.
220. Habash RWY. Electromagnetics—the uncertain health risks. *IEEE Potential* 2003a; 22: 23–26.
221. Habash RWY. Foreseeable health risk of electric and magnetic field residential exposure. *Energy Environ* 2003b; 14: 473–487.
222. Habash RWH, Brodsky LM, Leiss W, Krewski DK, Repacholi M. Health risk of electromagnetic fields. Part II: Evaluation and assessment of extremely low frequency fields. *Crit Rev Biomed Eng* 2003; 31: 197–254.
223. Elwood JM. Childhood leukemia and residential magnetic fields: are pooled analyses more valid than the original studies? *Bioelectromagnetics* 2006; 27: 112–118.

5 Radio Frequency Standards and Dosimetry

5.1 INTRODUCTION

The use of RF equipment such as mobile phones, microwave ovens and RF heaters, base stations, radar installations, telecommunications, and broadcast facilities has led to widespread human exposure to RFR, along with concerns about possible associations between RFR and adverse health outcomes, including cancer.

RF applications occupy a wide range of frequencies. For example, AM radio transmission uses 5–16 kHz, FM radio transmission uses 76–109 kHz, while 58–132 kHz and 8.8–10.2 MHz are used throughout the world for EAS, radio frequency identification (RFID), and other security systems. Cellular and personal communications use frequencies between 800 MHz and 2 GHz. Emerging wireless network-connected products and services may utilize frequencies up to 5 GHz. However, the 2.45 GHz frequency is reserved for ISM applications (mainly microwave cooking).

Scientists, engineers, technicians, and physicians have been apprehensive about the potential hazards of RFR since the Second World War. There have been repeated calls for measures and tools that reduce RF exposure. During the past few decades, people have been especially concerned about the safety of radar equipment in the workplace and microwave ovens at their homes. Currently, it is wireless communication equipment (mobile phones) cradled next to the heads of millions of users that are of greatest concern [1].

Recent advances in wireless communication technologies have focused attention on the possible health consequences of mobile phone use. To date, there is limited information on the health risks stemming from the use of wireless equipment. As more products and services are developed and used in everyday applications, the potential for human exposure to RFR will increase.

The interaction of RF fields with living systems can be considered at the molecular, sub-cellular, cellular, organ, or system level, as well as the entire body. Biological effects due to exposure to RFR are differentiated into three levels: (1) high-level (thermal) effects, (2) intermediate-level (athermal) effects, and (3) low-level (nonthermal) effects.

This chapter traces the development of major RF exposure guidelines including some of the uncertainties in the science underlying these guidelines. Following a survey of RF sources and exposure scenarios, we provide safety assessment for whole body and head phantoms including those of adults and children. Future developments in the fields of safety standards harmonization, engineering requirements, and dosimetric information are also discussed.

5.2   RF EXPOSURE GUIDELINES

Beginning in the eighteenth century, scientific organizations were formed not only to address societal needs and concerns but also to resolve scientific disagreements. In the second half of the nineteenth century and the first half of the twentieth century, a number of scientific and engineering organizations were formed to advise government agencies, industry, and others, with one of their primary tasks being the establishment of safety standards [2].

The development of protection guidelines is a complex process that starts from a comprehensive review of the scientific literature, including studies describing thermal and nonthermal effects, short- and long-term exposures, biological and health end points, and epidemiological and human studies. The next step is the identification of the critical effect, that is, the established adverse health effects that occur at the lowest level of exposure [3]. The exposure levels that are harmful, or are considered likely to be harmful, to human health are determined. Such levels for human exposure to EM fields are generally called MPE values, or reference levels. The frequency-dependent MPE is a suitable metric for exposure assessment and can be used in determining whether an exposure complies with the basic exposure restrictions.

Various quantities are utilized to express MPE limits, including magnetic flux density (T) for static and VLF fields, current density (A/m^2) for frequencies up to approximately 10 MHz, SAR for frequencies up to 10 GHz, and power density (W/m^2) for frequencies between 10 and 300 GHz.

5.2.1   MAJOR GUIDELINES

Guidelines recommending the limitation of RF exposure have been continually developing for over a decade. MPE values from seven different organizations were compared. Many countries develop their guidelines by either adopting or adapting the recommendations of major organizations such as the IEEE [4–7], the NRPB [8–10], the Federal Communications Commission (FCC) of the United States [11], the ICNIRP [12–14], the Chinese National RF Exposure Standard GB8702-1988, Health Canada [15], and the ARPANSA [16].

The differences in RF safety standards are due to different philosophical approaches to public health standards development, different scientific approaches and interpretations of the scientific data, and different jurisdictions in various countries [17]. The most commonly used safety standards at present are the ANSI/IEEE C95.1 [4–7] and ICNIRP [12–14]. The basic restrictions for both these standards are in terms of induced current density (or electric fields) at lower frequencies of up to a few megahertz and SAR at higher frequencies of up to a few GHz [18].

The exposure guidelines compared in this book are generally related in scope. All the guidelines include separate exposure limits for various ranges of frequencies (although the defined limits for frequency groups differ). Each differentiates whole-body from partial-body exposure, and considers exposure to multiple frequencies for comparison with the standard.

5.2.2 IEEE Guidelines

The IEEE standard was developed by the SCC28 under the sponsorship of the IEEE Standards Board and was submitted to the ANSI for recognition as an American standard.

5.2.2.1 IEEE Standard C95.1

The safety standards most widely used in the Unites States are the ANSI C95.1 guidelines. ANSI is a voluntary standards body which has served in its capacity as administrator and coordinator of the U.S. private sector voluntary standardization system for more than 80 years. Founded in 1918 by five engineering societies and three government agencies as the American Standards Association (ASA), ASA became the United States of America Standards Institute (USASI) in 1966. By 1974, USASI had become the American National Standards Institute.

The history of the C95.1 standards goes back to the 1940s and fear for the safety of military personnel working close to radars during World War II. In 1942, the U.S. Navy directed the Naval Research Laboratory to investigate the possible health effects of RFR. Other military agencies in the United States were also involved within a short period. Early results showed no reason to fear, but proposed that procedures should be put in place to avoid extensive exposure. No guidelines were endorsed. Immediately after the war, very little research was conducted on the bioeffects of RFR. In 1948 and the following years, a few researchers reported the formation of cataracts in dogs and other animals. During the 1950s, researchers reported concerns over other adverse health effects such as leukemia, brain tumors, heart problems, and headaches.

The industry was more interested in setting up guidelines for its employees. For example, in 1953, the Central Safety Committee of Bell Telephone Laboratories issued a bulletin that recommended reduction of the power density 100 W/cm^2 to a 30-dB safety margin. This led to a recommendation of 10 mW/cm^2. This figure was the first safety standard decided for a human being under RF exposure. In 1954, General Electric recommended a stricter standard by a factor of 100, at 1 mW/cm^2. In 1957, Bell Telephone developed a standard at 1 W/cm^2 for continuous exposure. However, the Bell Telephone standard allows for the high-exposure levels for shorter periods of time. The Bell standard limits were based on certain biological effects (especially cataracts), which may occur at this level. In 1958, General Electric adopted a 10-mW/cm^2 limit. However, the U.S. Air Force (USAF) adopted an upper limit of 10 mW/cm^2 through its first Tri-Service Conference held in 1957.

The IEEE C95.1 MPE limits are frequency- and time-dependent in controlled and uncontrolled environments, as shown in Table 5.1. The MPE limits were not intended to be final guidelines, but only the beginning of long-term research and investigation. The intention was to provide some kind of protection until enough data were available to set up solid safety guidelines.

These guidelines were approved by the IEEE in 1991 and were subsequently adopted by ANSI in 1992 as a replacement for the previous ANSI C95.1-1982. In April 1993, the FCC proposed using the ANSI/IEEE C95.1-1992 for evaluating environmental RF fields created by transmitters it licenses and authorizes.

TABLE 5.1

Maximum Permissible Exposure Limits for IEEE Standard C95.1

Frequency Range (MHz)	Electric Field (E)	Magnetic Field (H) (V/m)	Power Density (P) (A/m)	Averaging Time ($|E|^2$), S (mW/cm^2) (min)
Controlled Environments				
0.003–0.1	614	163	100; 1,000,000[a]	6
0.1–3.0	614	16.3/f	100; 10,000/f^{2a}	6
3–30	1824/f	16.3/f	900/f^2; 10,000/f^2	6
30–100	61.4	16.3/f	1.0; 10,000/f^2	6
100–300	61.4	0.163	1.0	6
300–3,000	—	—	f/300	6
3,000–15,000	—	—	10	6
15,000–300,000	—	—	10	616,000/$f^{1.2}$
Uncontrolled Environments				
0.003–0.1	614	163	100; 1,000,000[a]	6
0.1–1.34	614	16.3/f	100; 10,000/f^{2a}	6
1.34–3.0	823.8/f	16.3/f	180/f^2; 10,000/f^2	f^2/3
3–30	823.8/f	16.3/f	180/f^2; 10,000/f^2	30
30–100	27.5	158.3/$f^{1.668}$	0.2; 940,000/$f^{3.336}$	30
100–300	27.5	0.0729	0.2	30
300–3,000	—	—	f/1,500	30
3,000–15,000	—	—	f/1,500	90,000/f^2
15,000–300,000	—	—	10	616,000/$f^{1.2}$

Note: f is the frequency in MHz.

[a] Plane wave equivalent power density, not suitable for near-field region but useful for comparing them with the power density limits for the higher frequency ranges.

The maximum time-averaged SAR for IEEE C95.1 guidelines is 8 W/kg for six or more minutes for controlled environments and a corresponding value at 1.6 W/kg for exposure in uncontrolled environments for 30 or more minutes. Higher local SARs are permitted for shorter exposure periods.

The IEEE C95.1 guidelines require averaging the power level over time periods ranging from 6 to 30 minutes for power density calculations, depending on the frequency. The exposure limits for uncontrolled environments are lower than those for controlled environments. To compensate for that, the guidelines allow exposure levels in those environments to be averaged over much longer time periods (30 minutes). Time averaging is based on the concept that the human body may bear a greater rate of body heating (that is, a higher level of RF energy) for a shorter time than for a longer period. However, time averaging may not be appropriate in considerations of nonthermal effects of RF energy.

5.2.2.2 IEEE Standard 1528

In December 2003, the IEEE Standard 1528 was published [6]. It specifies protocols and test procedures for the measurement of the peak spatial-average SAR induced inside a simplified model of the head of users of certain handheld radio transceivers. These transceivers are intended to be used for personal wireless communications services, operate in the 300 MHz–3 GHz frequency range, and are intended to be operated while held against the ear. The results obtained by following the protocols specified in IEEE 1528 represent a conservative estimate of the peak spatial-average SAR induced in the head of a significant majority of persons, subject to measurement and other uncertainties that are defined in this standard. The results are representative of those expected during conditions of normal use of a handheld wireless device. IEEE 1528 does not set specific limits for exposures of users of cellular phones and other personal communication devices, but helps wireless device manufacturers and regulators assess compliance with the requirements of the FCC and similar government agencies internationally that limit exposure from personal communication devices.

5.2.2.3 IEEE C95.1-2005

This newly approved standard represents a complete revision of and replaces IEEE Standard C95.1-1991. This standard gives recommendations to prevent harmful effects in human beings exposed to EM fields in the frequency range from 3 kHz to 300 GHz. The recommendations are intended to apply to exposures in uncontrolled, as well as controlled environments. They are not intended to apply to the purposeful exposure of patients under the direction of practitioners of the healing arts. The induced and contact current limits of IEEE C95.1-1991 are modified in this edition. In addition, field strengths below which induced and contact currents do not have to be measured are specified [7].

In the frequency range from 100 kHz to 3 GHz, the new IEEE standard of 0.08 W/kg averaged over the whole body for the general public is based on restricting heating of the body during whole-body exposure. It is to be applied when an RF safety program is not available. The new basic restriction for localized exposure is 2 W/kg for most parts of the body. A basic restriction SAR of 4 W/kg is fixed for the extremities (arms and legs distal from the elbows and knees, respectively, including the fingers, toes, hands, and feet) and for pinnae. The value of SAR is obtained by averaging over some specified time period (e.g., 6–30 min) and by averaging over any 10 g of tissue (described as a tissue volume in the shape of a cube). The new IEEE standard established segregation of the pinnae or the external ears by relaxation of the aforementioned basic SAR restriction from 2 W/kg to 4 W/kg. The SAR value for the basic restriction for localized exposure has been increased from 1.6 W/kg averaged over any 1 g of tissue to 2 W/kg over any 10 g of tissue [19].

The new MPE in terms of power density is 2 W/m^2, between 30 and 400 MHz. It moves up from 2 to 10 W/m^2 between 400 and 2000 MHz. For frequencies greater than 2 GHz, the MPE is 10 W/m^2.

The new IEEE standard contains some of the characteristics of the ICNIRP guidelines, with few differences. The main similarities are basic restrictions in terms of a 2 W/kg SAR averaged over 10 g of tissues in the head and trunk and the reference levels (2–10 W/m^2) for certain frequency ranges. The major differences include the tissue mass and time period over which SAR values are to be averaged and the applicable frequency bands for the MPEs.

5.2.3 ICNIRP GUIDELINES

In 1992, the ICNIRP was chartered as the successor to International Radiation Protection Association (IRPA)/International Non-Ionizing Radiation Committee (INIRC). The ICNIRP's mission is to coordinate knowledge of protection against various nonionizing exposures in the development of internationally accepted recommendations.

In April 1998, the ICNIRP published guidelines (Table 5.2) for limiting RF exposure in the frequency range up to 300 GHz. Development of the guidelines was based on a quantitative relationship between exposure and adverse effects. Only established effects have been used as the basis for the recommended limitation of exposure.

The ICNIRP guidelines include a reduction factor of five in maximum SAR for the general public as opposed to occupational environments. The reason for this approach is the possibility that some members of the general public might be exceptionally sensitive to RFR. However, no detailed scientific evidence to justify this

TABLE 5.2
ICNIRP Protection Guidelines

Frequency Range	E-Field Strength	H-Field Strength (V/m)	B-Field (A/m)	Power Density (µT) (W/m²)
Occupational Exposure				
Up to 1 Hz		1.63×10^5	2×10^5	—
1–8 Hz	20,000	$1.63 \times 10^5/f^2$	$2 \times 10^5/f^2$	—
8–25 Hz	20,000	$2 \times 10^4/f$	$2.5 \times 10^4/f$	—
25–820 Hz	$500/f$	$20/f$	$25/f$	—
820 Hz–65 kHz	610	24.4	30.7	—
65 kHz–1 MHz	610	$1.6/f$	$2/f$	—
1–10 MHz	$610/f$	$1.6/f$	$2/f$	—
10–400 MHz	61	0.16	0.2	10
400 MHz–2 GHz	$3\,f^{0.5}$	$0.008\,f^{0.5}$	$0.01\,f^{0.5}$	$f/40$
2–300 GHz	137	0.36	0.45	50
General Public				
Up to 1 Hz	—	3.2×10^4	4×10^4	—
1–8 Hz	10,000	$3.2 \times 10^4/f^2$	$4 \times 10^4/f^2$	—
8–25 Hz	10,000	$4000/f$	$5000/f$	—
25–800 Hz	$250/f$	$4/f$	$5/f$	—
800 Hz–3 kHz	$250/f$	5	6.25	—
3–150 kHz	87	5	6.25	—
150 kHz–1MHz	87	$0.73/f$	$0.92/f$	—
1–10 MHz	$87/f^{0.5}$	$0.73/f$	$0.92/f$	—
10–400 MHz	28	0.073	0.092	2
400–2000 MHz	$1.375\,f^{0.5}$	$0.0037\,f^{0.5}$	$0.0046\,f^{0.5}$	$f/200$
2–300 GHz	61	0.16	0.2	10

additional safety factor is provided. The basic restriction for occupational exposure to EMF with frequencies up to 1 kHz is 10 mA/m^2, and above that it is frequency dependent. The value of 10 mA/m^2 was chosen as less than one-tenth of the value of the current density above. This is the same value recommended by NRPB in the United Kingdom.

For exposures received by the general public a reduction factor of five is applied, resulting in a basic restriction of 2 mA/m^2. In its clarification, the ICNIRP notes that compliance with this basic restriction may permit higher current densities in body tissues other than the CNS under similar exposure conditions.

The basic restriction for occupational exposure to EM fields with frequencies between 100 kHz and 10 GHz is 0.4 W/kg for whole-body SAR. Again, this is the same as the value recommended by the NRPB. For the general public, the reduction factor of five results in a basic restriction on whole-body SAR of 0.08 W/kg. The factor of five reduction also applies to the basic restriction on localized SAR (head and trunk), the values for those occupationally exposed and for the general public being 10 W/kg and 2 W/kg, respectively, averaged over any 10-g tissue. However, localized SAR values at limbs for those occupationally exposed and for the general public are 20 W/kg and 4 W/kg, respectively.

In 1999, the ICNIRP guidelines for the public were incorporated in a European Council Recommendation, which has been agreed in principle by all countries in the EU, including the United Kingdom. The ICNIRP standard is used in most European countries and is gaining acceptance in many other countries throughout the world outside of North America. These guidelines are recommended by the WHO and have been adopted by more than 35 countries.

5.2.3.1   CENELEC EN 50392:2004

In January 2004, the European Committee for Electrotechnical Standardization (CENELEC) released the European standard EN 50392:2004 to demonstrate the compliance of electronic and electrical apparatus with the basic restrictions related to human exposure to EM fields (0 Hz–300 GHz) [20]. This standard considers basic restrictions or reference levels on exposure of the general public related to electric, magnetic, and EM fields as well as induced and contact current. Generally, it contains: (1) compliance criteria, assessment methods, and reporting, (2) evaluation of compliance to limits, (3) characteristics and parameters of apparatus to be considered, (4) sources of multiple frequencies, and (5) information to be supplied with the apparatus.

5.2.3.2   EC Directive 2004/40/EC

On April 29, 2004, the Council of the European Parliament published Directive 2004/40/EC. This directive addresses the minimum health and safety requirements regarding the exposure of workers to the risks arising from EM fields. The directive follows the ICNIRP basic restrictions. It addresses risks due to known short-term adverse effects in the human body; however, it does not consider long-term effects.

The directive distinguishes between exposure limit values and action values. The exposure limit values (Table 5.3) must not be exceeded and are linked to physical variables that are directly related to effects on the body, such as current density in the CNS at low frequencies, the specific absorption rate of energy, and the power density at high frequencies. Because these variables are usually difficult to measure, the directive incorporates action values (Table 5.4) for easy-to-measure variables, such as the EMF outside the body. If the action values are not exceeded, then according to the directive it can be assumed that the exposure limit values will not be exceeded under normal circumstances. If the action values are exceeded, the employer must ensure that exposure values are reduced to below the action values or the employer must show that the exposure limit values are not exceeded. Exceeding limit values or action values does not necessarily result in an unsafe situation.

TABLE 5.3
Exposure Limit Values in Directive 2004/40/EC

Frequency Range	Current Density (J) for Head and Trunk (mA/m²) (rms)	Whole-Body Average SAR (W/kg)	Localized SAR (Head and Trunk) (W/kg)	Localized SAR (Limbs) (W/kg)	Power Density (S) (W/m²)
Up to 1 Hz	40	—	—	—	—
1–4 Hz	$40/f$	—	—	—	—
4–1000 Hz	10	—	—	—	—
1000 Hz–100 kHz	$f/100$	—	—	—	—
100 kHz–10 MHz	$f/100$	0.4	10	20	—
10 MHz–10 GHz	—	0.4	10	20	—
10–300 GHz	—	—	—	—	50

Note: No ceiling values for static magnetic fields. SAR values are 6 min time averages.

TABLE 5.4
Action Values in Directive 2004/40/EC

Frequency Range	Electric Field Strength E (V/m²)	Magnetic Field Strength H (A/m²)	Equivalent Plane Wave Power Density S (W/m²)	Contact Current I_c (mA)	Limb Induced Current I_L (mA)
0.1–1 MHz	610	$1.6/f$	—	40	—
1–10 MHz	$610/f$	$1.6/f$	—	40	—
10–110 MHz	61	0.16	10	40	100
110–400 MHz	61	0.16	10	—	—
400–2000 MHz	$3 f^{1/2}$	$0.008 f^{1/2}$	$f/40$	—	—
2–300 GHz	137	0.36	50	—	—

Modification of the directive may be proposed if new scientific information and collected data indicate that a change will not affect the level of protection of workers exposed to EM fields. The frequencies of interest published in the directive cover all eventualities, ranging from 0 Hz to 300 GHz, for static magnetic fields and EM fields. Compliance with this directive is mandatory from April 30, 2008. This directive will make it necessary for employers to introduce measures to protect workers from the risks associated with EM fields. The limits and action values are specified for measurement purposes along with recommendations concerning risk management, health surveillance, and information and training for those working in exposed conditions.

5.2.4 SAFETY FACTORS

Historically, scientists fixed a safety factor of 10, based on an exposure of 0.1 W/cm^2. The above figure took into account an average male weighting 70 kg and having a surface area of 3000 cm^2. Sometime later, Professor Herman Schwan, a pioneer researcher in the field at the University of Pennsylvania, noticed that the absorbing surface of the body is closer to 20,000 cm^2 rather than 3000 cm^2. He figured out that the pure effect of absorbed radiation was 20 times greater than the body could resolve. Therefore, the standard was lowered to 10 mW/cm^2, and this was the base for the C95.1 recommendations of 1966.

Currently, MPE values usually include a safety factor that results in permissible exposures at levels well below those where potentially hazardous effects may occur. The value of the safety factor reflects the extent of uncertainty about the lowest exposure level that could be hazardous, coupled with a desire to remain conservative with respect to health and safety. Improved knowledge about thresholds for hazardous effects may justify smaller safety factors [21]. Safety factors allow for extrapolating from animal studies to humans, heat dissipation in the body, uncertainties in determining the precise threshold, and the hypothesis that some people may be more sensitive than others. Safety factor values between 10 and 1000 are often used. However, most of the known exposure standards have chosen a value of 50 for the public environment.

5.2.5 INCORPORATING SPECIFIC ABSORPTION RATE

SAR, as a most biologically effective quantity used in protection guidelines and in extrapolating across species, cannot be directly measured. The level of electric field intensity E in volts per meter is calculated as a directly measurable exposure parameter that corresponds to basic exposure restrictions. SAR is the rate at which RF energy is absorbed by the tissue and thus is a good predictor of thermal effects. In the context of RF or microwaves, two alternatives are used, allowing the SAR evaluation from either the electric field or temperature measurement. Accordingly, SAR is defined as

$$\text{SAR} = \frac{\sigma |\text{E}|^2}{\rho} = c \frac{dT}{dt} \qquad (5.1)$$

where dT/dt is the time derivative of the temperature in kelvin per second (K/s), σ the electrical conductivity in siemens per meter (S/m), ρ the mass density in kilogram per cubic meter (kg/m^3), and c the specific heat in joules per kilogram per kelvin (J/kg/K). The unit of SAR is watts per kilogram (W/kg).

SAR calculations and estimates usually use many EM properties of biological tissues (e.g., complex dielectric constants and conductivity of different tissues) whose accuracy depends on their acquisition techniques, which are mostly *in vivo*.

There are two major types of SAR: (1) a whole-body average SAR and (2) a local (spatial) peak SAR when the power absorption takes place in a confined body region, as in the case of a head exposed to a mobile phone. Whole-body SAR measurements are significant in estimating elevations of the core body temperature. As SAR increases, the possibility of heating and, therefore, tissue damage also rises. The whole-body SAR for a given organism will be highest within a certain resonant frequency range, which is dependent on the size of the organism and its orientation relative to the electric and magnetic field vectors and the direction of wave propagation. For an average human, the peak whole-body SAR occurs in a frequency range of 60–80 MHz while the resonant frequency for a laboratory rat is about 600 MHz [22].

Both types of SAR are averaged over a specific period of time and tissue masses of 1 or 10 g (defined as a tissue volume in the shape of a cube). Averaging the absorption over a larger amount of body tissue gives a less reliable result. The 1-g SAR is a more precise representation of localized RF energy absorption and a better measure of SAR distribution. Local SAR is generally based on estimates from the whole-body average SAR. It incorporates substantial safety factors (e.g., 20).

The accepted safe occupational exposure whole-body SAR level is 0.4 W/kg (power density/mass) and the public exposure level is 0.08 W/kg, based on a SAR of 4 W/kg as the level at which adverse effects are said to be detected. A SAR of 4 W/kg can be compared to the measured threshold for stress protein synthesis in the ELF range, 2.6×10^{-7} J/m^3 (energy density/volume) by first converting to a per mass basis using an approximate tissue density of water, 10^3 kg/m^3, the major constituent of cells. In these units, the threshold for stress protein synthesis is 2.6×10^{-10} J/kg [23].

There are two local SAR safety limits applicable to RFR: 1.6 W/kg averaged over 1 g (SAR$_{1g}$) in North America and 2 W/kg averaged over 10 g (SAR$_{10g}$) developed by the ICNIRP and accepted for use in Europe, Australia, Japan, and other parts of the world. Whether 1.6 W/kg or 2 W/kg is a correct limit for RF exposure remains controversial. Table 5.5 shows SAR limits for various exposure guidelines.

Exposure to RFR from mobile phones is in the region close to the antenna, the near-field. However, exposure from other sources such as base stations is in the far field, which is often quantified in terms of power density, and expressed in units of watts per square meter. At lower frequencies, from about 0.1 to 10 MHz, the energy absorbed is less important than current density and total current, which can affect the nervous system. There is an overlap region at the upper part of this range where either current density or energy absorption rate is the limiting quantity. The MPE values at the lower frequencies are concerned with preventing adverse effects on the CNS and electric shock [24]. Exposure limits at these lower frequencies also involve numerous technical issues as well, but are not the focus of this paper.

TABLE 5.5
SAR Limits for RFR

Standard	Frequency Range	Whole-Body SAR (W/kg)		Local SAR in Head (W/kg)		Local SAR in Limbs (W/kg)	
		Public	Occupational	Public	Occupational	Public	Occupational
ARPANSA	100 kHz– 6 GHz	0.08 (6)	0.4 (6)	2 [10] (6)	10 [10] (6)	4 [10] (6)	20 [10] (6)
TTC/MPT	100 kHz– 6 GHz	0.04 (6)	0.4 (6)	2 [10] (6)	8 [10] (6)	—	—
Safety Code 6	100 kHz– 10 GHz	0.08 (6)	0.4 (6)	1.6 [1] (6)	8 [1] (6)	4 [10] (6)	20 [10] (6)
ICNIRP	100 kHz– 6 GHz	0.08 (6)	0.4 (6)	2 [10] (6)	10 [10] (6)	4 [10] (6)	20 [10] (6)
FCC	100 kHz– 6 GHz	0.08 (30)	0.4 (6)	1.6 [1]	8 [1] (6)	4 [10]+	20 [10] (6)+
NRPB	100 kHz– 6 GHz	0.4 (15)		10 [10] (6)		20 [100] (6)	
ANSI/IEEE	100 kHz– 6 GHz	0.08 (30)	0.4 (6)	1.6 [1] (30)	8 [1] (6)	4 [10] (30)+	20[10] (6)+

Note: ( ) Averaging time in minutes. [ ] Averaging mass in grams. + In hands, wrists, feet, and ankles.

5.3 MEASUREMENT SURVEYS

Dosimetry means measuring the dose of radiation emitted by a source. Dose measures that aspect of field exposure that is directly linked to the biological activity of the field, even though this aspect of the field may not directly cause the changes [25]. Quantitative analysis of SAR in the human body under EM radiation, including the evaluation of incident and internal RF fields, is referred to as RF dosimetry [26]. RF fields are either measured or calculated, depending upon the type and shape of the object [27].

Measurement surveys provide procedures that are implemented in developing programs to protect workers and the public from exposure to RF energy above the allowable limits, as well as to protect utilities from litigation or possible penalties. The first and foremost step is to survey any utility-owned or leased sites that have transmitters, heat sealers, induction units, or any other devices that emit RF energy to determine if hazards are present. Taking an inventory of all site hazards is essential to follow the correct course of compliance action. During this surveillance phase, it is not always possible to specify the safety of a site. The only expected result is to show whether the site is complying with the adopted exposure guideline. The aim of this phase is to identify the highest fields and the safety relief program required. In addition, periodic site surveys are needed when RF sources are replaced or changed—to identify the effects that these changes have on RF coverage. Once identified, remedial action may be recommended to reestablish a state of optimal performance and ensure a safer environment.

5.3.1 BASE TRANSCEIVER STATIONS

The rapid growth of mobile communication infrastructure has resulted in the installation of a large number of base transceiver stations (BTSs), which are mounted on freestanding towers, rooftops, or the sides of buildings. A BTS refers to the antennas and their associated electronic equipment (equivalent to a radio station). A BTS may contain more than one transmitter, with the output of each transmitter fed to the antenna on top of the tower. BTSs usually transmit between less than a watt to as high as 500 W per transmitter depending on the location and type of the antenna used for communication. While a typical BTS could have as many as 60–90 channels, not all of the channels would be expected to operate simultaneously, therefore reducing overall radiation.

The installation of BTS antennas frequently raises concerns about their human health impacts and safety, mostly for people who live in the vicinity of these sites. There might be circumstances where people could be exposed to fields greater than the MPE values. Power density in the radiation beam from the antenna decreases with increasing distance. However, actual radiation level at a given site is a function of several factors, such as output power of the antenna, direction of transmission, attenuation due to obstacles or walls, and scattering from buildings and trees. Because of building attenuation, levels of power density inside buildings at corresponding distances from the BTS antenna would be from 10 to 20 times smaller than the outside. It is only in specific areas on the rooftop, depending on the proximity to the antenna, that the exposure levels are higher than those allowed by the RF protection guidelines. Accordingly, access to such locations should be restricted. Therefore, measurements in rooms exactly below roof-mounted antennas show power density levels lower than those of the rooftop locations. This depends on the construction material. The level of power densities behind sector antennas is hundreds of times less than in front. Therefore, levels are too low in rooms located behind sector antennas. Figure 5.1 illustrates the conditions of RFR around a BTS.

5.3.1.1 Shielding

To shield base station antennas, resistive plates based on the utilization of resistive material [28,29] are designed and installed on both sides of the antenna horizontally

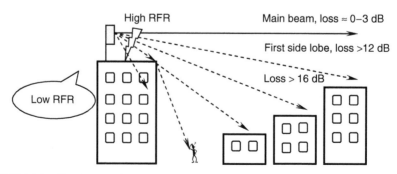

FIGURE 5.1 Conditions of RFR around a BTS.

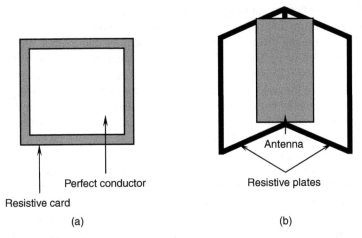

Perfect conductor

Resistive card

Resistive plates

Antenna

(a)   (b)

FIGURE 5.2   (a) Resistive plate. (b) Implementation of resistive plates around a BTS antenna.

to act as reflecting surfaces. These plates reflect the energy of the far end part of the main lobe and the side lobes from the overlapping regions to the angular regions that require more energy. The advantages of the resistive plates are that the edges are treated with resistive material and edge diffractions, and their associated multipath signals can be minimized. Hsiao et al. [30] experimentally implemented the resistive plates. All the side lobes and part of the main lobe that covers beyond the designated regions will be reduced and will therefore reduce the coverage overlapping between adjacent sectors. Figure 5.2a shows a resistive plate while Figure 5.2b shows its implantation to enhance the performance of the BTS antenna.

5.3.1.2 Exposure Levels

The exposure situation around a typical BTS can be computed easily. The field strength data can then be analyzed with respect to possible conflicts with the available guidelines for limiting RF exposure. In general, the maximum exposure levels near the base of a typical BTS antenna are, really, lower than all recommended safety limits. These maximum exposure levels may occur only at limited distances close to the base of the BTS antenna. Typical safety distances for BTS range from 1 to 5 m for one RF carrier in the direction of the main beam of the antenna. It is difficult to specify a typical BTS since the configuration (i.e., service, power output, frequencies, antenna configuration, etc.) may vary considerably [31].

Measurements near typical BTSs have mostly shown that radiation levels in publicly accessible areas are well below the widely promulgated guidelines [32–39]. Nevertheless, residents living close to BTSs are especially concerned that this radiation might be harmful [40]. Bernardi et al. [34] indicated that the highest exposure could occur on nearby buildings in the direct path of the antenna's main path. However, there may be circumstances where workers could be exposed to RF energy higher than the MPE values, generally on rooftops and close to antennas. The study provided theoretical evidence to suggest that the presence of reflecting and scattering structures, such as building walls, can have a profound influence on both the exposure and the power deposition inside the human body. For example, a subject standing on a rooftop at a distance of 8 m from the base of an antenna, operating with 21 channels at a radiated power of 7.5 watts per channel, would be exposed to spatial average and maximum incident power density of 0.6 and 1.3 W/m^2. If the human subject (1.8 m in height, with shoes), is facing the BTS antenna, a maximum SAR of 28 mW/kg, averaged over 1 g, would be found in the head. A corresponding average SAR of 0.63 mW/kg would be obtained for the whole body. If the same subject stands 2 m away from the building wall, on a balcony located 30 m away, facing the antenna on the building next door, the maximum SAR in the head would be 69 mW/kg, and the SAR would be 2.4 mW/kg for the whole-body average. This means an increase of more than twofold in SAR.

Radon et al. [41] investigated the feasibility and reliability of personal dosimetry. Twenty-four hour exposure assessment was carried out in 42 children, 57 adolescents, and 64 adults using the Maschek dosimeter prototype. Self-reported exposure to mobile phone frequencies were compared with the dosimetry results. In addition, dosimetry readings of the Maschek device and those of the Antennessa DSP-090 were compared in 40 subjects. Self-reported exposures were not associated with dosimetry readings. The measurement results of the two dosimeters were in moderate agreement. The authors concluded: "Personal dosimetry for exposure to mobile phone base station might be feasible in epidemiologic studies. However, the consistency seems to be moderate."

A report by the Advisory Group on Nonionizing Radiation of the NRPB [42] gives advice on possible health effects of TETRA. The report concluded that "although areas of uncertainty remain about the biological effects of low level RF radiation in general, including modulated signals, current evidence suggests that it is unlikely that the special features of the signals from TETRA mobile terminals and repeaters pose a hazard to health."

5.3.2 BROADCAST STATIONS

Broadcast stations are usually located near densely populated areas so that large audiences can receive the signals. The radiation patterns from broadcast antennas are not as highly collimated as those from other RF sources such as dish antennas used for satellite earth stations. Therefore, exposure to main-beam radiation intensities near the broadcast antenna is possible, especially if individuals are at eye level with the antenna bays (e.g., residents of high-rise buildings). Measurements near broadcast stations have shown significant differences in readings indoors and outdoors, as well as at home and away. Exposures encountered by the public were well below the recommended MPE values [43,44].

5.3.3 TRAFFIC RADAR DEVICES

Radiation levels associated with traffic radar devices vary according to the particular make and model of the radar gun. Usually radiation intensity drops to safe levels at distances of several meters from the antenna. Exposure to radiation from radar above the safety limits is most likely in the immediate vicinity of the antenna when it is stationary. A number of studies have been conducted concerning potential operator exposure to RFR emitted by traffic radars. Most of these studies measured some features of the emitted radiation intensity, and some of them measured levels of exposure at other locations away from the aperture of the antenna [45–50].

5.3.4 RF Heaters and Sealers

RF ovens, dryers, sealers, and heaters provide the flexibility and speed to heat, dry, and cure a vast spectrum of products with demonstrated increase in productivity at lower costs. Such devices have been among the major sources of employee RF over-exposure. RF operators experience an almost whole-body exposure where, depending on the machine and the task, different parts of the body (hands, head, and chest) will obtain the highest exposure. Several studies [51–55] show that safe limits for RF energy from such devices are often exceeded for operators. In the frequency range of such equipment, fields may penetrate the human body and cause heating of internal tissues. Workers nearby may be unaware of their exposure to RF fields, because the fields can penetrate deeply into the human body without activating the heat sensors located in the skin.

5.3.5 Microwave Ovens

Given the popularity of microwave ovens, care must be taken to avoid exposure to the microwaves that heat and cook food. The main concern is leakage from the oven door. Surveys carried out to evaluate RF leakage levels from used microwave ovens [56–58] found that no models emitted microwave radiation in excess of the maximum allowed leakage (5 mW/cm^2). The levels of leakage were all well below the requirements of the regulations.

5.3.6 RF Environmental Levels

In the 1970s, the U.S. Environmental Protection Agency (EPA) measured environmental field intensities at chosen locations in 15 U.S. cities. RFR levels were measured at sites near to single or multiple RF emitters, for example, at the bases of transmitter towers and at the upper stories (including the roof) of tall buildings or hospital complexes in the vicinity of transmitter towers. Janes et al. [59] and Tell and Mantiply [60] presented the results for those cities (a total of 486 sites). Those results were also summarized in Hankin [61] and EPA [62]. The exposure levels for all cities were largely below the MPE values. The major contributions to those exposure values were from FM radio and TV stations. This data is still used today as there have been no further measurements of RFR levels.

Hondou [63] found that when hundreds of mobile phones emit radiation, their total power is comparable to a microwave oven or a satellite broadcasting station and this level can reach the reference level for general public exposure (ICNIRP guideline) in daily life. This is caused by the fundamental properties of EM fields, namely, reflection and additivity. However, Toropainen [64] applied radio-engineering principles to estimate the power density and SAR levels versus the number of mobile phones in screened environments occupied by humans. The author concluded that it is unlikely that exposure levels are exceeding the safe limits recommended by the ICNIRP due to multiple mobile phones users in trains, elevators, cars, or similar environments.

5.3.7   MAGNETIC RESONANCE IMAGING AND SPECTROSCOPY SYSTEMS

Magnetic resonance imaging and spectroscopy systems are used in diagnostic medicine and display images in a format similar to computed tomography (CT). Images of the body may be acquired and viewed with submillimeter resolution in the axial, coronal, or other planes. Applications of MRI are emerging in the areas of cardiology, neuroscience, image-guided surgery, and other minimally invasive procedures. Many safety issues, however, remain as possible concerns.

The proliferation of high field (1–3 T), very high field (3–7 T), and ultra high field (above 7 T) whole-body MRIs calls for a review of the safety literature that can guide future studies of critical health related issues [65]. A number of computational reports have predicted the possibility of high SAR levels at high frequencies and formation of regions of high RF intensity (hot spots) at higher field strengths [66–68].

5.4   PERSONAL SAFETY ASSESSMENT

Determination of SAR or induced electric fields or current densities at lower frequencies is very cumbersome for use in the field for real-life exposure situations [18]. Of particular interest at the present time are two sources of exposure: wireless base stations, especially in metropolitan and urban settings, and mobile phones. The estimation of SAR or electric fields may be carried out theoretically or experimentally.

5.4.1   WHOLE-BODY PHANTOMS

Dosimetry can be studied by evaluating devices with a dummy model called phantom. A phantom is a device that simulates the size, contours, and electrical characteristics of human tissue at normal body temperature. It is composed of a mannequin (solid shell) cut in half and filled with tissue-equivalent synthetic material solution, which has electrical properties of tissues. The phantom is typically set up in relation to other SAR measurement equipment. Measured pieces of equipment for this set up include a robot arm and miniature isotropic electric field probe. A device is positioned against the mannequin operating at full power while the computer-controlled probe inserted into the tissue maps the electric fields inside. Computer algorithms determine the maximum electric field and then calculate a 1-g or 10-g average over a body to give a SAR value.

Whole-body phantoms made of plastic human-shaped bags [69] filled with homogenous gels representing the average of electrical properties of human tissues (dielectric constants and conductivities) are not very portable and certainly are incapable of providing full information on SAR distributions [18]. Several investigations were performed to estimate the RF fields to which human subjects were to be exposed [69–72]. Allen et al. [73] reported the dosimetry performed to support an experiment that measured physiological responses of volunteer human subjects exposed to the resonant frequency for a seated human adult at 100 MHz. The dosimetry plan required measurement of transmitter harmonics, stationary probe drift, field strengths as a function of distance, electric and magnetic field maps at 200, 225, and 250 cm from the dipole antenna, and SAR measurements using a human phantom. Whole body averaged SARs of 0.26, 0.39, and 0.52 W/kg result for the 4, 6, and

8 mW/cm^2 exposures. SAR values are just under, at, and just over the IEEE/ANSI C95.1 exposure standard [4–7] of 0.4 W/kg. The authors also presented theoretical predictions of SAR using the finite difference time domain (FDTD) method. The FDTD results predicted higher localized SAR in the head, spinal column, and the highest SAR in the ankle.

Nagaoka et al. [74] developed realistic high-resolution whole-body voxel models for Japanese adult males and females of average height and weight. The developed models consist of cubic voxels of 2 mm on each side; the models are segmented into 51 anatomic regions. The adult female model was the first of its kind in the world and both are the first Asian voxel models (representing average Japanese) that enable numerical evaluation of EM dosimetry at high frequencies of up to 3 GHz. The authors described and calculated the basic SAR characteristics of the developed models for the VHF/UHF bands using the FDTD method.

5.4.2 In-Head Assessments

RFR is significant from mobile handsets because of the presence of the phone-transmitting antenna close to the head, neck, and hand of the user. The extent of exposure to RF energy from a mobile phone depends on the power of the signal the device transmits. Usually mobile phones transmit power in the range of 0.2 W to 0.6 W. Such power is limited by the cellular system (number of cells) and manufac-turer specifications (design of the cellular phones casing, chassis length, electronic circuitry, channel access technique, antenna geometry, etc. [75]). The second-generation (2G) systems employ the TDMA technique. Under TDMA, subscribers share the radio spectrum in time domain, in which each user has full power during a defined time slot. The GSM standard employs the TDMA technique with eight time slots. This means that the transmitter is only switched on for an eighth of the time. Therefore, the maximum average power output is 0.25 W for a 900 MHz GSM phone. Eight GSM phone users can share a pair of 200 kHz wideband channels, because each user is given access only to a single time slot of 576 microsecond (μs) duration in a 4.6 millisecond (ms) frame that is repeated 217 times a second (s). This 217-Hz cycle of power pulses is in the range of the normal bioelectrical functions both in and between cells, so it may induce low-frequency power surges causing health problems. The 900-MHz RF carrier, with its lower average power output, likely does not cause health problems. Third-generation (G3) systems make use of code division multiple access (CDMA) technique, in which all data are continuously transported at the same time, with a special code attached so that only the intended receivers can decode the messages.

High dosimetric precision requires the application of numerical and experimen-tal methods. Anatomical human head models based on MRI or other techniques must be used for numerical evaluation. High resolutions (<1 mm) are essential to resolve functional subregions of the brain, e.g., the thalamus. Experimental methods are required to verify the simulations and to identify the possible shortcomings of the numerical model [76].

Mobile phones yield numerically modeled brain SARs, which often exceed the 1.6 W/kg or 2 W/kg limits. This amount of power is less than the body's normal resting metabolic output power [77]. However, manufacturers should always be interested in reducing brain SAR as much as possible, not only because of possible health effects, but also to increase the battery lifetime (the energy deposited in the brain drains the battery without any functional communication task).

Dosimetry of mobile phones targets SAR generated in the human head due to RFR, or the temperature rise due to SAR as a heat source. The energy absorbed in the head is mainly due to electric fields induced by the magnetic fields generated by currents flowing through the feed point, along the antenna and the body of the phone. The RF energy is scattered and attenuated as it propagates through the tissues of the head, and maximum energy absorption is expected in the more absorptive high-water-content tissues near the surface of the head.

The local peak SARs differ depending on many factors, such as the antenna type, antenna radiation efficiency, antenna inclination with the head, distance of antenna from head, effect of the hand holding the handset, and the structural accuracy and resolution of the head model. Therefore, values of SARs are a function of various conditions set by each investigator. In other words, SAR is a result of a complex physical phenomenon of reactive coupling of the whole radiating structure with the human tissue. A significant contributor to the uncertainty in estimating SAR is the absence of a standard tissue averaging technique of the local SAR values over 1 or 10 g.

Experimental dosimetry for cellular telephones held against models of the head is more advanced, and automated SAR measurement systems have been set up for determination of the 1- and 10-g peak SARs needed for compliance testing of personal wireless devices [78–80].

5.4.2.1 Adult Size Heads

During the past few years, a considerable number of dosimetrical studies have been performed for calculating or measuring power absorbed in phantoms simulating human heads exposed to RFR (Table 5.6). It is evident that many SAR values exceeded the MPE values [78,81–89]. However, the temperature rise is far too small to have any lasting effects. Temperature measurements are significant only in case of high SARs. Increases in temperature (0.03–0.19°C) are much lower than the threshold temperature for neuron damage (4.5°C for more than 30 min), cataract induction (3–5°C), and physiological effects (1–2°C) [82,86,87,90]. Therefore, the temperature rise caused by mobile phone exposure has no effect on the temperature-controlling functions of the human brain. In fact, the thermostabilizing effect of brain perfusion often prevents temperature increase.

Moneda et al. [91] verified by means of numerical calculation that the higher the frequency the more superficial is the absorption. The numerical application manifests that the eyes, despite their small volume, absorb a considerable amount of the incident RFR, especially when the antenna is in front of the head, which is the most typical configuration related to use of 3G mobile phones. Another important issue raised by the authors is the enhancement of the hot spot near the center of the brain as the size of the head is reduced, which points to potential hazards to children using mobile phones.

Bahr et al. [92] designed an exposure system for investigation of volunteers during simulated GSM and wide code division multiple access (WCDMA) mobile phones. It was shown that the SAR distribution of the antenna exhibited similar characteristics to mobile phones with an integrated antenna. The 10 g averaged localized SAR, normalized to an antenna input power of 1 W and measured in the flat phantom area, amounted to 7.82 mW/g (900 MHz) and 10.98 mW/g (1966 MHz). The simulated SAR_{10g} in the visible human head model agreed with measured values to within 20%. A variation of the antenna rotation angle results in an SAR_{10g} change below 17%. The increase of the antenna distance by 2 mm with respect to the human head leads to a SAR_{10g} change of 9%.

5.4.2.2 Child Size Heads

There have been a limited number of studies that address the issue of a possible difference in sensitivity between adults and children [93]. Only model studies have been conducted into how EM waves propagate in children's size heads, relative to those of adults [94,95]. Gandhi et al. [94] reported that the deposition of EM energy in children's heads is higher than that in adults. However, Schonborn et al. [95] demonstrated Gandhi's conclusion to be incorrect. They calculated SAR for three different models of the head, namely for an adult, a 3-year-old, and a 7-year-old child. These models were obtained from actual MRI scans. The authors showed that no difference exists between their three models in terms of absorption of EM fields. However, these calculations use the same dielectric parameters for all ages. The effect of using an age-dependent magnitude for these parameters is unknown, assuming that they undergo significant changes between the age of 3 and adulthood. Moreover, it has been known that these model calculations are associated with uncertainties of up to 30% for 10-g average SAR values [96]. It is expected that effects of age-related changes in dielectric parameters, if any, fall within this uncertainty.

Based on Japanese children's statistical data on external shapes of heads, Wang and Osamu [97] developed two kinds of children's models from a Japanese adult head model. Using the children's head models, they calculated the local peak SAR under the same conditions as those previously employed by Gandhi et al. [94] and Schonborn et al. [95]. Compared to the local peak SAR in the adult head model, they found a considerable increase in the children's heads when they fixed the output power of the monopole-type antenna, but no significant differences when they fixed the effective current of the dipole-type antenna. This finding suggests that the contradictory conclusions drawn by the above two groups may be due to the different conditions in their numerical peak SAR calculations.

Bit-Babik et al. [98] tested several human head models and found that penetration depths for children and adults are about the same. This finding is consistent with other recent publications [99–102]. However, De Salles et al. [103] found that 1-g-SAR calculated for children is higher than that for the adults. When using a 10-year-old child model, SAR values more than 60% higher than those for adults were obtained.

TABLE 5.6
Summary of SAR Levels and Temperature Rise in Human Head

Investigator	Description of Source	SAR (W/kg)	Temperature Rise
Dimbylow (1994) [81]	900 MHz: $\lambda/4$; 600 mW;1.8 GHz; $\lambda/4$; 125 mW; calculated	For 900 MHz $SAR_{1g} = 2.17$; $SAR_{10g} = 1.82$ For 1.8 GHz $SAR_{1g} = 0.7$; $SAR_{10g} = 0.48$	—
Balzano et al. (1995) [78]	Motorola: 800–900 MHz; 600 mW and 2 W; measured	For analog (600 mW) Classic antenna: $SAR_{1g} = 0.2$–0.4; Flip antenna: $SAR_{1g} = 0.9$–1.6; Extended antenna: $SAR_{1g} = 0.6$–0.8 For GSM (2 W) Classic antenna: $SAR_{1g} = 0.09$–0.2; Flip antenna: $SAR_{1g} = 0.2$–0.3; Extended antenna: $SAR_{1g} = 0.1$–0.2	—
Anderson and Joyner (1995) [82]	AMPS phones; 600 mW; 800/900 MHz	SAR in the eye: 0.007–0.21; Metal-framed spectacles enhanced SARs in the eye by 9–29%; SAR in brain: 0.12–0.83	Eye: 0.022°C due to SAR of 0.21 W/kg Brain: 0.034°C due to SAR of 0.83 W/kg
Okoniewski and Stuchly (1996) [83] Lazzi and Gandhi (1998) [84]	Handset; 1W; 915 MHz; $\lambda/4$; calculated Handset; Helical antenna 600 mW; 835 MHz 125 mW; 1900 MHz; calculated and measured	$SAR_{1g} = 1.9$; $SAR_{10g} = 1.4$ $SAR_{1g} = 3.90$ (calculated); $SAR_{1g} = 4.02$ (measured); $SAR_{1g} = 0.15$ (calculated); $SAR_{1g} = 0.13$ (measured)	— —

Reference	Exposure conditions	SAR	Temperature
Gandhi et al. (1999) [85]	AMPS phones; 600 mW; 800/900 MHz; calculated and measured	$SAR_{1g} > 1.6$ unless antennas are carefully designed and placed further away from the head	—
Van Leeuwen et al. (1999) [86]	Mobile phones; 250 mW; calculated	$SAR_{10g} = 1.6$	0.11°C
Wang and Fujiwara (2000) [26]	Portable phone: 900 MHz; 600 mW; helical antenna; calculated	$SAR_{1g} = 2.10$; $SAR_{10g} = 1.21$	—
Bernardi et al. (2000) [87]	AMPS phones; 600 mW; 900 MHz; calculated	$SAR_{1g} = 2.2$–3.7	Ear: 0.22–0.43°C; Brain: 0.08–0.19°C
Van de Kamer and Lagendijk (2002) [88]	Dipole antenna; 250 mW; 900 MHz; calculated	Cubic $SAR_{1g} = 1.72$; Arbitrary $SAR_{1g} = 2.55$; Cubic $SAR_{10g} = 0.98$; Arbitrary $SAR_{10g} = 1.73$	—
McIntosh et al. (2005) [89]	Plane wave; 10 W/m^2; 100–3000 MHz; calculated	With the presence of a metallic plate in the head of RF-exposed worker SAR reaches 7.67 W/kg at 200 MHz, and 4.50 W/kg at 2500 MHz	1°C
Bahr et al. (2006) [92]	GSM and WCDMA; 1 W; 900 MHz and 1966 MHz; calculated and measured	The 10 g averaged localized SAR measured in the flat phantom area amounted to 7.82 mW/g (900 MHz) and 10.98 mW/g (1966 MHz)	—

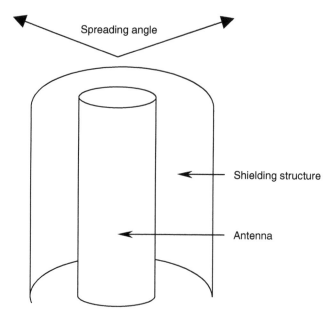

FIGURE 5.3   Shielding structures for mobile antennas.

5.4.2.3   Shielding for Mobile Antennas

It is known that magnetic materials are good for shielding structures because the magnetic near-field is the major cause of SAR [30]. Monopole antennas that are widely used in mobile phones are shielded by a finite and cylindrical shielding structure of magnetic material, as shown in Figure 5.3. The finite cylindrical sheet centered at the antenna position has a properly determined spreading angle so that only the near-field on the side of the human brain can be reduced, and the SAR is also reduced correspondingly.

5.5   FUTURE DEVELOPMENT

The level of safety is the domain of regulators and others who derive their authority from a number of laws and statutes. The scientific community, the media, and ultimately the general public are often presented with contradictory information on the validity of standards originating from a variety of governmental and advisory organizations [2]. When scientists have considerable evidence of the health risks at high-intensity levels, yet minimal evidence of health risks at low levels, they have difficulty defining the safe levels. Current exposure guidelines are based on a scientific assessment of the relevant literature and may offer protection against the established health hazards of RF energy, which are thermal in nature. However, many research investigations of low-power exposure have shown some biological effects which may lead to serious health consequences, including neurological, cardiological and hormonal disorders, breakdown of the BBB, DNA damage, cancers, diabetes, and asthma. Children, who are subject to such exposure through mobile phones and wireless base stations, have brains and nervous systems that are still developing; they might be vulnerable.

5.5.1 HARMONIZATION OF SAFETY STANDARDS

Most of the RF standards reviewed have similar basic restrictions and almost similar MPE values. These similarities are related, in part, to the various dosimetric models used to relate field strengths to the basic restrictions. A comprehensive set of safety standards for all kinds of exposure to all frequency bands of RFR is not practical or probable. There are still many questions related to (1) main parameters such as SAR levels, duration of exposure, pulse effects, exposure geometry, modulation technique, and type of effect (thermal or nonthermal); (2) differences in absorption of RF energy by humans of different sizes and orientations; (3) complexity of measuring exposures, models, and statistical methods employed; and (4) incomplete discussion of research concerning possible long-term health effects. Although laboratory and epidemiological studies are available to address the likelihood of long-term effects, these data are not clearly described or specified in the standards. These questions require answers to define levels at which harmful effects can occur.

Do these exposure guidelines need to be reconsidered? It might be necessary because the guidelines are still intended basically to deal with thermal effects, not with energy at lower levels. However, during the past few years there have been around 200 studies that suggest there may be health risks of RFR even at levels too low to cause heating of body tissue [104,105]. There is not widespread acceptance of this fact in the scientific community, although many such studies were included in the ICNIRP review. The reason is attributed to the fact that the literature on nonthermal effects is complex and the validity of the reported effects is poorly established. One reviewer [106] concludes: "Many reported effects find conventional explanation or simply disappear when follow-up studies are conducted under better controlled conditions." Nevertheless, the existence of health effects at low-level RFR should not be entirely ignored until more decisive information is provided through current and future research programs.

In addition, the guidelines were developed based on research studies conducted during and prior to the 1980s when many of the current-day sources of RF energy (such as mobile phones) were not widely available. For example, the IEEE/ANSI C95.1-1992 standard did not include any studies published after the 1980s. However, the most recent review of literature for the purpose of formulating exposure guidelines has been undertaken by the ICNIRP [12–14].

Another important issue is international harmonization, which refers to an international attempt to get various standard-setting bodies, health agencies, national governments, and international organizations to coordinate on health and safety standards for RFR. This does not necessarily mean that the world will have only one accepted RF standard, but it does mean that the basis for the differences is known. While the new IEEE (IEEE C95.1-2005) standard and the current ICNIRP exposure guidelines possess some similarities as a step toward harmonization, they are still far from harmonized. International harmonization of exposure guidelines would be a desirable goal. This process should be accomplished through better techniques for SAR estimation, less uncertainty in exposure assessment, and greater reliability in biological and epidemiological results. In this regard, Osepchuk and Petersen [107] state: "The trend toward international harmonization of standards, at the moment, faces barriers posed by the regulations and rationales inherited from the Russian era. Many international meetings and the spread of electronic communication technologies will help eventually reach into Eastern Europe and the former communist countries. This will help in the movement toward international harmonization of standards."

5.5.2   ENGINEERING REQUIREMENTS AND DOSIMETRIC INFORMATION

Many published studies suffer from inappropriate engineering implementations and a lack of dosimetric information. Therefore, basic engineering and dosimetric requirements to conduct scientifically sound experiments investigating biological effects or health consequences should be implemented. Negovetic et al. [108] outlines specific recommendations from a four-day workshop dedicated to an interdisciplinary exploration of engineering requirements and quality assurance in the main field of bioelectromagnetics. Consensus on the following points was reached:

- Since effects are expected to be small, the likelihood of evoking effects should be maximized; that is, maximum exposure levels close to the thermal threshold, minimum noise level, optimized modulation, etc. should be adopted.
- The setup must be designed in such a way as to enable the intended experiments according to standard protocol, meeting all dosimetric needs and avoiding any EMI/EMC issues. Since protocols differ from end point to end point, setups cannot be standardized.
- Blinding of the exposure is a plus for any setup but mandatory for human provocation studies. Regarding *in vitro* and *in vivo* experiments, at least evaluation should be blinded.
- True sham exposure is mandatory. Incubator controls and positive controls will depend on the experiment.
- In general, close collaboration between biological/medical and engineering parties is required throughout the design phase of exposure setups. The dosimetry characterization of the exposure should include the distribution of SAR in space and time, including the distribution of temperature increase or at least the maximum temperature increase if it is negligibly small from a biological point of view. The minimum requirements regarding SAR information should include whole-body average, spatial peak averaged over appropriate masses, and organ average. A two-step procedure is appropriate, that is, (1) characterization of the field distribution on the macro level (macrodosimetry) from which (2) microdosimetry data (i.e., at the cellular or subcellular levels) can then be derived.
- An important part of dosimetry is the analysis of uncertainty and variation. Uncertainty describes the uncertainty of the determined mean value of the exposure distribution (e.g., cell and time or animal and time). Variation describes the variations from the mean as a function of change during the exposure (e.g., position, different dielectric parameters, etc.). Uncertainties and variations should be provided for whole-body, spatial peak, as well as tissue-specific SAR values.

- Dosimetry should be based on numerical dosimetry. In general, numerical dosimetry must be verified by experimental measurements, the agreement between which must be within the combined uncertainty of both techniques. Numerical dosimetry also constitutes an essential part in the development and optimization of exposure setups.
- The current commercially available numerical tools are sufficient for dosimetric studies. Since most dosimetric evaluation involves greatly nonhomogenous structures, FDTD was defined as the most suitable technique.

Further dosimetric studies are required, especially in areas related to numerical modeling of the energy absorbed in models of the human head, measurement of electrical properties of various head tissues, and modeling the relationship between SAR and temperature elevation to predict potential hazards associated with specific RF exposure conditions.

REFERENCES

1. Habash RWH, Brodsky LM, Leiss W, Krewski DK, Repacholi M. Health risk of electromagnetic fields, Part II: Evaluation and assessment of radio frequency radiation. *Crit Rev Biomed Eng* 2003; 31: 197–254.
2. Moghissi AA, Straja SR, Love BR. The role of scientific consensus organizations in the development of standards. *Health Phys* 2003; 84: 533–537.
3. Vecchia P. The approach of ICNIRP to protection of children. *Bioelectromagnetics* 2005; 7 (Suppl): S157–S160.
4. IEEE. Safety levels with respect to human exposure to radio frequency electromagnetic fields, 3 kHz to 300 GHz. *IEEE Standard C95.1-1991*, 1992.
5. IEEE. Standard for safety levels with respect to human exposure to radio frequency electromagnetic fields, 3 kHz to 300 GHz. *IEEE Standard C95.1-1991*, 1999.
6. IEEE. Recommended practice for determining the peak spatial-average specific absorption rate (SAR) in the human head from wireless communications devices. *IEEE Standard 1528-2003*, 2003.
7. IEEE. Standard for safety levels with respect to human exposure to radio frequency electromagnetic fields, 3 kHz to 300 GHz. *IEEE Standard C95.1-2005*, 2006.
8. NRPB. Board statement on restrictions on human exposure to static and time-varying electromagnetic fields. National Radiological Protection Board. Doc NRPB, 4(5), Chilton, Didcot, Oxon, UK, 1993.
9. NRPB. ICNIRP guidelines for limiting exposure to time-varying electric, magnetic and electromagnetic fields (up to 300 GHz). Advice on aspects of implementation in the UK. National Radiological Protection Board. Doc NRPB, 10(2), Chilton, Didcot, Oxon, UK, 1999.
10. NRPB. Review of the scientific evidence for limiting exposure to electromagnetic fields (80–300 GHz). National Radiological Protection Board. Doc NRPB, 15(2), Chilton, Didcot, Oxon, UK, 2004.
11. FCC. Guidelines for evaluating the environmental effects of radio frequency radiation. Federal Communications Commission, 96-326, Washington, DC, 1996.
12. ICNIRP. Guidelines for limiting exposure to time-varying electric, magnetic, and electromagnetic fields (up to 300 GHz). *Health Phys* 1998; 74: 494–522.
13. ICNIRP. Responses to questions and comments on ICNIRP. *Health Phys* 1998; 75: 438–439.
14. ICNIRP. General approach to protection against non-ionizing radiation. *Health Phys* 2002; 82: 540–548.

15. Safety Code 6. Limits of human exposure to radiofrequency electromagnetic fields in the frequency range from 3 kHz to 300 GHz. Environmental Health Directorate, Health Protection Branch, Health Canada, Canada, 1999.
16. ARPANSA. Maximum exposure levels to radiofrequency fields—3 kHz–300 GHz. Radiation Protection Series No. 3. Australian Radiation Protection and Nuclear Safety Agency, Australia, 2002.
17. Chou CK. Basic problems of diversely reported biological effects of radio frequency fields. *Radiats Biol Radioecol* 2003; 43: 512–518.
18. Gandhi OP. Electromagnetic fields: human safety issues. *Annu Rev Biomed Eng* 2002; 4: 211–234.
19. Lin JC. Update of IEEE radio frequency exposure guidelines. *IEEE Microw Mag* 2006; 7: 24–28.
20. CENELEC EN 50392:2004-01. Generic standard to demonstrate the compliance of electronic and electrical apparatus with the basic restrictions related to human exposure to electromagnetic fields (0 Hz to 300 GHz), European Committee for Electromechanical Standardization, 2004.
21. Sheppard AR, Kavet RR, David C. Exposure guidelines for low frequency electric and magnetic fields: report from the Brussels workshop. *Health Phys* 2002; 83: 324–332.
22. Durney CH, Massoudi H, Iskander MF. Radiofrequency radiation dosimetry handbook. Brooks AFB, TX: USAF School of Aerospace Medicine, Aerospace Medical Division: USAFSAM-TR-85-73, 1986.
23. Blank M, Goodman R. Comment: a biological guide for electromagnetic safety: the stress response. *Bioelectromagnetics* 2004; 25: 642–646.
24. Erdreich LS, Klauenberg BJ. Radio frequency radiation exposure standards: considerations for harmonization. *Health Phys* 2001; 80: 430–439.
25. Repacholi MH, Greenebaum B. Interaction of static and extremely low frequency electric and magnetic fields with living systems: health effects and research needs. *Bioelectromagnetics* 1999; 20: 133–160.
26. Wang J, Fujiwara O. Dosimetric evaluation of human head for portable telephones. *Electr Comm Japan* 2000; E85-Part I: 12–22.
27. Durney CH, Christensen DA. *Basic Introduction to Bioelectromagnetics*. Boca Raton, FL: CRC Press, 1999.
28. Beyerle PA, Gupta IJ. A resistive edge treated Gregorian subreflector for a dual reflector compact range measurement system. Technical Report 721223-8, The Ohio State University ElectroScience Laboratory, Columbus, OH, 1990.
29. Handel CS. Low frequency modification of a dual chamber compact range. MS Thesis. The Ohio State University, Columbus, OH, 1997.
30. Hsiao Y-T, Tuan S-H, Chou H-T, Wang J-S. Applications of shielding techniques to enhance the antenna performance of mobile communications and reduce SAR induction in the human head. *Electromagnetics* 2005; 25: 343–361.
31. Habash RWY. *Electromagnetic Fields and Radiation: Human Bioeffects and Safety*. New York: Marcel Dekker, 2001.
32. Thansandote A, Gajda GB, Lecuyer DW. Radiofrequency radiation in five Vancouver schools: exposure standards not exceeded. *Can Med Ass J* 1999; 160: 1311–1312.
33. Mann SM, Cooper TG, Allen SG, Blackwell RP, Lowe AJ. Exposure to radio waves near mobile phone base stations. National Radiation Protection Board, UK, 2000.
34. Bernardi P, Cavagnaro M, Pisa S, Piuzzi E. Human exposure to radio-base station antennas in urban environment. *IEEE Trans Microw Theory Tech* 2000; 48: 1996–2002.
35. Silvi AM, Zari A, Licitra G. Assessment of the temporal trend of the exposure of people to electromagnetic fields produced by base stations for mobile telephones. *Radiat Prot Dosim* 2001; 97: 387–390.

36. Anglesio L, Benedetto A, Bonino A, Colla D, Martire F, Saudino Fusette S, d'Amore G. Population exposure to electromagnetic fields generated by radio base stations: evaluation of the urban background by using provisional model and instrumental measurements. *Radiat Prot Dosim* 2001; 97: 355–358.

37. Cooper J, Marx B, Buhl J, Hombach V. Determination of safety distance limits for a human near a cellular base station antenna, adopting the IEEE standard or ICNIRP guidelines. *Bioelectromagnetics* 2002; 23: 429–443.

38. Van Wyk MJ, Bingle M, Meyer FJC. Antenna modeling considerations for accurate SAR calculations in human phantoms in close proximity to GSM cellular base station antennas. *Bioelectromagnetics* 2005; 26: 502–509.

39. Henderson, SI, Bangay MJ. Survey of RF exposure levels from mobile telephone base stations in Australia. *Bioelectromagnetics* 2006; 27: 73–76.

40. Sandstrom M, Wilen J, Oftedal G, Hansson MK. Mobile phone use and subjective symptoms. Comparison of symptoms experienced by users of analogue and digital mobile phones. *Occup Med (Lond)* 2001; 51: 25–35.

41. Radon K, Spegel H, Meyer N, Klein J, Brix J, Wiedenhofer A, Eder H, Praml G, Schulze A, Ehrenstein V, von Kries R, Nowak D. Personal dosimetry of exposure to mobile telephone base stations? An epidemiologic feasibility study comparing the Maschek dosimeter prototype and the Antennessa DSP-090 system. *Bioelectromagnetics* 2006; 27: 77–81.

42. NRPB. Possible health effects from Terrestrial Trunked Radio (TETRA). Report of an Advisory Group on Non-ionising Radiation. National Radiological Protection Board. Doc NRPB, 12(2), Chilton, Didcot, Oxon, UK, 2001.

43. Hocking B, Gordon I, Grain H, Hatfield G. Cancer incidence and mortality and proximity to TV towers. *Med J Aust* 1996; 65: 601–605.

44. McKenzie DR, Yin Y, Morrell S. Childhood incidence of acute lymhoblastic leukaemia and exposure to broadcast radiation in Sydney—a second look. *Aust NZ J Pub Health* 1998; 22: 360–367.

45. Baird RC, Lewis RL, Kremer DP, Kilgore SB. Field strength measurements of speed measuring radar units. NBSIR 81-2225, National Bureau of Standards, Washington, DC, 1981.

46. Fisher PD. Microwave exposure levels encountered by police traffic radar operators. MSU-ENGR-91-007, Michigan State University, Michigan, IL, 1991.

47. Fisher PD. Microwave exposure levels encountered by police traffic radar operators. *IEEE Trans Electromagn Compat* 1993; 35: 36–45.

48. Lotz WG, Rinsky RA, Edwards RD. Occupational exposure of police officers to microwave radiation from traffic radar devices. National Institute for Occupational Safety and Health (NIOSH), PB95-261350, USA, 1995.

49. Balzano Q, Bergeron JA, Cohen J, Osepchuk JM, Petersen RC, Roszyk LM. Measurement of equivalent power density and RF energy deposition in the immediate vicinity of a 24-GHz traffic radar antenna. *IEEE Trans Electromagn Compat* 1995; 37: 183–191.

50. Fink JM, Wagner JP, Congleton JJ, Rock JC. Microwave emissions from police radar. *Am Ind Hyg Assoc J* 1999; 60: 770–776.

51. Stuchly MA, Repacholi MH, Lecuyer D, Mann R. Radiation survey of dielectric (RF) heaters in Canada. *J Microw Power* 1980; 15: 113–121.

52. Bini M, Checcucci A, Ignesti A, Millanta L, Olmi R, Rubino N, Vanni R. Exposure of workers to intense RF electric fields that peak from plastic sealers. *J Microw Power* 1986; 21: 33–40.

53. Olsen RG, Griner TA, Van Matre BJ. Measurement of RF current and localized SAR near a shipboard RF heat sealer. In: Blank M, Editor. *Electricity and Magnetism in Biology and Medicine*. San Francisco, CA: San Francisco Press, pp. 927–929, 1993.

54. Gandhi OP, Wu D, Chen JW, Conover DL. Induced current and SAR distributions for a worker model exposed to an RF dielectric heater under simulated workplace conditions. *Health Phys* 1997; 72: 236–42.
55. Wilén J, Hörnsten R, Sandström M, Bjerle P, Wiklund U, Stensson O, Lyskov E, Mild KH. Electromagnetic field exposure and health among RF plastic sealer operators. *Bioelectromagnetics* 2004; 25: 5–15.
56. Moseley H, Davison M. Radiation leakage levels from microwave ovens. *Ann Occup Hyg* 1989; 33: 653–654.
57. Matthes R. Radiation emission from microwave ovens. *J Radiol Prot* 1992; 12: 167–172.
58. Thansandote A, Lecuyer DW, Blais A, Gajda GB. Compliance of before-sale microwave ovens to the Canadian radiation emitting devices regulations. 32nd Microwave Power Symposium Proceedings. July 14–16, Ottawa, Ontario, Canada, 1997.
59. Janes DE, Tell RA, Athey TW, Hankin NN. Radiofrequency radiation levels in urban areas. *Radio Sci* 1977; 12: 49–56.
60. Tell RA, Mantiply ED. Population exposure to VHF and UHF broadcast radiation in the United States. *Proc IEEE* 1980; 68: 6–12.
61. Hankin NN. The radiofrequency radiation environment: environmental exposure levels and RF radiation emitting sources, U.S. EPA Technical Report EPA 520/1-85-014, 1985.
62. EPA. Federal radiation protection guidance; proposed alternatives for controlling public exposure to radiofrequency radiation; notice of proposed recommendations. Environmental Protection Agency (EPA), *Federal Register* (Part II) 51 (146): 27318–27339, 1986.
63. Hondou T. Rising level of public exposure to mobile phones: accumulation through additivity and reflectivity. *J Phys Soc Japan* 2002; 71: 432–435.
64. Toropainen A. Human exposure by mobile phones in enclosed areas. *Bioelectromagnetics* 2003; 24: 63–65.
65. Kangarlu A, Robitaille P-ML. Biological effects and health implications in magnetic resonance imaging. *Concepts Magn Reson* 2000; 12: 321–359.
66. Gandhi OP, Chen XB. Specific absorption rates and induced current densities for an anatomy-based model of the human for exposure to time-varying magnetic fields of MRI. *Magn Reson Med* 1999; 41: 816–823.
67. Collins CM, Smith MB. Signal-to-noise ratio and absorbed power as functions of main magnetic field strength, and definition of "90" RF pulse for the head in the birdcage coil. *Magn Reson Med* 2001; 45: 684–691.
68. Kangarlu A, Shellock FG, Chakeres DW. 8.0 Tesla human MR system: temperature changes associated with radiofrequency-induced heating of a head phantom. *J Magn Reson Imag* 2003; 17: 220–226.
69. Olsen RG, Griner TA. Outdoor measurements of SAR in a full-size human model exposed to 29.2 MHz near-field irradiation. *Bioelectromagnetics* 1989; 10: 162–171.
70. Adair ER, Kelleher SA, Mack GW, Morocco TS. Thermophysiological responses of human volunteers during controlled whole-body radio frequency exposure at 450 MHz. *Bioelectromagnetics* 1998; 19: 232–245.
71. Adair ER, Cobb BL, Mylacraine KS, Kelleher SA. Human exposure at two radio frequencies (450 and 2450 MHz): similarities and differences in physiological response. *Bioelectromagnetics* 1999; 20: 12–20.
72. Adair ER, Mylacraine KS, Cobb BL. Partial-body exposure of human volunteers to 2450 MHz pulsed or CW fields provokes similar thermoregulatory responses. *Bioelectromagnetics* 2001; 22: 246–259.
73. Allen SJ, Adair ER, Mylacraine KS, Hurt W, Ziriax J. Empirical and theoretical dosimetry in support of whole body resonant RF exposure (100 MHz) in human volunteers. *Bioelectromagnetics* 2003; 24: 502–509.

74. Nagaoka T, Watanabe S, Sakurai K, Kunieda E, Watanabe S, Taki M, Yamanaka. Development of realistic high-resolution whole-body voxel models of Japanese adult males and females of average height and weight, and application of models to radio-frequency electromagnetic-field dosimetry. *Phys Med Biol* 2004; 49: 1–15.

75. Kivekäs O, Ollikainen J, Lehtiniemi T, Vainikainen P. Effect of the chassis length on the bandwidth, SAR, and efficiency of internal mobile phone antennas. *Microw Optical Tech Lett* 2003; 36: 457–462.

76. Kuster N, Schuderer J, Christ A, Futter P, Ebert S. Guidance for exposure design of human studies addressing health risk evaluations of mobile phones. *Bioelectromagnetics* 2004; 25: 524–529.

77. Moulder JE, Erdreich LS, Malyapa RS, Merritt J, Pickard WF, Vijayalaxmi. Cell phones and cancer: what is the evidence for a connection? *Radiat Res* 1999; 151: 513–531.

78. Balzano Q, Garay O, Manning TJ Jr. Electromagnetic energy exposure of simulated users of portable cellular telephones. *IEEE Trans Veh Tech* 1995; 44: 390–403.

79. Schmid T, Egger O, Kuster N. Automated E-field scanning system for dosimetric assessments. *IEEE Trans Microw Theory Tech* 1996; 44: 105–113.

80. Yu Q, Gandhi OP, Aronsson M, Wu D. An automated SAR measurement system for compliance testing of personal wireless devices. *IEEE Trans Electromagn Compat* 1999; 4: 234–245.

81. Dimbylow PJ. FDTD calculations at the SAR for a dipole closely coupled to the head at 900 MHz and 1.9 GHz. *Phys Med Biol* 1993; 38: 361–368.

82. Anderson V, Joyner KH. Specific absorption rate levels measured in a phantom head exposed to radio frequency transmissions from analog hand-held mobile phones. *Bioelectromagnetics* 1995; 16: 60–69.

83. Okoniewski M, Stuchly MA. A study of the handset antenna and human body interaction. *IEEE Trans Microw Theory Tech* 1996; 44: 1855–1864.

84. Lazzi G, Gandhi OP. On modeling and personal dosimetry of cellular telephone helical antennas with the FDTD code. *IEEE Trans Antennas Propag* 1998; 46: 525–529.

85. Gandhi OP, Lazzi G, Tinniswood A, Yu QS. Comparison of numerical and experimental methods for determination of SAR and radiation patterns of handheld wireless telephones. *Bioelectromagnetics* 1999; 20: 93–101.

86. Van Leeuwen GM, Lagendijk JJ, Van Leersum BJ, Zwamborn AP, Hornsleth SN, Kotte AN. Calculation of change in brain temperatures due to exposure to a mobile phone. *Phys Med Biol* 1999; 44: 2367–2379.

87. Bernardi P, Cavagnaro M, Pisa S, Piuzzi E. Specific absorption rate and temperature increases in the head of a cellular-phone user. *IEEE Trans Microw Theory Tech* 2000; 48: 1118–1125.

88. Van de Kamer JB, Lagendijk JJ. Computation of high-resolution SAR distributions in a head due to a radiating dipole antenna representing a hand-held mobile phone. *Phys Med Biol* 2002; 47: 1827–1835.

89. McIntosh RL, Anderson V, McKenzie RJ. A numerical evaluation of SAR distribution and temperature changes around a metallic plate in the head of a RF exposed worker. *Bioelectromagnetics* 2005; 26: 377–388.

90. Chen H-Y, Yang H-P. Temperature increase in human heads due to different models of cellular phones. *Electromagnetics* 2006; 26: 439–459.

91. Moneda AP, Ioannidou MP, Chrissoulidis DP. Radio-wave exposure of the human head: analytical study based on a versatile eccentric spheres model including a brain core and a pair of eyeballs. *IEEE Trans Biomed Eng* 2003; 50: 667–676.

92. Bahr A, Dorn H, Bolz T. Dosimetric assessment of an exposure system for simulating GSM and WCDMA mobile phone usage. *Bioelectromagnetics* 2006; 27: 320–327.

93. Van Rongen E, Roubos EW, van Aernsbergen LM, Brussaard G, Havenaar J, Koops FB, Van Leeuwen FE, Leonhard HK, van Rhoon GC, Swaen GM, van de Weerdt RH, Zwamborn AP. Mobile phones and children: is precaution warranted? *Bioelectromagnetics* 2004; 25: 142–144.

94. Gandhi OP, Lazzi G, Furse CM. Electromagnetic absorption in the human head and neck for mobile telephones at 835 and 1900 MHz. *IEEE Trans Microw Theory Tech* 1996; 44: 1884–1897.

95. Schonborn F, Burkhard M, Kuster N. Differences in energy absorption between heads of adults and children in the near field of sources. *Health Phys* 1998; 74: 160–168.

96. Nikita KS, Cavagnaro M, Bernardi P, Uzunoglu NK, Pisa S, Piuzzi E, Sahalos JN, Krikelas GI, Vaul JA, Excell PS, Cerri G, Chiarandini S, De Leo R, Russo P. A study of incertainties in modeling antenna performance and power absorption in the head of a cellular phone user. *IEEE Trans Microw Theory Tech* 2000; 48: 2676–2685.

97. Wang J, Osamu F. Comparison and evaluation of electromagnetic absorption characteristics in realistic human head models of adult and children for 900-MHz mobile telephones. *IEEE Trans Microw Theory Tech* 2003; 51: 966–971.

98. Bit-Babik G, Guy AW, Chou CK, Faraone A, Kanda M, Gessner A, Wang J, Fujiwara Q. Simulation of exposure and SAR estimation for adult and child heads exposed to RF energy from portable communication devices. *Radiat Res* 2005; 163: 580–590.

99. Christ A, Kuster N. Differences in RF energy absorption in the heads of adults and children. *Bioelectromagnetics* 2005; 26: S31–S44.

100. Wiart J, Hadjem A, Gadui N, Bloch I, Wong MF, Pradier A, Lautru D, Hanna VF, Dale C. Modeling of RF head exposure in children. *Bioelectromagnetics* 2005; 26: S19–S30.

101. Beard BB, Kainz W, Ohnishi T, Takahiro I, Watanabe S, Fujiwara O, Wang J, Bit-Babik G, Faraone A, Wiart J, Christ A, Kuster N, Lee A-K, Kroeze H, Siegbahn M, Keshvari J, Abrishamkar H, Simon W, Manteuffel D, Nikoloski N. Comparisons of computed mobile phone induced SAR in the SAM phantom to that in anatomically correct models of the human head. *IEEE Trans Electromagn Compat* 2006; 48: 397–407.

102. Keshvari J, Kwshvari R, Lang S. The effect of increase in dielectric values on specific absorption rate (SAR) in eye and head tissues following 900, 1800, and 2450 MHz radio frequency (RF) exposure. *Phys Med Biol* 2006; 51: 1463–1477.

103. De Salles AA, Bulla G, Fernandez Rodrigues CE. Electromagnetic absorption in the head of adults and children due to mobile phone operation close to the head. *Electromag Biol Med* 2006; 25: 349–360.

104. Michaelson SM, Elson EC. Interaction of nonmodulated and pulse modulated radio frequency fields with living matter: experimental results. In: Polk C, Postow E, Editors. *Handbook of Biological Effects of Electromagnetic Fields*. Boca Raton, FL: CRC Press, pp. 435–534, 1996.

105. Postow E, Swicord M. Modulated fields and "window" effects. In: Polk C, Postow E, Editors. *Handbook of Biological Effects of Electromagnetic Fields*. Boca Raton, FL: CRC Press, pp. 435–533, 1996.

106. Foster KR. Thermal and nonthermal mechanisms of interaction of radio-frequency energy with biological systems. *IEEE Trans Plasma Sci* 2000; 28: 15–23.

107. Osepchuck JM, Petersen RC. Historical review of RF exposure standards and the International Committee on Electromagnetic Safety (ICES). *Bioelectromagnetics* 2003; 24: S7–S16.

108. Negovetic S, Samaras T, Kuster N. EMF health risk research: lessons learned and recommendations for the future. Workshop in Monte Verita, Nov. 20–25, 2005.

6 Bioeffects and Health Implications of Radiofrequency Radiation

6.1 INTRODUCTION

Significant concern has been raised about possible health effects from exposure to RFR, especially after the rapid introduction of mobile phones. Parents are especially concerned with the possibility that RFR emissions from mobile phones and base stations erected in or near homes and schools might have health impact on children.

While mobile communications are advancing, the idea of health effects from cellular phones is quickly becoming the focus of much research. There have been few scientific studies of this new service and there is limited information on whether the radiation emitted by cellular equipment poses a risk to human health. For many researchers, the findings are confirming the observations made over the years of the effects of low-level energy on living systems: They believe that small amounts of energy when delivered in the right way can have the same effect as a massive dose of chemicals. Others just do not see the threat.

It is important to distinguish between biological and physiological effects and health effects. A biological effect occurs when exposure to EM fields causes some noticeable or detectable physiological change in a living system. Such an effect may sometimes, but not always, lead to an adverse health effect, which means a physiological change that exceeds normal range for a brief period of time. It occurs when the biological effect is outside the normal range for the body to compensate, and therefore leads to some detrimental health condition. Health effects are often the result of biological effects that accumulate over time and depend on exposure dose. For example, if an effect of EM exposure has been noticed on cultured cells, this does not necessarily mean that the exposure will lead to adverse effect for the health of the organism as a whole. In general, the number of cellular and animal studies in the literature is large due to the large number of cellular processes and systems that may possibly be affected by RFR [1].

The permanent problem in the controversy of health risk is the limited knowledge about the fact that very specific fields interacting with our bodies can have critical effects on our health. These effects vary throughout populations as some are affected to a greater degree than others. This is related to our physical and biochemical differences.

The potential for exposure to RFR resulting in adverse health outcomes has been the subject of intensive investigation. In this chapter, we examine epidemiological, cellular and animal, and human evidences on possible health effects associated with RFR. Important areas of research that need further investigation including risk for children are also highlighted.

6.2 EPIDEMIOLOGICAL STUDIES

During the past 30 years, there have been a number of epidemiological studies analyzing health effects of RF exposure. Epidemiological studies are of primary importance in health risk assessment. There have been a number of epidemiological studies analyzing health effects of RF exposure. With the increased interest in wireless networks and the safety concerns of this emerging technology, it can be expected that there will be more studies in the future.

6.2.1 OCCUPATIONAL EXPOSURE STUDIES

Occupational or controlled environments represent areas in which people are exposed to RFR as a result of their employment. The various health risks, including cancers, have been examined in occupational RF exposure studies. These include investigations involving radar and military personnel [2–5], police officers using traffic radar devices [6,7], amateur radio operators [8,9], and telephone operators [10,11]. A few epidemiological studies [12,13] have been performed with operators in industrial settings to assess specific problems that may arise such as RF burns and burns from contact with thermally hot surfaces; numbness in hands and fingers; disturbed or altered tactile sensitivity; eye irritation; and warming and leg discomfort.

While some positive results have been reported in occupational studies of RFR, these studies provide no consistent evidence of an association between RFR and adverse health effects.

6.2.1.1 Navy Personnel and Military Workers

Robinette et al. [14] conducted a study of mortality results on males who had served in the U.S. Navy during the Korean War. They selected 19,965 equipment-repair men who had occupational exposure to RFR. They also chose 20,726 naval equipment-operation men who, by their titles, had lower occupational exposure to RFR as a control group. The researchers studied mortality records for 1955–1974, in-service morbidity for 1950–1959, and morbidity for 1963–1976 in Veterans Administration hospitals. Although exposures in the high-exposure group were assumed as 1 mW/cm², the three high-exposure categories included occasions of exposure in excess of 10 mW/cm². As a result, there were 619 deaths (3.1%) from all causes in the exposed group versus 579 deaths (2.8%) in the age-specific general white male population. The death rate from trauma was higher in the exposed than the control group, 295 (1.5%) versus 247 (1.2%). No difference in cancer mortality or morbidity was seen among the high- and low-exposure groups.

Szmigielski [3] showed strong association between RF exposure and several types of cancer (including brain cancer and cancer of the alimentary canal) in a cohort of about 120,000 Polish military personnel, of whom 3% had worked with RF heat sealers. Exposure was determined from assessments of field levels at various locations. The study did not consider the length of time at the location, the nature of the job, or the number of cases observed.

Groves et al. [15] have reported the outcome of a 40-year follow-up of mortality due to cancer and other causes in the same group of Navy personnel during the Korean War. The results were similar to those of Robinette et al. [14] confirming that radar exposure had little effect on mortality.

6.2.1.2   Traffic Radar Devices

Davis and Mostofi [6], in a brief communication, reported six cases of testicular cancer in police who used handheld radars between 1979 and 1991 among a cohort of 340 police officers employed at two police departments within contiguous counties in the north-central United States. The six cases had been employed as police officers as their primary lifetime occupation, and all had been exposed to traffic radar on a routine basis. The mean length of service prior to testicular-cancer diagnosis was 14.7 years, the mean age at diagnosis was 39 years, and all had used radar at least 4.5 years before the diagnosis.

Finkelstein [7] presented the results of a retrospective cohort cancer study among 22,197 officers employed by 83 Ontario police departments. The standardized incidence ratio (SIR) for all tumor sites was 0.90. There was an increased incidence of testicular cancer (SIR = 1.3) and melanoma skin cancer (SIR = 1.45). No information about individual exposures to radar devices was provided.

6.2.1.3   RF Heat Sealers

Lagorio et al. [12] reported higher cancer mortality among Italian plasticware workers exposed to RFR generated by dielectric heat sealers for the period 1962–1992. Six types of cancers were found in the exposed group. The standardized mortality ratio (SMR) analysis was applied to a small cohort of 481 women workers, representing 78% of the total person-years at risk. Mortality from malignant neoplasms was slightly elevated, and increased risk of leukemia was detected. The all-cancer SMR was higher among women employed in the sealing. Exposure assessment was based on the time assigned on jobs. Exposure to RFR was based on a previous survey, which showed that the radiation exceeded 1 mW/cm^2. The work area also included exposure to chemicals associated with cancer (solvents and vinyl chloride), which may have an impact on the result.

6.2.1.4   Telecom Operators

In Norway, Tynes et al. [10] studied breast cancer incidence in female radio and telegraph operators with potential exposure to light at night, RFR (405 kHz to 25 MHz), and ELF fields (50 Hz). The researchers linked the Norwegian Telecom cohort of female radio and telegraph operators working at sea to the Cancer Registry of Norway to conduct their study. The cohort consisted of 2619 women who were certified to work as radio and telegraph operators. The incidences of all cancers were not significant, but an excess risk was seen for breast cancer. They noted that these women were exposed to light at night, which is known to decrease melatonin levels, an expected risk factor for breast cancer.

6.2.2   Public Exposure Studies

Studies of public exposure to RFR have focused on two common RF field sources: radio and TV transmitters and mobile phone use.

6.2.2.1   Radio and TV Transmitters

Populations residing near telecommunications broadcasting installations tend to have the highest nonoccupational RF exposures [16]. An association between proximity of residences to TV towers and increased incidence of childhood leukemia was found in an Australian study conducted by Hocking et al. [17]. The researchers studied the leukemia incidence among people living close to TV towers (exposed group) and compared this to the incidence among those living further out from the towers (unexposed or control group). People were assigned to one of the two groups based on data from the New South Wales Cancer Registry and their accompanying address. The Hocking study concluded that there was a 95% increase in childhood leukemia associated with proximity to TV towers. No such association was found between RFR emitted by the TV towers and adult leukemia. McKenzie et al. [18] repeated the Hocking study, using more accurate estimates of RFR at the same area and at the same time period. They found increased childhood leukemia in one area near the TV antennas, but not in other similar areas near the same TV antennas. They found no significant correlation between RF exposure and the rate of childhood leukemia. They also found that much of the "excess childhood leukemia" reported by the Hocking study occurred before high-power 24-hour TV broadcasting had started.

In Italy, Michelozzi et al. [19,20] conducted a small area study to investigate a cluster of leukemia near a high-power radio transmitter in a peripheral area of Rome. The leukemia mortality within 3.5 km (5863 inhabitants) was higher than expected. The excess was due to a significantly higher mortality among men (seven cases were observed). Also, the results showed a significant decline in risk with distance from the transmitter, only among men, but no association for women, and a nonsignificant decrease in risk for both sexes combined. For childhood leukemia, based on eight cases, there was a significant trend of risk decreasing with distance.

Burch et al. [16] study demonstrated the feasibility of using global positioning system (GPS) and geographic information system (GIS) technologies to improve RF exposure assessment and reduce exposure misclassification. They found that proximity, elevation, line of sight, alternate sources, and temporal variability each contributed to RF exposure and should be evaluated in future investigations of the potential health effects of RF broadcasting in human populations.

6.2.2.2   Mobile and Cordless Phones

Most of the mobile phone studies (Table 6.1) show no increased incidences of brain tumors among mobile phone users (analog or digital). Furthermore, there was no relationship between brain tumor incidences and duration of mobile phone use. Hardell et al. [21–23] studied more than 200 brain tumor patients aged 20–80 years in two regions in Sweden. In the first study, Hardell et al. [21] conducted a case-control study (1994–1996) using patients diagnosed with brain tumors who were alive at the time the study commenced. Mobile phone usage and the type of phone (analog or digital) were determined by questionnaire. Dose–response assessment provided no evidence of an association between RFR and brain cancer. However, the small number of cases and the short period of exposure to RFR from mobile phones limit the opportunity to identify an increased risk. The second and third studies [22,23] were similar in design to the previous study and covered a wide range of exposures from other RF sources in addition to mobile phones. An association between the use of analog phones and benign brain tumors for >1 year (OR = 1.3), for >5 years (OR = 1.4), and >10 years (OR = 1.8) was reported. A multivariate analysis revealed no statistical significance and lower risk for the >5 years (OR = 1.1) latencies.

Hardell et al. [24] conducted another case-control study of patients with malignant or benign cranial tumors diagnosed in Sweden from 1997 to 2000. They used a postal questionnaire supplemented by phone interviews. Information on mobile phones was divided into analog (450 or 900 MHz), digital, and cordless phones. The analysis assessed type of phone, duration of use, time since first use, and site, history, and laterality of tumor. A small, but statistically significant, increased risk of any type of brain tumor was seen with the use of analog phones (OR = 1.3, 95% CI = 1.02–1.6), increasing to 1.4 with more than 5 years latency and 1.8 with over 10 years latency. For digital phones, there was no increased risk. For cordless phones, there was no association in general (OR = 1.0, 0.8–1.2). The highest risk was for acoustic neurinoma (OR = 3.5, 95% CI = 1.8–6.8) with the use of analog phones. In a following paper [25] based on modified analysis of the data for malignant tumors already presented in the previous paper [24], the authors concluded that a significantly increased risk was seen with ipsilateral use of analog phones. Data on acoustic neuroma, and benign and malignant brain tumors from the previous studies [24,25] were reported [26,27] with different analysis. The results show increased incidence of acoustic neuroma compared to other brain tumors in the Swedish Cancer Registry between 1980 and 1998.

Recently, Hardell et al. [28] found for all studied phone types an increased risk for brain tumors, mainly acoustic neuroma and malignant brain tumors. Contrary to the previous studies, Hardell et al. [29] did not find evidence that the use of cellular or cordless phones increases the risk of testicular cancer.

A question that is urgent to address is the potential for greater biological effects from RF fields in young age groups. Hardell et al. [30–32] have found some indication for higher risk of brain tumors in persons with first use of cellular or cordless phones before the age of 20 years compared with older ages.

Adaptive power control (APC) gives a difference in power output from mobile phones between urban and rural areas due to regulations of the emissions by the distance to the base stations. Using Statistics Sweden, Hardell et al. [33] divided place of residence into groups based on population density. A clear effect was seen for digital phone users with highest risk in rural areas, OR = 3.2, 95% CI = 1.2–8.4, compared with in urban areas, OR = 0.9, 95% CI = 0.6–1.4, using >5 year latency period. The power output is highest in rural areas, so the results indicate a dose–response effect.

TABLE 6.1
Summary of Epidemiological Studies of Mobile Phones and Cancer Risk

Investigator	Description	Risk Measure	Outcome
Brain Tumors			
Hardell et al. (1999) [21]	PBC: Sweden (1994–1996); (GSM/NMT phones); 209 brain tumor cases; 425 controls	OR = 0.98 (0.69–1.41); same side of the head: OR = 2.42 (0.97–6.05)	Right brain tumors for users who used the phone at their right ear. Stronger for temporal or occipital localization of the tumor on right side (only for analog phones). Temporal or occipital localization of the tumor on the same side as phone use for left side use.
Muscat et al. (2000) [34]	CC: USA (1994–1998); 469 brain cancer; 422 controls	OR = 0.85 (0.6–1.2)	No significant association between primary brain cancer and years of mobile phone use, number of hours of use per month, or the cumulative number of hours of use.
Inskip et al. (2001) [36]	CC: USA (1994–1998); 489 glioma; 197 meningiomad; 96 acoustic neuroma; 799 controls	OR = 1.0 (0.6–1.5); glioma: 0.9 (0.5–1.6); meningioma: 0.2 (0.3–1.7); acoustic neuroma: 1.4 (0.6–3.5).	The results do not support the existence of an association between mobile phone use and certain cancers (glioma, meningioma, or acoustic neuroma). There was no difference for side of head.
Auvinen et al. (2002) [38]	CC: Finland (1996); 398 brain tumors; 198 gliomas; 34 salivary gland; 5 controls per case	Brain tumor: OR = 1.3 (0.9–1.8); salivary gland: OR = 1.3 (0.4–4.7); gliomas: OR = 2.1 (1.3–3.4) (analog); gliomas: OR = 1.0 (0.5–2.0) (digital)	No clear association between use of mobile phones and risk of cancer has been provided. Gliomas were associated with the use of analog but not digital phones.
Muscat et al. (2002) [35]	CC: USA (1997–1999); 90 cases of acoustic neuroma; 86 controls	Up to 60 h of use: OR = 0.7 (0.2–0.6); 3–6 years of use: OR = 1.7 (0.5–5.1)	Although there was an elevated risk with 3 or more years of phone use, these longer-term users were also the most infrequent users, and there was no association with cumulative use.
Hardell et al. (2002a) [24]	CC: Sweden (1997–2000); 1303 brain tumor cases and controls	For >1 year latency, analog: OR = 1.3 (1.02–1.6); digital: OR = 1.0 (0.8–1.2); cordless: OR = 1.0 (0.8–1.2); acoustic neuroma: OR = 3.5 (1.8–6.8)	Significant association for analog and cordless phones and all tumors. No evidence of dose–response by duration of phone use.
Hardell et al. (2003) [24]	CC: Sweden (1997–2000); 1429 cases; 1470 controls; questionnaire	For cordless: OR = 1.5; for analog phone: OR = 3.7	Some of the statistically significant results are surprising. For instance, OR for cordless phones for astrocytomas of 1.5 is unusual, given that cordless phones, which use extremely low power in Sweden, have never been implicated in brain tumors.

Hardell et al. (2002b) [25]	CC: Sweden (1997–2000); malignant tumors; 588 cases; 581 controls	Analog: OR = 1.85 (1.16–2.96); cordless: OR = 1.46 (0.96–2.23)	Statistically significant results for analog and cordless phones. Multivariate analysis not significant. No increased risk with longer duration, except for cordless.
Hardell et al. (2003) [27]	CC: Sweden (1960–1979); vestibular schwannoma (VS).	For >1year latency, analog: OR = 3.45 (1.77–6.76); digital: OR = 1.21 (0.66–2.22); cordless: OR = 1.03 (0.62–1.72)	A significant increased risk for VS was found for analog phone users. Digital and cordless phones also revealed an increased but not significant risk.
Warren et al. (2003) [39]	CC: USA (1995–2000); 18 cases; 192 controls; intratemporal facial nerve (IFN) tumor	OR = 0.6 (0.2–1.9)	Regular cellular telephone use does not appear to be associated with a higher risk of IFN tumor development. The short duration of widespread cellular telephone use precludes definite exclusion as a risk for IFN tumor development
Lonn et al. (2004) [41]	PBC: Sweden (1999–2002); 148 case; 604 controls	Overall OR = 1.0 (0.6–1.5); 10 years OR = 1.9 (0.9–4.1)	No increased risk of acoustic neuroma related to short-term mobile phone use after a short latency period. Data suggest an increased risk of acoustic neuroma associated with mobile phone use of at least 10 years' duration.
Lonn et al. (2005) [40]	CC: Sweeden (2000–2002); 499 glioma cases and 320 meningioma cases; 956 controls	OR = 0.8 (95% CI 0.6, 1.0) for glioma, and 0.7 (0.5, 0.9) for meningioma	Data do not support the hypothesis that mobile phone use is related to an increased risk of glioma or meningioma.
Takebayashi et al. (2006) [42]	CC: Japan (2000–2004); 101 acoustic neuroma; 192 controls	OR = 0.73 (0.43–1.23)	No significant increase of acoustic neuroma risk was observed.
Melanoma of the Eye			
Stang et al. (2001) [44]	CC: Germany; (1994–1997); uveal melanoma; 118 case; 475 control.	OR = 3.0 (1.4–6.3)	Association between RF exposure from mobile phones and uveal melanoma.

Note: OR: odds ratio; CC: case control; CE: case ecological; PBC: population-based control.

Other studies have failed to find a relationship between phone use and the location and incidence of brain tumors [34,35–43]. Two studies examining association between uveal melanoma (a rare form of cancer of the eye) and exposure to RFR have found no relationship between this cancer and mobile phone use [37,44].

Overall, the results indicate that mobile phone use does not increase the risk of brain cancer. Only Hardell's group in Sweden [21–33] has reported an association between analog phone use and brain tumors. Their results have found no support in the investigation of other researchers. It is also doubtful whether results for analog phone users can be extrapolated to digital phone users.

6.2.3 SUMMARY OF EPIDEMIOLOGICAL STUDIES

Most of epidemiological studies have many methodological shortcomings, including deficiencies in size, design, analysis, bias, multiple comparisons, exposure control and assessments, and consistency of results. Based on the above criteria, more weight may be given to the few epidemiological studies with acceptable design and analysis, large number of cases, and minimized potential bias [8,9,34,36,45,46] and longer follow-up time [14]. Most of these studies do not show statistically significant association between RFR and cancer. Further studies are underway to evaluate potential carcinogenic effects of exposure from long-term usage of mobile phones and other RF sources.

Elwood [47] reviewed epidemiological studies of RFR and cancer. He concludes, "The epidemiological results fall short of the strength and consistency of evidence that is required to come to a conclusion that RF emissions are a cause of human cancer. Although the epidemiological evidence in total suggests no increased risk of cancer, the results cannot be unequivocally interpreted in terms of cause and effect. The results are inconsistent, and most studies are limited by lack of detail on actual exposures, short follow-up periods, and the limited ability to deal with other relevant factors. In some studies, there may be substantial biases in the data used."

Schuz et al. [48] investigated cancer risk among Danish cellular phone users who were followed for up to 21 years (1982–2002). The authors found no evidence for an association between tumor risk and cellular phone use among either short-term or long-term users.

In summary, the epidemiologic evidence is not strong enough to the level required to conclude that RFR are a likely cause of one or more types of human cancer. This is attributed to weak design of the studies, lack of detail on actual exposures, limitations of the ability of studies to deal with other likely factors, and in some cases there might be biases in the data used. The current epidemiologic evidence justifies further research to clarify the situation. Moreover, since there are only a few epidemiological studies that examine the health risks associated with exposure to RFR, research at the cellular and animal level is needed to better understand this relationship.

6.3 CELLULAR AND ANIMAL STUDIES

Cellular studies play a supporting task in health risk assessment. Cellular model systems are good candidates for testing the plausibility of mechanistic hypotheses and investigating the ability of RFR to have synergistic effects with agents of known biological activity. They are significant to the optimal design of animal and epidemiological studies. On the other hand, animal studies are used when it is unethical or impossible to perform studies on humans and have the advantage that experimental conditions can be thoroughly controlled.

6.3.1 GENETIC TOXICOLOGY

Genotoxicity does not have a clear cancer endpoint or any other adverse health outcome; however, there is the possibility that genotoxic effects on cells might lead to adverse health effects such as cancer or other diseases. Studies in this regard have been performed at a variety of levels including damage to DNA *in vitro* or *in vivo*, damage to chromosomes, induction of sister chromatid exchange (SCE), and induction of phenotypic mutations. A good number of laboratory experiments have been conducted to assess possible genotoxic effects of broad range of RF frequencies at a variety of levels of biological complexity. Many of the studies found no evidence for any direct genotoxic or mutagenic effects of RFR at different power densities [49–68]. However, investigations at the University of Washington, Seattle [69–71], reported an increase in DNA single- and double-stranded breaks in rat brain cells at whole-body SAR levels of 0.6 and 1.2 W/kg, which are lower than the MPE values. Their observations aroused significant interest because of the possible implications with respect to carcinogenesis. Based on these data, two more studies [72] were performed on human glioblastoma cells and rat brains using the same SAR levels. However, there was no increased DNA damage. Moreover, Hossmann and Hermann [73] suggest that the experiments by Lai and Singh used peak power that was much higher than the mean power, which may have accounted for the observed DNA damage.

Tice et al. [74], as a part of a comprehensive investigation of the potential genotoxicity of RF signals emitted by mobile phones, demonstrated that, under extended exposure conditions, RFR from mobile phones at an average SAR of at least 5 W/kg is capable of inducing chromosomal damage in human lymphocytes.

Similar findings were reported by d'Ambrosio et al. [75] when radiating human cells to 1748 MHz at 5 W/kg, and Mashevich et al. [76] when radiating human lymphocytes to continuous 830 MHz RF energy at SAR in the range 1.6–8.8 W/kg for 72 h. These results demonstrate that RFR has a genotoxic effect.

In a review, Verschaeve and Maes [77] concluded that: "According to a great majority of papers, RF fields, and mobile telephone frequencies in particular, are not genotoxic: they do not induce genetic effects *in vitro* and *in vivo*, at least under nonthermal conditions, and do not seem to be teratogenic (cause birth defects) or to induce cancer."

The Royal Society of Canada Expert Panel Report [78,79] reviewed the subject and concluded that: "A large number of laboratory studies of the potential health effects of RF fields have focused on genotoxicity, including studies of tumorigenesis, promotion, progression, altered cell proliferation, and DNA damage. The great majority of these studies have failed to demonstrate genotoxic effects due to exposure to RF fields."

The UK Independent Expert Group on Mobile Phones (IEGMP) [80] summarized the situation as follows: "The balance of evidence, from both *in vitro* and *in vivo* experiments, indicates that neither acute nor chronic exposure to RF fields increased mutation or chromosomal aberration frequencies when temperatures are maintained within physiological limits. This suggests that RF exposure is unlikely to act as a tumor initiator."

Meltz [81] reviewed the *in vitro* literature pertinent to the issue of the possible induction of toxicity, genotoxicity, and transformation of mammalian cells due to RF exposure. The author concludes, "The weight of evidence available indicates that, for a variety of frequencies and modulations with both short and long exposure times, at exposure levels that do not (or in some instances do) heat the biological sample such that there is a measurable increase in temperature, RF exposure does not induce (a) DNA strand breaks, (b) chromosome aberrations, (c) sister chromatid exchange (SCEs), (d) DNA repair synthesis, (e) phenotypic mutation, or (f) transformation (cancer-like changes)." The author further concludes, "While there is limited experimental evidence that RF exposure induces micronuclei formation, there is abundant evidence that it does not. There is some evidence that RF exposure does not induce DNA excision repair, suggesting the absence of base damage."

Overall, it may be clear at the moment that low levels of exposure to RF fields do not cause genotoxic damage.

6.3.2 Cell Function

6.3.2.1 Cell Proliferation

Disturbance of the normal cell cycle is a possible sign of uncontrolled cell growth, or cancer. Czerska et al. [82] reported an increased proliferation of cells exposed to 2.45-GHz RFR at SAR of 1 W/kg when the radiation was pulsed. CW RFR increased proliferation only when absorbed energy was high enough to induce heating. Other investigators reported increased and decreased cell proliferation rates after applying RFR of various SARs [83–85]. In contrast, d'Ambrosio et al. [75] found no significant changes in cell distribution or cell proliferation in cells exposed to 1748 MHz, either CW or phase only modulated wave gaussian minimum shift keying (GMSK), for 15 min.

6.3.2.2 Intracellular Calcium

Granfield et al. [86] studied whether exposure to simulated GSM mobile phone signals influences the concentration of calcium or calcium signaling patterns in single cells. The authors estimated the intracellular calcium concentration ($[Ca^{2+}]_i$) in the human lymphocyte cell line, Jurkat, exposed to 915-MHz, 2-W/kg RFR. The results indicated that there is no clear indication that RFR from mobile phones is associated with any changes in calcium levels or calcium signaling in lymphocytes, although an alteration in the frequency of calcium oscillations was noted in activated cells exposed to pulsed wave (PW) RFR. However, Guisasola et al. [87] found that 64-MHz RFR, associated with turbo spin echo MRI, resulted in a significant increase in $[Ca^{2+}]_i$ in human embryonic lung cells, L-132. Exposure to MRI related static and gradient fields showed no effect on $[Ca^{2+}]_i$.

6.3.2.3 Ornithine Decarboxylase

ODC is an important enzyme for the role it plays in regulating cell growth through synthesis of polyamines necessary for protein and DNA synthesis. ODC is an enzyme activated during carcinogenesis. Increased ODC activity is an indication for cancer. It is believed that low-level modulated RFR can affect intracellular activities of enzymes. Byus et al. [88] reported evidence of RFR effects on the activity of ODC, as well as on ODC messenger RNA levels and polyamine export in a number of cultured cell lines after exposure to 450 MHz modulated at 16-Hz (1 mW/cm^2) RFR. The effect was noted for certain modulations of the carrier wave illustrating the window effect (an effect that occurs at some combination of exposure conditions, but not at a nearby slightly different set of conditions). Penafiel et al. [89] reported an increase in ODC activity in L929 cells after irradiation to 835-MHz RFR at SAR of approximately 2.5 W/kg. The results depended upon the type of modulation employed. Amplitude-modulated frequencies of 16 and 60 Hz produced a transient increase in ODC activity that reached a peak at 8 h of exposure and returned to control levels after 24 h of exposure. Paulraj and Behari [85] also reported increased ODC levels after exposure for 2 h/day for 35 days to 2.45-GHz RFR at SAR of 0.1 W/kg.

6.3.3   HORMONAL SECRETION

An area attracting attention as a likely potential mechanism for RFR intervention in living organisms is consideration of a cancer-promoting effect of RFR by altered circadian rhythms of pineal activity and melatonin release. Several investigations examined to what extent hormonal secretion is influenced by RFR. Exposure at up to 0.3 W/kg did not disturb the normal circadian profile of melatonin of the hypothalamo–pituitary–adrenal axis [90,91]. However, Stark et al. [92] conducted a pilot study to investigate the influence of RFR at 3–30 MHz on salivary melatonin concentration in dairy cattle. Two commercial dairy herds at two farms were compared, one located at a distance of 500 m (exposed), the other at a distance of 4 km (unexposed) from a RF transmitter. A chronic melatonin reduction effect seemed unlikely. On the first night of reexposure after the transmitter had been off for three days, the difference in salivary melatonin concentration between the two farms was statistically significant, indicating a two- to sevenfold increase of melatonin concentration in the exposed cows.

6.3.4   ANIMAL CANCER EXPERIMENTS

As RF exposure is not considered to be directly carcinogenic, research should be aimed particularly toward its possible promotional and co-promotional effects. Different animal studies have been reported whose designs are suitable for describing brain carcinogenesis or brain tumor promoting effects of RF energy. It is evident from the literature that only a few studies [93–95] suggest an increased incidence of tumors as a result of exposure to high-level SAR. However, Utteridge et al. [96] could not replicate the increase in lymphoma in either normal mice or in the same lymphoma-prone mice reported in Repacholi et al. [94]. Other studies using SARs at modest levels have shown no increase in cancer induction or tumor development rates [97–111].

Heynick et al. [112] reviewed studies on cancer and related effects from exposure to EM fields in the nominal frequency range of 3 kHz to 300 GHz. They concluded that: "The preponderance of published epidemiologic and experimental findings does not support the supposition that *in vivo* or *in vitro* exposures to such fields are carcinogenic."

Overall, there is little evidence to suggest that RFR is carcinogenic. However, the few positive results, including those reported by Repacholi et al. [94], merit further investigation.

6.3.5 NONCANCER ANIMAL STUDIES

6.3.5.1 Morphological and Physiological Effects

While most experimental studies focus on carcinogenesis, tumor promotion, and mutagenic effects, noncancer effects also need to be considered. RFR may induce other effects. These include morphological and physiological changes [113–115]. According to Adey [113] and Adey et al. [114], RF carriers sinusoidally modulated at ELF fields can induce changes to the CNS. However, Tsurita et al. [116] found no significant morphological changes of the brain in group of rats exposed for 2–4 weeks to a 1439-MHz (2 W/kg) TDMA signal. The exposure period was 2 or 4 weeks.

6.3.5.2 Testicular Function and Development

Bol'shakov et al. [117] studied the combined effect of 460-MHz RFR and increased (up to 40°C) temperature on Drosophila embryos of definite age. The results of the study indicated that RFR did not produce any effect on development of the Drosophila. In addition, Dasdag et al. [118] found no evidence suggesting an adverse effect of mobile phone exposure on measures of testicular function or structure in rats confined in plexiglass cages when mobile phones were placed 0.5 cm under the cages. Mobile phones were activated 20 min per day (7 days a week) for 1 month.

6.3.5.3 Cataracts

RFR can induce cataracts if the exposure intensity and the duration are sufficient. Lesions in the cornea, degenerative changes in cells of the iris and retina, and changed visual functions were reported by Kues and Monahan [119] and Kues et al. [120] in nonhuman primates after frequent exposures to RFR (CW 2.45 GHz at SAR of 0.26 W/kg) and at 60 GHz and power density of 10 mW/cm^2 [121]. However, many studies on the ocular effect of RFR on animals have reported no effects, despite the fact that most studies employed exposure levels greatly in excess of those seen with mobile phones [122–125].

6.3.5.4 Behavioral Effects

Changes in learning behavior occurred after RF exposure at SAR of 1.2 W/kg [126] and 2.5 W/kg [127]. Lai et al. [128] observed retarded learning of a task in rats exposed to 2.45 GHz. Bornhausen and Scheingraber [129] found that exposure *in utero* to the GSM (900 MHz, 217 Hz pulse-modulated RFR; 17.5 and 75 mW/kg) field did not induce any measurable cognitive deficits in exposed Wistar rats during pregnancy. Dubreuil et al. [130] noted that head-only exposure of rats to 900 MHz pulsed RFR (SAR of 1 or 3.5 W/kg) for 45 min had no effect on learning. Also, Yamaguchi et al. [131] suggest that the exposure to a pulsed 1439-MHz TDMA field at levels about four times stronger than emitted by mobile phones (SAR of 7.5 W/kg or 25 W/kg for either 1 h daily for 4 days or for 4 weeks) does not affect the learning and memory processes in rats when there are no thermal effects.

6.3.5.5   Blood–Brain Barrier

RFR-induced breakdown of the BBB has been studied either alone or in combination with magnetic fields. Many authors agree that exposure to RFR increases BBB disruption *in vivo* [132–137]. However, other studies have not found RFR-induced disruption of the BBB [138–141]. Most of the studies conclude that high-intensity RFR is required to alter the permeability of the BBB. Salford et al. [142] have shown that extremely low doses of GSM radiation can cause brain damage in rats. The authors report nerve damage following a single 2-h exposure at a SAR of 2 mW/kg. They showed that RFR can impair the BBB, but they add that the chemicals that leak through the BBB probably damage neurons in the cortex, the hippocampus, and the basal ganglia of the brain. The cortex is close to the surface of the skull, while the basal ganglia are much deeper.

For more details, see the review on this subject by D'Andrea et al. [143]. The authors concluded, "Effects of RF exposure on the BBB have been generally accepted for exposures that are thermalizing. Low level exposures that report alterations of the BBB remain controversial. Exposure to high levels of RF energy can damage the structure and function of the nervous system. Much research has focused on the neurochemistry of the brain and the reported effects of RF exposure. Research with isolated brain tissue has provided new results that do not seem to rely on thermal mechanisms."

6.4   CLINICAL STUDIES

Human laboratory studies allow RF effects to be studied on humans with control of experimental parameters.

6.4.1   Perception and Auditory Response

In 1960, based on a series of human and animal studies, Frey [144] concluded that very low-level microwave pulses trigger the auditory nerve, resulting in the subject hearing buzzes or clicks when the head was exposed to short (less than 70 µs) microwave pulses of various repetition rates. This has been called auditory phenomena or RF hearing. These sounds, e.g., buzzes, clicks, tones, vary as a function of the modulation. Many studies have been published over the years, especially those conducted by Dr. Chou and his colleagues investigating RF hearing [145,146]. They originally presented the RF-induced auditory phenomena as an example of RF interaction that has been widely accepted as a weak field effect. Although the hypothesis of direct nervous system stimulation was proposed, the alternative is that RF auditory or hearing effect does not occur from an interaction of RFR with the auditory nerves or neurons. Instead, the RF pulse, upon absorption by soft tissues in the head, launches a thermoelastic wave of acoustic pressure that travels by bone conduction to the inner ear and activates the cochlear receptors via the same mechanism as normal hearing.

Kellenyi et al. [147] found that a 15-min exposure to GSM phone radiation caused an increase in auditory brainstem response in the exposed side of human subjects. However, Hietanen et al. [148] indicated that none of the individuals tested with analogue Nordic mobile Telephony (NMT) phone (900 MHz) or GSM phones (900 and 1800 MHz) could distinguish real RF exposure from sham exposure.

Microwave hearing is a proven low-level microwave effect (at the threshold level, the temperature rise from each microwave pulse is a millionth of a degree Celsius). Although the temperature rise is very small, the mechanism is still thermal in nature. Since hearing microwave pulses is similar to hearing very weak acoustic sound, the response is not considered adverse to human health [149]. For more details on this subject, see the review by Elder and Chou [150]. The authors concluded, "The auditory response has been shown to be dependent upon the energy in a single pulse and not on average power density. The weight of evidence of the results of human, animal, and modeling studies supports the thermoelastic expansion theory as the explanation for the RF hearing phenomenon. RF-induced sounds involve the perception via bone conduction of thermally generated sound transients, that is, audible sounds are produced by rapid thermal expansion resulting from a calculated temperature rise of only 5×10^{-6}°C in tissue at the threshold level due to absorption of the energy in the RF pulse. The hearing of RF-induced sounds at exposure levels many orders of magnitude greater than the hearing threshold is considered to be a biological effect without an accompanying health effect."

6.4.2 THERMOREGULATORY RESPONSES

Thermoregulation, or the maintenance of a fairly steady body temperature even under a variety of external conditions, is important to humans because each body has a preferred temperature at which functioning is optimal. These external conditions can include changes in temperature, vapor pressure, air velocity, exposure to radiation including RFR, and insulation among other factors that affect the temperature of the skin. Adair et al. [151] exposed two different groups of volunteers to 2450 MHz CW (two females, five males) and PW (65 s pulse width, 10^4 pps; three females, three males) RF fields. They measured thermophysiological responses of heat production and heat loss under a standardized protocol (30 min baseline, 45 min RF or sham exposure, 10 min baseline), conducted in three ambient temperatures (24, 28, and 31°C). At each temperature average power density studied was 0, 27, and 35 mW/cm^2 (SAR = 0, 5.94, and 7.7 W/kg). Mean data for each group showed minimal changes in core temperature and metabolic heat production for all test conditions and no reliable differences between CW and PW exposure. Local skin temperatures showed similar trends for CW and PW exposure that were power density-dependent; only the skin temperature of the upper back (facing the antenna) showed a reliably greater increase during PW exposure than during CW exposure. Local sweat rate and skin blood flow were both temperature and power density-dependent and showed greater variability than other measures between CW and PW exposures; this variability was attributable primarily to the characteristics of the two subject groups.

Adair and Black [152] reviewed the literature concerned with physiological thermoregulatory responses of humans and laboratory animals in the presence of RF fields. They stated, "The conclusion is inescapable that humans demonstrate far superior thermoregulatory ability over other tested organisms during RF exposure at, or even above current human exposure guidelines."

6.4.3   Ocular Effects

The cornea and lens are the parts of the eye most exposed to RFR at high levels by their surface location and because heat produced by RFR is more effectively removed from other eye regions by blood circulation. Early investigations of RFR effects on the eye focused on the parameters of power density and duration of exposure required to produce cataracts in the lens of the eye. Hirsch and Parker [153] reported the first RFR-induced human cataract. However, Cleary and Pasternak [154] found more subclinical lens changes in a group of 736 microwave workers than in 559 controls, but no cataracts or decrease in visual acuity were noted. The exact conditions under which these changes may occur in humans are a subject of argument [155,156].

One related modeling study of the human eye by Hirata et al. [157] showed that 5 mW/cm^2, the MPE value for occupational environments [158], caused a temperature change in the lens less than 0.3°C at frequencies from 0.6 to 6 GHz. This small temperature change is overestimated because the eye model was thermally isolated from the head and did not consider the effect of blood flow. Therefore, RFR much in excess of currently allowable exposure limits would be required to produce cataracts in human beings and exposures below the cataractogenic level would be expected to cause other effects in other parts of the eye and face.

Reviews of the literature of RFR-induced cataracts [159–162] have concluded that clinically significant ocular effects, including cataracts, have not been confirmed in human populations exposed for long periods of time to low-level RFR.

6.4.4   Brain Function

The close placement of RFR sources such as mobile phones to the user's head has elevated possibilities of interference with brain activities. While many studies have addressed this issue, they have only investigated the short-term effects of RF exposure. The studies that have considered the effects of RFR on numerous brain functions include slow brain potentials (SP) [163–166], cognitive function in humans including shortening of reaction times after exposure to RF signal [167–172], sleep and sleep encephalograms [173–175], brain function, especially in tasks requiring attention and manipulation of information in working memory [168,169,176,177], electroencephalogram (EEG) activity [165,169,178–182], brain potential and activity [183,184], and attentional capacity [185–189]. The above studies have demonstrated mixed results. The findings suggest that some aspects of cognitive functions and measures of brain physiology may be affected without offering a uniform view. These include changes in memory tasks, response patterns, normal sleeping EEG patterns, and other brain functional changes. Several studies have demonstrated improved cognitive functions in volunteers exposed to RFR in the frequency range of mobile phones.

Subjective symptoms such as dizziness, disorientation, nausea, headache, and other unpleasant feelings such as a burning sensation or a faint pain might be a direct result of RFR, although such symptoms are very general and may have many other causes. Wilén et al. [190] made use of the information about prevalence of symptoms, calling time per day, and number of calls per day from a previous epidemiological study [191] and combined it with measurements of the SAR of the specific mobile phone used by each person included in the above study. Two new exposure parameters have been devised: specific absorption per day (SAD) and specific absorption per call (SAC). The results indicated that SAR values >0.5 W/kg may be an important factor for the prevalence of some of the subjective symptoms, especially in combination with long calling times per day.

Hamblin and Wood [192] compared the findings of the main studies that have examined the effects of GSM mobile phone RF emissions on human brain activity and sleep variables. They concluded, "Although, in general, outcomes have been inconsistent and comparison between individual studies is difficult, enhanced electroencephalogram alpha-band power has been noted in several of the studies, a phenomenon also observed in some animal studies."

In another review of the literature, Hossmann and Hermann [73] concluded, "At present, there is little evidence that pulsed or continuous microwave exposure at power and frequencies related to mobile communication could interfere with the functional and structural integrity of the brain. Under experimental conditions, most of the positive results so far could be attributed to thermal effects. Such effects are unlikely to occur during regular use of mobile telephones because the total emitted power is far too low to raise whole body temperature, and because local elevations of brain temperature, if present, would be prevented by the thermostabilizing effect of the circulating blood."

D'Andrea et al. [193] reviewed the literature concerning RF exposure and behavioral and cognitive effects. They concluded, "Reports of change of cognitive function (memory and learning) in humans and laboratory animals are in the scientific literature. Mostly, these are thermally mediated effects, but other low level effects are not so easily explained by thermal mechanisms. The phenomenon of behavioral disruption by microwave exposure, an operationally defined rate decrease (or rate increase), has served as the basis for human exposure guidelines since the early 1980s and still appears to be a very sensitive RF bioeffect. Nearly all evidence relates this phenomenon to the generation of heat in the tissues and reinforces the conclusion that behavioral changes observed in RF exposed animals are thermally mediated. Such behavioral alteration has been demonstrated in a variety of animal species and under several different conditions of RF exposure. Thermally based effects can clearly be hazardous to the organism and continue to be the best predictor of hazard for *Homo sapiens*. Nevertheless, similar research with man has not been conducted. Although some studies on human perception of RF exist, these should be expanded to include a variety of RF parameters."

Despite the absence of serious outcomes, a priority may be given for further research to study the effect of RFR on brain functions. As yet, human studies of cognitive performance and EEG focused on the consequences of short-term exposure. Following a group of new mobile phone users over time could be a right approach to address the issue of long-term exposure. Special attention should be directed toward children because their developing nervous systems are more sensitive to RFR.

6.4.5 CARDIOVASCULAR DISEASES

Both acute and long-term effects have been investigated. One author reported that most studies showed no acute effect on blood pressure, heart rate, or ECG waveform; others reported subtle effects on the heart rate.

Braune et al. [194] reported that exposure of human volunteers to RFR of mobile phones (GSM 900-MHz, 2-W, 217-Hz frame repetition rate) increased the sympathetic efferent activity, with increases in the resting blood pressure between 5 and 10 mm Hg. However, Braune et al. [195] repeated their study and summarized that RFR had no effect on the outcomes. They claimed that their 1998 finding of increased blood pressure in mobile phone users was due to an artifact in the design of the original study.

Mann et al. [196] did not find any effect on the autonomic control of heart rate by applying weak-pulsed RFR emitted by digital mobile phones during sleep in healthy humans. However, Parazzini et al. [197] observed weak interaction between some heart rate variability parameters and RF exposure from a 900 MHz mobile phones at the maximum allowed power. This effect seems to be gathered around the sympathetic response to stand.

Black and Heynick [198] reviewed the subject and concluded, "Cardiovascular tissue is not directly affected adversely in the absence of significant radiofrequency electromagnetic fields (RFEMF) heating or electric currents. The regulation of blood pressure is not influenced by ultra high frequency (UHF) RFEMF at levels commonly encountered in the use of mobile communication devices."

6.4.6 MELATONIN

RFR effect on melatonin has been studied in a few human studies. Wang [199] found that workers who were highly exposed to RFR had a dose–response increase in serotonin, and hence indicates a reduction in melatonin. According to Burch et al. [200], frequent mobile phone use may be associated with reduced daytime melatonin production. Also, Burch et al. [201] reported that mobile phone use of <25 min per day was associated with a drop in melatonin. In contrast, de Seze et al. [90,91], Radon et al. [202], and Bortkiewicz et al. [203] found no evidence of RFR-related effects on melatonin secretion.

The interpretation of the available data from all types of studies suffers from differences in exposure parameters. Also, there is little evidence that RFR from mobile phones promotes carcinogenesis by depressing melatonin.

6.5 CONCLUDING REMARKS AND FUTURE RESEARCH

A significant uncertainty exists in the interpretation of most of the studies. The current evidence from epidemiological, laboratory, and clinical research indicates that environmental RFR does not cause cancer or other diseases. But there is now some evidence that effects on biological functions, including those of the brain, may be induced by RFR at levels comparable to those associated with the use of mobile phones. There is, as yet, no evidence that these biological effects lead to health hazards but currently only limited data are available [1].

Two large reviews [77,204] concluded that RFR below the existing MPE values is not directly genotoxic. In the review of cancer studies, the IEGMP [80] of the UK concluded, "Some individual experimental studies have suggested that RFR can initiate tumor formation, enhance the effects of known carcinogens or promote the growth of transplanted tumors. However, in some of these studies, the intensity was high enough to produce thermal effects. The balance of evidence, both *in vitro* and *in vivo* experiments, indicates that neither acute nor chronic exposure to RFR increases mutation or chromosomal aberration frequencies when temperatures are maintained within physiological limits."

The Swedish Radiation Protection Authority supports the commonly accepted view that RF energy, at least under levels of power emitted by mobile phones, is not genotoxic and cannot directly damage DNA, and is thus unlikely to be an initiator. Hence the risk of cancer from a thermal or nonthermal mechanism would be one that, if anything, promotes tumor growth. Nevertheless, there is no convincing evidence from animal experiments or epidemiologic research that RF signals can promote tumor growth or induce genetic effects [205]. However, there might be effects under extended exposure conditions or at high-level SARs.

It is important to note that modulated or pulsed RFR seems to be more effective in producing an effect. It can also elicit a different effect, especially on brain function, when compared with CW RFR of the same characteristics. Many studies supporting this fact have been summarized throughout this Chapter. Juutilainen and de Seze [206] reviewed this matter extensively.

Experimental investigations of weak ELF field (including RFR-ELF field associated with mobile phones) effects on human physiology have yielded some evidence of an effect in a number of different areas, such as heart rate variability, sleep disturbance, and melatonin suppression [207]. In general, there have been inconsistencies in results between experiments due to various experimental protocols and exposure characteristics. Adair [208] reviewed this subject and by using biophysical criteria, demonstrated that it is unlikely that low-intensity fields can generate significant physiological consequences.

6.5.1 RISK FOR CHILDREN

An important area of research that needs further investigation is health risk associated with children's use of mobile phones. Following recommendations from the IEGMP [80], the UK government published a brochure recommending that children up to the age of about 16 years should minimize the use of mobile phones. The IEGMP notes that the head and nervous system continue to develop until about 16 years of age. The density of synapses reaches adult level around puberty and skull thickness and brain size reach adult levels around ages 14–15 years. Because of higher tissue conductivity (higher water content and ion concentrations), children may absorb more energy from a given mobile phone than do adults.

Health Council of the Netherlands [209] advocates against the IEGRP recommendation. The Council feels there is no reason to recommend the children should restrict the use of mobile phones as much as possible. In this regard, we feel that children's use of mobile phones is a critical area of research that needs further dosimetrical and laboratory investigations.

A WHO conference concluded that: "There was a consensus that, from present knowledge, the ICNIRP (1998) guidelines appear to incorporate sufficient safety factors in their general public limits to be protective of children. However, given the uncertainty about effects in children, the use of measures that reduce their exposure, in addition to the adoption of international standards, seems appropriate" [210].

6.5.2 RESEARCH

At this point, it appears that RFR may pose a human health risk only at moderately high levels of exposure. Most environmental exposures to RFR, such as those from mobile phones, are relatively low, although measurable. The detection of biological responses at such low-exposure levels will require either large-scale population based studies with the sensitivity to identify small risks, should they exist, or sophisticated assays employing sensitive biomarkers of exposure and biological effects.

Although there is already a large body of literature on health risks of RFR, below we list some areas likely to prove fruitful in enhancing our knowledge of the above subject. Additional research into both the risk of RFR exposure and long-term epidemiology studies to further our understanding of the health effects of RFR is encouraged. Among other research, the following areas of inquiry would be useful: (1) changing patterns of wireless communication usage and exposure of different parts of the human body, (2) biophysical interaction mechanisms to explain observed *in vitro* and *in vivo* effects at field levels to which the public is exposed, (3) improved dosimetric models of RF energy deposition in children of different ages and pregnant women with appropriate models of the human thermoregulatory responses (e.g., inner ear, head, eye, trunk, embryo, and foetus), (4) *in vitro* and *in vivo* research to obtain reproducible results on previously reported genetic and carcinogenic effects, (5) experimental studies to clarify possible effects related to circulating melatonin, sleep disruption, heart rate, learning, and memory, (6) clinical studies focusing on cognitive, behavioral, and physiological effects on the CNS (especially in children, whose nervous systems remain under development), (7) epidemiological studies to investigate the highest exposure levels encountered and to individual exposure versus time, incorporating reliable dosimetry in the design. Collectively, this information will strengthen the scientific basis on which a more complete assessment of RFR health risks can be made [1].

Because risk assessment has advanced greatly since many of the standards for both occupational and population exposures were developed, reexamination of those standards by the related organizations would be helpful. Additionally, efforts are needed to better understand public perception of RFR risks, which may assist setting up risk communication strategies that lead to the management of health risks (see Chapter 7).

In conclusion, the use of RF equipment and services is likely to expand greatly over the coming years. It is therefore important to continue research to further our knowledge of any potential health risks that might result from different levels and pathways of exposure.

REFERENCES

1. Habash RWH, Brodsky LM, Leiss W, Krewski DK, Repacholi M. Health risk of electromagnetic fields. Part II: Evaluation and assessment of radio frequency radiation. *Crit Rev Biomed Eng* 2003; 31: 197–254.
2. Garland FC, Shaw E, Gorham ED, Garland CF, White MR, Sinsheimer PJ. Incidence of leukemia in occupations with potential electromagnetic field exposure in United States Navy personnel. *Am J Epidemiol* 1990; 132: 293–303.
3. Szmigielski S. Cancer morbidity in subjects occupationally exposed to high frequency (radiofrequency and microwave) electromagnetic radiation. *Sci Total Environ* 1996; 180: 9–17.
4. Reeves GI. Review of extensive workups of 34 patients overexposed to radiofrequency radiation. *Aviat Space Environ Med* 2000; 71: 206–215.
5. Richter E, Berman T, Ben-Michael E, Laster R, Westin JB. Cancer in radar technicians exposed to RF/microwave radiation: sentinel episodes. *Int J Occup Environ Health* 2000; 6: 187–193.
6. Davis RL, Mostofi FK. Cluster of testicular cancer in police officers exposed to hand-held radar. *Am J Ind Med* 1993; 24: 231–233.
7. Finkelstein MM. Cancer incidence among Ontario police officers. *Am J Ind Med* 1998; 34: 157–162.
8. Milham S Jr. Increased mortality in amateur radio operators due to lymphatic and hematopoietic malignancies. *Am J Epidemiol* 1988; 127: 50–54.
9. Milham S Jr. Mortality by license class in amateur radio operators. *Am J Epidemiol* 1988b; 128: 1175–1176.
10. Tynes T, Hannevik M, Andersen A, Vistnes AI, Haldorsen T. Incidence of breast cancer in Norwegian female radio and telegraph operators. *Cancer Causes Control* 1996; 7: 197–204.
11. Grajewski B, Schnorr TM, Reefhuis J, Roeleveld N, Salvan A, Mueller CA, Conover DL, Murray WE. Work with video display terminals and the risk of reduced birthweight and pattern birth. *Am J Ind Med* 1997; 32: 681–688.
12. Lagorio S, Rossi S, Vecchia P, De Santis M, Bastianini L, Fusilli M, Ferrucci A, Desideri E, Comba P. Mortality of plastic-ware workers exposed to radiofrequencies. *Bioelectromagnetics* 1997; 18: 418–421.
13. Irgens A, Kruger K, Ulstein M. The effect of male occupational exposure in infertile couples in Norway. *J Occup Environ Med* 1999; 41: 1116–1120.
14. Robinette CD, Silverman C, Jablon S. Effects upon health of occupational exposure to microwave radiation. *Am J Epidemiol* 1980; 112: 39–53.
15. Groves F, Page W, Gridley G, Lisimaque L, Stewart P, Tarone R, Gail M, Boice J, Beebe G. Cancer in Korean War Navy technicians—mortality survey after forty years. *Ann Epidemiol* 2002; 12: 488–534.
16. Burch JB, Clark M, Yost MG, Fitzpatrick CTE, Bachand AM, Ramaprasad J, Rei JS. Radio frequency nonionizing radiation in a community exposed to radio and television broadcasting. *Environ Health Perespec* 2006; 114: 248–253.
17. Hocking B, Gordon I, Grain H, Hatfield G. Cancer incidence and mortality and proximity to TV towers. *Med J Aust* 1996; 65: 601–605.
18. McKenzie DR, Yin Y, Morrell S. Childhood incidence of acute lymphoblastic leukemia and exposure to broadcast radiation in Sydney—a second look. *Aust NZ J Pub Health* 1998; 22: 360–367.
19. Michelozzi P, Ancona C, Fusco D, Forastiere F, Perucci CA. Risk of leukemia and residence near a radio transmitter in Italy. *Epidemiology* 1998; 9: S354.

20. Michelozzi P, Ancona C, Kirchmayer U, Forastiere F, Biggeri A, Barca A, Perucci CA. Adult and childhood leukemia near a high-power radio station in Rome, Italy. *Am J Epidemiol* 2002; 155: 1096–1103.

21. Hardell L, Nasman A, Pahlson A, Hallquist A, Mild KH. Use of cellular telephones and the risk for brain tumors: a case-control study. *Int J Oncol* 1999; 15: 113–116.

22. Hardell L, Nasman A, Pahlson A, Hallquist A. Case-control study on radiology work, medical X-ray investigations, and use of cellular telephones as risk factors for brain tumors. *Med Gen Med* 2000; 2: E2.

23. Hardell L, Mild KH, Pahlson A, Hallquist A. Ionizing radiation, cellular telephones and the risk for brain tumors. *Eur J Cancer Prev* 2001; 10: 523–529.

24. Hardell L, Hallquist A, Mild KH, Carlberg M, Pahlson A, Lilja A. Cellular and cordless telephones and the risk for brain tumors. *Eur J Cancer Prev* 2002; 11: 377–386.

25. Hardell L, Mild KH, Carlberg M. Case-control study on the use of cellular and cordless phones and the risk for malignant brain tumours. *Int J Rad Ecol* 2002; 78: 931–936.

26. Hardell L, Mild KH, Carlberg M. Further aspects on cellular and cordless phones and brain tumours. *Int J Oncol* 2003; 22: 399–407.

27. Hardell L, Mild KH, Carlberg M, Carlberg M, Hallquist A, Pahlson A. Vestibular schwannoma, tinnitus and cellular telephones. *Neuroepidemiology* 2003; 22: 124–129.

28. Hardell L, Mild KH, Carlberg M, Soderqvist F. Tumour risk associated with use of cellular telephones or cordless desktop telephones. *World J Surg Oncol* 2006a 4: 74.

29. Hardell L, Carlberg M, Ohlson C-G, Westberg H, Eriksson M, Hansson Mild K. Use of cellular and cordless telephones and risk of testicular cancer. *Int J Androl* 2006; 30: 115–122. (online early article).

30. Hardell L, Hansson Mild K, Carlberg M, Hallquist A. Cellular and cordless telephones and the association with brain tumours in different age group. *Arch Environ Health* 2004; 59: 132–137.

31. Hardell L, Carlberg M, Hansson Mild K. Pooled analysis of two case-control studies on the use of cellular and cordless telephones and the risk of benign tumours diagnosed during 1997–2003. *Int J Oncol* 2006; 28: 509–518.

32. Hardell L, Hansson Mild K, Carlberg M. Pooled analysis of two case-control studies on use of cellular and cordless telephones and the risk for malignant brain tumours diagnosed in 1997–2003. *Int Arch Occup Environ Health* 2006; 79: 630–639.

33. Hardell L, Carlberg M, Hansson Mild K. Use of cellular telephones and brain tumour risk in urban and rural areas. *Occup Environ Med* 2005; 62: 390–394.

34. Muscat JE, Malkin MG, Thompson S, Shore RE, Stellman SD, McRee D, Neugut AI, Wynder EL. Handheld cellular telephone use and risk of brain cancer. *J Am Med Ass* 2000; 284: 3001–3007.

35. Muscat JE, Malikin MG, Shore RE, Thompson S, Neugut AI, Stellman SD, Bruce J. Handheld cellular telephones and risk of acoustic neuroma. *Neurology* 2002; 58: 1304–1306.

36. Inskip PD, Tarone RE, Hatch EE, Wilcosky TC, Shapiro WR, Selker RG. Cellular telephone use and brain tumors. *N Eng J Med* 2001; 344: 79–86.

37. Johansen C, Boice JD Jr, McLaughlin JK, Christensen HC, Olsen JH. Mobile phones and malignant melanoma of the eye. *Br J Cancer* 2002; 86: 348–349.

38. Auvinen A, Hietanen M, Luukkonen R, Koskela RS. Brain tumors and salivary gland cancers among cellular telephone users. *Epidemiology* 2002; 13: 356–359.

39. Warren HG, Prevatt AA, Daly KA, Antonelli PJ. Cellular telephone use and risk of intratemporal facial nerve tumour. *Laryngoscope* 2003; 113: 663–667.

40. Lonn S, Ahlbom A, Hall P, Feychting M. Long-term phone use and brain tumor risk. *Am J Epidemiol* 2005; 161: 526–535.

41. Lonn S, Ahlbom A, Hall P, Feychting M. Mobile phone use and the risk of acoustic neuroma. *Epidemiology* 2004; 15: 653–659.
42. Takebayashi T, Akiba S, Kikuchi Y, Taki M, Wake K, Watanabe S, Yamaguchi N. Mobile phone use and acoustic neuroma risk in Japan. *Occup Environ Med* 2006; 63: 802–807.
43. Roosli M, Michel G, Kuehni CE, Spoerri A. Cellular telephone use and time trends in brain tumour mortality in Switzerland from 1969 to 2002. *Eur J Cancer Prev* 2007; 16: 77–82.
44. Stang A, Anastassiou G, Ahrens W, Bromen K, Bornfeld N, Jöckel KH. The possible role of radiofrequency radiation in the development of uveal melanoma. *Epidemiology* 2001; 12: 7–12.
45. Kheifets L, Repacholi M, Saunders R, van Deventer E. Sensitivity of children to EMF. *Pediatrics* 2005; 115: e303–e313.
46. Neubauer G, Feychting M, Hamnerius Y, Kheifets L, Kuster N, Ruiz I, Schuz J, Uberbacher R, Wiart J, Roosli M. Feasibility of future epidemiological studies on possible health effects of mobile phone base stations. *Bioelectromagnetics* 2007; 28: 224–230.
47. Elwood JM. Epidemiological studies of radio frequency exposures and human cancer. *Bioelectromagnetics* 2003; 24: S63–S73.
48. Schuz J, Jacobsen R, Olsen JH, Boice Jr JD, McLaughlin JK, Johansen C. Cellular telephone use and cancer risk: update of nationwide Danish cohort. *J Nat Cancer Inst* 2006; 98: 1707–1713.
49. Dhahi SJ, Habash RWH, Alhafid HT. Lack of mutagenic effects on conidia of aspergillus amstelodami irradiated by 8.7175 GHz microwaves. *J Microwave Power* 1982; 17: 346–351.
50. Meltz ML, Walker KA, Erwin DN. Radiofrequency (microwave) radiation exposure of mammalian cells during UV-induced DNA repair synthesis. *Radiat Res* 1987; 110: 255–266.
51. Meltz ML, Eagan P, Erwin DN. Absence of a mutagenic interaction between microwaves and mitomycin C in mammalian cells. *Environ Mol Mutagen* 1989; 13: 294–303.
52. Meltz ML, Eagan P, Erwin DN. Proflavin and microwave radiation: absence of a mutagenic interaction. *Bioelectromagnetics* 1990; 11: 149–157.
53. Kerbacher JJ, Meltz ML, Erwin DN. Influence of radiofrequency radiation on chromosome aberrations in CHO cells and its interaction with DNA-damaging agents. *Radiat Res* 1990; 123: 311–319.
54. Malyapa RS, Ahern EW, Straube WL, Moros EG, Pickard WF, Roti JL. Measurement of DNA damage after exposure to 2450 MHz electromagnetic radiation. *Radiat Res* 1997; 148: 608–617.
55. Malyapa R S, Ahern EW, Straube WL, Moros EG, Pickard WF, Roti JL. Measurement of DNA damage after exposure to electromagnetic radiation in the cellular communication frequency band (835.62 and 847.74 MHz). *Radiat Res* 1997; 148: 618–627.
56. Vijayalaxmi, Natarajan M, Meltz ML, Wittler MA. Proliferation and cytogenetic studies in human blood lymphocytes exposed in vitro to 2450 MHz radiofrequency radiation. *Int J Radiat Biol* 1997; 72: 751–757.
57. Vijayalaxmi, Leal BZ, Szilagyi M, Prihoda TJ, Meltz ML. Primary DNA damage in human blood lymphocytes exposed in vitro to 2450 MHz radiofrequency radiation. *Radiat Res* 2000; 153: 479–486.
58. Vijayalaxmi, Bisht KS, Pickard WF, Meltz ML, Roti Roti JL, Moros EG. Chromosome damage and micronucleus formation in human blood lymphocytes exposed in vitro to radiofrequency radiation at a cellular telephone frequency (847.74 MHz, CDMA). *Radiat Res* 2001; 156: 430–432.

59. Vijayalaxmi, Leal BZ, Meltz ML, Pickard WF, Bisht KS, Roti Roti JL, Straube WL, Moros EG. Cytotoxic studies in human blood lymphocytes exposed in vitro to radiofrequency radiation at a cellular telephone frequency (835.62 MHz, FDMA). *Radiat Res* 2001; 155: 113–121.

60. Gos P, Eicher B, Kohli J, Heyer W-D. No Mutagenic or recombinogenic effects of mobile phone fields at 900 MHz in the yeast saccharomyces cerevisiae. *Bioelectromagnetics* 2000; 21: 515–523.

61. Li L, Bisht KS, LaGroye I, Zhang P, Straube WL, Moros EG, Roti Roti JL. Measurement of DNA damage in mammalian cells exposed in vitro to radiofrequency fields at SARs of 3–5 W/kg. *Radiat Res* 2001; 156: 328–332.

62. Takahashi S, Inaguma S, Chao Y-M, Imaida K, Wang J, Fujiwara O, Sherai T. Lack of mutation induction with exposure to 1.5 GHz electromagnetic near fields used for cellular phones in brains of big blue mice. *Cancer Res* 2002; 2: 1956–1960.

63. Bisht KS, Moros EG, Straube WL, Baty JD, Roto Roti JL. The effect of 835.62 MHz FDMA or 847.74 MHz CDMA modulated radiofrequency radiation on the induction of micronuclei in C3H 10T1/2 cells. *Radiat Res* 2002; 157: 506–515.

64. McNamee JP, Bellier PV, Gajda GB, Miller SM, Lemay EP, Lavallee BF, Marro L, Thansandote A. DNA damage and micronucleus induction in human leukocytes after acute in vitro exposure to a 1.9 GHz continuous-wave radiofrequency field. *Radiat Res* 2002a; 158: 523–533.

65. McNamee JP, Bellier PV, Gajda GB, Lavallee BF, Lemay EP, Marro L, Thansandote A. DNA damage in human leukocytes after acute in vitro exposure to a 1.9 GHz pulse–modulated radiofrequency field. *Radiat Res* 2002b; 158: 534–537.

66. Zeni O, Chiavoni AS, Sannino A, Antolini A, Forigo D, Bersani F, Scarfì MR. Lack of genotoxic effects (micronucleus induction) in human lymphocytes exposed in vitro to 900 MHz electromagnetic fields. *Radiat Res* 2003; 160: 152–158.

67. Sakuma N, Komatsubara Y, Takeda H, Hirose H, Sekijima M, Nojima T, Miyakoshi J. DNA strand breaks are not induced in human cells exposed to 2.1425 GHz band CW and W-CDMA modulated radiofrequency fields allocated to mobile radio base stations. *Bioelectromagnetics* 2006; 27: 51–57.

68. Chemeris NK, Gapeyev AB, Sirota NP, Gudkova O Yu, Tankanag AV, Konovalov IV, Buzoverya ME, Suvorov VG, Logunov VA. Lack of direct DNA damage in human blood leukocytes and lymphocytes after in vitro exposure to high power microwave pulses. *Bioelectromagnetics* 2006; 27: 197–203.

69. Lai H, Singh, NP. Acute low-intensity microwave exposure increases DNA single-strand breaks in rat brain cells. *Bioelectromagnetics* 1995; 16: 207–210.

70. Lai H, Singh NP. Single and double strand DNA breaks in rat brain cells after acute exposure to radiofrequency electromagnetic radiation. *Int J Radiat Biol* 1996; 69: 513–521.

71. Lai H, Carino MA, Singh NP. Naltrexone blocks RFR-induced DNA double strand breaks in rat brain cells. *Wireless Net* 1997; 3: 471–476.

72. Malyapa RS, Ahern EW, Bi C, Straube WL, La Regina M, Pickard WF, Roti JL. DNA damage in rat brain cells after in vivo exposure to 2450 MHz electromagnetic radiation and various methods of euthanasia. *Radiat Res* 1998; 149: 637–645.

73. Hossmann K-A, Hermann DM. Effects of electromagnetic radiation of mobile phones on the central nervous system. *Bioelectromagnetics* 2003; 24: 49–62.

74. Tice RR, Hook GG, Donner M, McRee D, Guy AW. Genotoxicity of radiofrequency signals. I. Investigation of DNA damage and micronuclei induction in cultured human blood cells. *Bioelectromagnetics* 2002; 23: 113–126.

75. D'Ambrosio G, Massa R, Scarfi MR, Zeni O. Cytogenic damage in human lymphocytes following GMSK modulated microwave exposure. *Bioelectromagnetics* 2002; 23: 7–13.

76. Mashevich M, Folkman D, Kesar A, Barbul A, Korenstein R, Jerby E, Avivi E. Exposure of human peripheral blood lymphocytes to electromagnetic fields associated with cellular phones leads to chromosomal instability. *Bioelectromagnetics* 2003; 24: 82–90.

77. Verschaeve L, Maes A. Genetic, carcinogenic and teratogenic effects of radiofrequency fields. *Mutat Res* 1998; 410: 141–165.

78. Royal Society of Canada. A review of the potential health risks of radiofrequency fields from wireless telecommunication devices. Expert Panel Report, Ottawa, Canada, 1999.

79. Krewski D, Byus CV, Glickman BW, Lotz WG, Mandeville R, McBride ML, Prato FS, Weaver DF. Potential health risks of radiofrequency fields from wireless telecommunication devices. *J Toxicol Environ Health* 2001; 4: 1–143.

80. IEGMP. Mobile phones and health. *Independent Expert Group on Mobile Phones.* Chilton, Didcot, Oxon, UK: National Radiological Protection Board, 2000.

81. Meltz ML. Radiofrequency exposure and mammalian cell toxicity, genotoxicity, and transformation. *Bioelectromagnetics* 2003; 24: S196–S213.

82. Czerska EM, Elson EC, Davis CC, Swicord ML, Czerski P. Effects of continuous and pulsed 2450-MHZ radiation on spontaneous lymphoblastoid tranformation of human lymphocytes in vitro. *Bioelectromagnetics* 1992; 13: 247–259.

83. Kwee S, Raskmark P. Changes in cell proliferation due to environmental non-ionizing radiation: microwave radiation. *Bioelectrochem Bioenerg* 1998; 44: 251–255.

84. Velizarov S, Raskmark P, Kwee, S. The effects of radiofrequency fields on cell proliferation are non-thermal. *Bioelectrochem Bioenerg* 1999; 48: 177–180.

85. Paulraj R, Behari J. The effect of low-level continuous 2.45 GHz waves on enzymes of the developing rat brain. *Electromag Biol Med* 2002; 21: 221–231.

86. Granfield CG, Wood AW, Anderson V, Menezes KG. Effects of mobile phones type signals on calcium levels within human leukemic T-cells (Jurkat cells). *Int J Radiat Biol* 2001; 77: 1207–1217.

87. Guisasola C, Desco M, Millán O, Villanueva FJ, García-Barreno P. Biological dosimetry of magnetic resonance imaging. *J Magn Reson Imag* 2002; 15: 584–590.

88. Byus CV, Kartum K, Pieper S, Adey WR. Increased ornithine decarboxylase activity in cultured cells exposed to low energy modulated microwave fields and phorbol ester tumor promoters. *Cancer Res* 1988; 48: 4222–4226.

89. Penafiel M, Litovitz T, Krause D, Desta A, Mullins JM. Role of modulation on the effect of microwaves on ornithine decarboxylase activity in L929 cells. *Bioelectromagnetics* 1997; 18: 132–141.

90. De Seze R, Fabbro-Peray P, Miro L. GSM radiocellular telephones do not disturb the secretion of antepituitary hormones in humans. *Bioelectromagnetics* 1998; 19: 271–278.

91. De Seze R, Ayoub J, Peray P, Miro L, Touitou Y. Evaluation in humans of the effects of radiocellular telephones on the cercadian patterns of melatonin secretion, a chronobiological rhythm marker. *J Pineal Res* 1999; 27: 237–242.

92. Stark KD, Krebs T, Altpeter E, Manz B, Griot C, Abelin T. Absence of chronic effect of exposure to short-wave radio broadcast signal on salivary melatonin concentrations in dairy cattle. *J Pineal Res* 1997; 22: 171–176.

93. Szmigielski S, Szudzinski A, Pietraszek A, Bielec M, Janiak M, Wrembel JK. Accelerated development of spontaneous and benzopyeous and benzopyrene-induced skin cancer in mice exposed to 2450-MHz microwave radiation. *Bioelectromagnetics* 1982; 3: 179–191.

94. Repacholi MH, Basten A, Gebski V, Noonan D, Finnie J, Harris AW. Lymphomas in Eμ-Pim1 transgenic mice exposed to pulsed 900 MHz electromagnetic fields. *Radiat Res* 1997; 147: 631–640.

95. Trosic I, Busljeta I, Kasuba V, Rozgaj R. Micronucleus induction after whole-body microwave irradiation of rats. *Mut Res* 2002; 521: 73–79.

96. Utteridge TD, Gebski V, Finnie JW, Vernon-Roberts B, Kuchel TR. Long-term exposure of Eμ-Pim1 transgenic mice to 898.4 MHz microwaves does not increase lymphoma incidence. *Radiat Res* 2002; 158: 357–364.

97. Chou C-K, Guy AW, Kunz LL, Johnson RB, Crowley JJ, Krupp JH. Long-term, low-level microwave irradiation of rats. *Bioelectromagnetics* 1992; 13: 469–496.

98. Wu RW, Chiang H, Shao BJ, Li NG, Fu WD. Effects of 2.45 GHz microwave radiation and phorbol ester 12-O-tetradecanoylphorbol-13-acetate on dimethylhydrazine-induced colon cancer in mice. *Bioelectromagnetics* 1994; 15: 531–538.

99. Toler JC, Shelton WW, Frei MR, Merritt JH, Stedham MA. Long-term low-level exposure of mice prone to mammary tumors to 435 MHz radiofrequency radiation. *Radiat Res* 1997; 148: 227–234.

100. Imaida K, Taki M, Watanabe S, Kamimura Y, Ito T, Yamaguchi T, Ito N, Shirai T. The 1.5 GHz electromagnetic near-field used for cellular phones does not promote rat liver carcinogenesis in a medium-term liver bioassay. *Jap J Cancer Res* 1998; 89: 995–1002.

101. Frei MR, Berger RE, Dusch SJ, Guel V, Jauchem JR, Merritt JH, Stedham M. Chronic exposure of cancer-prone mice to low-level 2450 MHz radiofrequency radiation. *Bioelectromagnetics* 1998; 19: 20–31.

102. Adey WR, Byus CV, Cain CD, Higgins RJ, Jones RA, Kean CJ, Kuster N, MacMurray A, Stagg RB, Zimmerman G, Haggren W. 1999. Spontaneous and nitrosourea-induced primary tumors of the central nervous system in Fischer 344 rats chronically exposed to 836 MHz modulated microwaves. *Radiat Res* 1999; 152: 292–302.

103. Adey WR, Byus CV, Cain CD, Higgins RJ, Jones RA, Kean CJ, Kuster N, MacMurray A, Stagg RB, Zimmerman G. Spontaneous and nitrosourea-induced primary tumors of the central nervous system in Fischer 344 rats exposed to frequency-modulated microwave fields. *Cancer Res* 2000; 60: 1857–1863.

104. Zook BC, Simmens SJ. The effects of 860 MHz radiofrequency radiation on the induction or promotion of brain tumours and other neoplasms in rats. *Radiat Res* 2001; 55: 572–583.

105. Mason PA, Walters TJ, DiGiovanni J, Beason CW, Jauschem JR, Dick EJ, Mahajan K, Dusch SJ, Shields BA, Merritt JH, Murphy MR, Ryan KL. Lack of effect of 94 GHz radio-frequency radiation exposure in an animal model of skin carcinogenesis. *Carcinogenesis* 2001; 22: 1701–1708.

106. Jauchem JR, Ryan KL, Frei MR, Dusch SJ, Lehnert HM, Kovatch RM. Repeated exposure of C3H/HeJ mice to ultra-wideband electromagnetic pulses: lack of effects on mammary tumors. *Radiat Res* 2001; 155: 369–377.

107. Heikkinen P, Kosma V-M, Hongisto T, Huuskonen H, Hyysalo P, Komulainen H, Kumlin T, Lang S, Puranen L, Juutilainen J. Effects of mobile phone radiation on X-ray induced tumorigenesis in mice. *Radiat Res* 2001; 156: 775–785.

108. Heikkinen P, Kosma V-M, Alhonens L, Huuskonen H, Kumlin T, Laitinen JT, Lang S, Puranen L, Juutilainen J. Effects of mobile phone radiation on UV-induced skin tumourigenesis in ornithine decarboxylase transgenic and non-transgenic mice. *Int J Radiat Biol* 2003; 79: 221–233.

109. Bartsch H, Bartsch C, Seebald E, Deerburg F, Dietz K, Bollrath L, Meeke D. Chronic exposure to a GSM-like signal (mobile phone) does not stimulate the development of DMBA-induced mammary tumors in rats: results of three consecutive studies. *Radiat Res* 2002; 157: 183–190.

110. Vijayalaxmi, Sasser L, Morris JE, Wilson BW, Anderson LA. Genotoxic potential of 1.6 GHz wireless communication signal: in vivo two-year bioassay. *Radiat Res* 2003; 159: 558–564.

111. La Regina M, Moros EG, Pickard WF, Straube WL, Baty J, Roti Roti JL. The effect of chronic exposure to 835.62 MHz FDMA or 847.74 MHz CDMA radiofrequency radiation on the incidence of spontaneous tumours in rats. *Radiat Res* 2003; 160: 143–151.

112. Heynick LN, Johnston SA, Mason PA. Radio frequency electromagnetic fields: cancer, mutagenesis, and genotoxicity. *Bioelectromagnetics* 2003; 24: S74–S100.

113. Adey WR. Tissue interactions with nonionizing electromagnetic fields. *Physiol Rev* 1981; 61: 435–514.

114. Adey WR, Bawin SM, Lawrence AF. Effects of weak amplitude modulated microwave fields on calcium efflux from awake cat cerebral cortex. *Bioelectromagnetics* 1982; 3: 295–307.

115. Pacini S, Ruggiero M, Sardi I, Aterini S, Gulisano F. Exposure to global system for mobile communication (GSM) cellular phone radiofrequency alters gene expression, proliferation, and morphology of human skin fibroblasts. *Oncol Res Anti-Cancer Drug Design* 2002; 13: 19–24.

116. Tsurita G, Nagawa H, Ueno S, Watanabe S, Taki M. Biological and morphological effects on the brain after exposure of rats to a 1439 MHz TDMA field. *Bioelectromagnetics* 2000; 21: 364–371.

117. Bol'shakov MA, Kniazeva IR, Evdokimov EV. Effects of 460 MHz microwave radiation on Drosophila embryos under raised temperature. *Radiatsionnaia Biologiia Radioecologiia* 2002; 42: 191–193.

118. Dasdag S, Akdag MZ, Aksen F, Ylmaz F, Bashan M, Dasdag MM, Celik MS. Whole body exposure of rats to microwaves emitted from a cell phone does not affect the testes. *Bioelectromagnetics* 2003; 24: 182–188.

119. Kues HA, Monahan JC. Microwave-induced changes to the primate eye. *Johns Hopkins APL Tech Digest* 1992; 13: 244–254.

120. Kues HA, Monahan JC, D'Anna SA, McLeod DS, Lutty GA, Koslov S. Increased sensitivity of the non-human primate eye to microwave radiation following ophthalmic drug pretreatment. *Bioelectromagnetics* 1992; 13: 379–393.

121. Kues HA, D'Anna SA, Osiander R, Green WR, Monahan JC. Absence of ocular effects after either single or repeated exposure to 10 mW/cm^2 from a 60 GHz CW source. *Bioelectromagnetics* 1999; 20: 463–473.

122. Carpenter RL. Ocular effects of microwave radiation. *Bull NY Acad Med* 1979; 55: 1048–1057.

123. Guy AW, Kramar PO, Harris CA, Chou CK. Long-term 2450-MHz CW microwave irradiation of rabbits: methodology and evaluation of ocular and physiologic effects. *J Microwave Power* 1980; 15: 37–44.

124. Kamimura Y, Saito K-I, Saiga T, Amenyima Y. Effect of 2.45 GHz microwave irradiation on monkey eyes. *IEICE Trans Comm* 1994; E77-B: 762–765.

125. Lu S-T, Mathur SP, Stuck B, Zwick H, D'Andrea H, Zeriax JM, Merritt JH, Lutty G, McLeod DS, Johnson M. Effects of high peak power microwaves on the retina of the Rhesus monkey. *Bioelectromagnetics* 2000; 21: 439–454.

126. D'Andrea JA, Gandhi OP, Lords JL, Durney CH, Johnson CC, Astle L. Physiological and behavioral effects of exposure to 2450 MHz microwaves. *J Microw Power* 1980; 14: 351–362.

127. De Lorge JO, Ezell CS. Observing responses of rats exposed to 1.28- and 5.62-GHz microwaves. *Bioelectromagnetics* 1980; 1: 183–198.

128. Lai H, Horita A, Guy AW. Microwave irradiation affects radial-arm maze performance in the rat. *Bioelectromagnetics* 1994; 15: 95–104.

129. Bornhausen M, Scheingraber H. Prenatal exposure to 900 MHz, cell-phone electromagnetic fields had no effect on operant-behavior performances of adult rats. *Bioelectromagnetics* 2000; 21: 566–574.

130. Dubreuil D, Jay T, Edeline JM. Does head-only exposure to GSM-900 electromagnetic fields affect the performance of rats in spatial learning tasks? *Behav Brain Res* 2002; 129: 203–210.

131. Yamaguchi H, Tsurita G, Ueno S, Watanabe S, Wake K, Taki M, Nagawa H. 1439 MHz pulsed TDMA fields affect performance of rats in a T-maze task only when body temperature is elevated. *Bioelectromagnetics* 2003; 24: 223–230.

132. Frey AH, Feld SR, Frey B. Neural function and behaviour: defining the relationship. *Ann New York Acad Sci* 1975; 247: 433–439.

133. Sutton CH, Carrol FB. Effects of microwave-induced hyperthermia on the blood–brain barrier of the rat. *Radiat Sci* 1979; 14: 329–334.

134. Lin JC, Lin MF. Microwave hyperthermia-induced blood–brain barrier alterations. *Radiat Res* 1982; 89: 77–87.

135. Neubauer C, Phelan AM, Kues H, Lange DG. Microwave irradiation of rats at 2.45 GHz activates pinocytotic-like uptake of tracer by capillary endothelial cells of cerebral cortex. *Bioelectromagnetics* 1990; 11: 261–268.

136. Persson BRR, Salford LG, Brun A, Eberhardt JL, Malmgren L. Increased permeability of the blood–brain barrier induced by magnetic and electromagnetic fields. *Ann New York Acad Sci* 1992; 649: 356–358.

137. Persson BRR, Salford RLG, Brun A. Blood–brain barrier permeability in rats exposed to electromagnetic fields used in wireless communication. *Wireless Net* 1997; 3: 455–461.

138. Ward TR, Ali J. Blood–brain barrier permeation in the rat during exposure to low-power 1.7-GHz microwave radiation. *Bioelectromagnetics* 1981; 2: 131–143.

139. Fritze K, Wiessner C, Kuster N, Sommer C, Gass P, Hermann DP, Kiessling M, Hossmann K-A. Effect of GSM microwave exposure on the genomic response of the rat brain. *Neuroscience* 1997; 81: 627–639.

140. Finnie JW, Blumbergs PC, Manavis J, Utteridge TD, Gebski V, Swift JG, Vernon-Roberts B, Kuchel TR. Effect of global system for mobile communication (GSM)-like radiofrequency fields on vascular permeability in mouse brain. *Pathology* 2001; 33: 338–340.

141. Finnie JW, Blumbergs PC, Manavis J, Utteridge TD, Gebski V, Davies RA, Vernon-Roberts B, Kuchel TR. Effect of long-term mobile communication microwave exposure on vascular permeability in mouse brain. *Pathology* 2002; 34: 344–347.

142. Salford LG, Brun AE, Eberhardt JL, Malmgren L, Persson BRR. Nerve cell damage in mammalian brain after exposure to microwaves from GSM mobile phones. *Environl Health Perspec* 2003; 111: 881–883.

143. D'Andrea JA, Chou CK, Johnston SA, Adair ER. Microwave effects on the nervous system. *Bioelectromagnetics* 2003; 24: S107–S147.

144. Frey AH. Auditory system response to radio frequency energy. *Aeromed Acta* 1961; 32: 1140–1142.

145. Chou CK, Guy AW, Foster KR, Galambos R, Justesen DR. Holographic assessment of microwave hearing. *Science* 1980; 209: 1143–1144.

146. Chou CK, Guy AW. Auditory perception of radio–frequency electromagnetic fields. *J Acous Soc Am* 1982; 71: 1321–1334.

147. Kellenyi L, Thuroczy G, Faludy B, Lenard L. Effects of mobile GSM radiotelephone exposure on the auditory brainstem response (ABR). *Neurobiology* 1999; 7: 79–81.

148. Hietanen M, Hämäläinen A-M, Husman T. Hypersensitivity symptoms associated with exposure to cellular telephones: no causal link. *Bioelectromagnetics* 2002; 23: 264–270.

149. Chou C-K. Thirty-five years in bioelectromagnetics research. *Bioelectromagnetics* 2007; 28: 3–15.

150. Elder JA, Chou CK. Auditory response to pulsed radiofrequency energy. *Bioelectromagnetics* 2003; 24: S162–S173.

151. Adair ER, Mylacraine KS, Allen SJ. Thermophysiological consequences of whole body resonant RF exposure (100 MHz) in human volunteers. *Bioelectromagnetics* 2003; 24: 489–501.

152. Adair ER, Black DR. Thermoregulatory responses to RF energy absorption. *Bioelectromagnetics* 2003; 24: S17–S38.
153. Hirsch FB, Parker JT. Bilateral opacities occurring in a technician operating a microwave generator. *Am Med Ass Arch Ind Hyg* 1952; 6: 512–517.
154. Cleary SF, Pasternack BS. Lenticular changes in microwave workers: a statistical study. *Arch Environ Health* 1966; 12: 23–29.
155. Lin JC. Health aspects of radio and microwave radiation. *J Environ Pathol Toxicol* 1979; 2: 1413–1432.
156. Michaelson SM, Lin JC. *Biological Effects and Health Implications of Radio Frequency Radiation*. New York: Plenum Press, 1987.
157. Hirata A, Matsuyama S, Shiozawa T. Temperature rises in the human eye exposed to EM waves in the frequency range 0.6–6 GHz. *IEEE Trans Electromagc Compat* 2000; 42: 386–393.
158. FCC. *Guidelines for Evaluating the Environmental Effects of Radio Frequency Radiation*. Washington, DC: Federal Communications Commission, 1996.
159. Tengroth BM. Cataractogenesis induced by RF and MW energy. In: Grandolfo M, Michaelson SM, Rindi, A, Editors. *Biological Effects and Dosimetry of Nonionizing Radiation*. New York: Plenum Press, 1983.
160. Elder JA. Special senses: cataractogenic effects. In: Elder JA, Cahill DF, Editors. *Biological Effects of Radiofrequency Radiation*. Environmental Protection Agency Report, EPA-600/8-83-026F: 5-64-5-68. Washington, DC: Environmental Protection Agency, 1984.
161. Elder JA. Ocular effects of radio frequency radiation. IEEE Subcommittee 28.4 White Paper, 2001.
162. Elder JA. Ocular effects of radiofrequency energy. *Bioelectromagnetics* 2003; 24: S148–S161.
163. Freude G, Ullsperger P, Eggert S, Ruppe I. Effects of microwaves emitted by cellular phones on human slow brain potentials. *Bioelectromagnetics* 1998; 19: 384–387.
164. Freude G, Ullsperger P, Eggert S, Ruppe I. Microwaves emitted by cellular telephones affect human slow brain potentials. *Eur J App Physiol* 2000; 81: 18–27.
165. Krause CM, Sillanmäki L, Koivisto M, Haggqvist A, Saarela C, Revonsuo A, Hämäläinen H. Effects of electromagnetic field emitted by cellular phones on the EEG during a memory task. *NeuroReport* 2000; 11: 761–764.
166. Krause CM, Sillanmäki L, Koivisto M, Häggqvist A, Saarela C, Revonsuo A, Laine M, Hämäläinen H. Effects of electromagnetic fields emitted by cellular phones on the electroencephalogram during a visual working memory task. *Int J Radiat Biol* 2000; 76: 1659–1667.
167. Preece AW, Iwi G, Davies-Smith A, Wesnes K, Butler S, Lim E, Varey A. Effect of a 915-MHz simulated mobile phone signal on cognitive function in man. *Int J Radiat Biol* 1999; 75: 447–456.
168. Koivisto M, Revonsuo A, Krause C, Haarala C, Sillanmaki L, Laine M, Hamalainen H. Effect of 902 MHz electromagnetic field emitted by cellular telephones on response times in humans. *NeuroReport* 2000; 11: 413–415.
169. Koivisto M, Krause C, Revonsuo A, Laine M, Hämäläinen H. The effects of electromagnetic field emitted by GSM phones on working memory. *NeuroReport* 2000; 11: 1641–1643.
170. Haarala C, Aalto S, Hautzel H, Julkunen L, Rinne JO, Laine M, Krause B, Hämäläinen H. Effects of a 902 MHz mobile phone on cerebral blood flow in humans: a PET study. *NeuroReport* 2003; 14: 2019–2023.
171. Haarala C, Björnberg L, Ek M, Laine M, Revonsuo A, Koivisto M, Hämäläinen H. Effect of a 902 MHz electromagnetic field emitted by mobile phones on human cognitive function: a replication study. *Bioelectromagnetics* 2003; 24: 283–288.

172. Zwamborn APM, Vossen SHJA, van Leersum BJAM, Ouwens MA, Makel WN. Effects of global communication system radio-frequency fields on well being and cognitive functions of human subjects with and without subjective complaints. Netherlands Organization for Applied Scientific Research (TNO). FEL-03-C148, 2003.

173. Mann K, Röschke J. Effects of pulsed high-frequency electromagnetic fields on human sleep. *Neuropsychobiology* 1996; 33: 41–47.

174. Wagner P, Röschke J, Mann K, Hiller W, Frank C. Human sleep under the influence of pulsed radiofrequency electromagnetic fields: a polysomnographic study using standardized conditions. *Bioelectromagnetics* 1998; 19: 199–202.

175. Borbely AA, Huber R, Graf T, Fuchs B, Gallmann E, Achermann P. Pulsed high-frequency electromagnetic field affects human sleep and sleep encephalogram. *Neurosci Lett* 1999; 275: 207–210.

176. Koivisto M, Haarala C, Krause CM, Revonsuo A, Laine M, Hamalainen H. GSM phone signal does not produce subjective symptoms. *Bioelectromagnetics* 2001; 22: 212–215.

177. Smythe J, Costall B. Mobile phone use facilitates memory in male, but not female, subjects. *NeuroReport* 2003; 14: 243–246.

178. Röschke J, Mann K. No short term effects of digital mobile radio telephone on the awake human electroencephalogram. *Bioelectromagnetics* 1997; 18: 172–176.

179. Hietanen M, Kovala T, Hamalainen MA. Human brain activity during exposure to radiofrequency fields emitted by cellular phones. *Scand J Work Environ Health* 2000; 26: 87–92.

180. Huber R, Graf T, Cote KA, Wittman L, Gallmann MD, Schuderer J, Kuster N, Borbély AA, Achermann P. Exposure to pulsed high-frequency electromagnetic field during waking affects human sleep EEG. *NeuroReport* 2000; 11: 3321–3325.

181. Huber R, Treyer V, Borbely AA, Schuderer J, Gottselig JM, Landolt HP, Werth E, Berthold T, Kuster N, Buck A, Achermann P. Electromagnetic fields, such as those from mobile phones, alter regional cerebral blood flow and sleep and waking EEG. *J Sleep Res* 2002; 11: 289–295.

182. Croft R, Chandler J, Burgess A, Barry R, Williams J, Clarke A. Acute mobile phone operation affect neural function in humans. *Clin Neurophysiol* 2002; 113: 1623–1632.

183. Lebedeva NN, Sulimov AV, Sulimova OP, Korotkovskaya TI, Gailus T. Investigation of brain potentials in sleeping humans exposed to the electromagnetic field of mobile phones. *Crit Rev Biomed Eng* 2001; 29: 125–133.

184. Lebedeva NN, Sulimov AV, Sulimova OP, Kotrovskaya TI, Gailus T. Cellular phone electromagnetic field effects on bioelectric activity of human brain. *Crit Rev Biomed Eng* 2000; 28: 323–337.

185. Lee TMC, Ho SMY, Tsang LYH, Yang SYC, Li LSW, Chan CCH. Effect on human attention of exposure to the electromagnetic field emitted by mobile phones. *NeuroReport* 2001; 12: 729–731.

186. Lee TMC, Lam P-K, Lee LTS, Chan CCH. The effect of the duration of exposure to the electromagnetic field emitted by mobile phones on human attention. *NeuroReport* 2003; 14: 1361–1364.

187. Petrides M. Exposure to electromagnetic fields by using cellular telephones and its influence on the brain. *NeuroReport* 2000; 11: 3321–3325.

188. Petrides M. Use of cellular telephones and performance on tests of attention. *NeuroReport* 2001; 12: A21.

189. Edelstyn N, Oldershaw A. The acute effects of exposure to the electromagnetic field emitted by mobile phones on human attention. *NeuroReport* 2002; 13: 119–121.

190. Wilén J, Sandström M, Mild KH. Subjective symptoms among mobile phone users—a consequence of absorption of radiofrequency fields? *Bioelectromagnetics* 2003; 24: 152–159.

191. Sandström M, Wilén J, Oftedal G, Mild KH. Mobile phone use and subjective symptoms. Comparison of symptoms experienced by users of analogue and digital mobile phones. *Occup Med* 2001; 51: 25–35.

192. Hamblin DL, Wood AW. Effects of mobile phone emissions on human brain activity and sleep variables. *Int J Radiat Biol* 2002; 78: 659–669.

193. D'Andrea JA, Adair ER, de Lorge JO. Behavioral and cognitive effects of microwave exposure. *Bioelectromagnetics* 2003; 24: S39–S62.

194. Braune S, Wrocklage C, Raczek J, Gailus T, Lücking CH. Resting blood pressure increase during exposure to a radiofrequency electromagnetic field. *Lancet* 1998; 351: 1857–1858.

195. Braune S, Riedel A, Schulte-Monting J, Raczek J. Influence of a radiofrequency electromagnetic field on cardiovascular and hormonal parameters of the autonomic nervous system in healthy individuals. *Radiat Res* 2002; 158: 352–356.

196. Mann K, Roschke J, Connemann B, Beta H. No effects of pulsed high-frequency electromagnetic fields on heart rate variability during human sleep. *Neuropsychobiology* 1998; 38: 251–256.

197. Parazzini M, Ravazzani P, Tognola G, Thuroczy G, Molnar FB, Sacchettini A, Ardesi G, Mainardi LT. Electromagnetic fields produced by GSM cellular phones and heart rate variability. *Bioelectromagnetics* 2007; 28: 122–129.

198. Black DR, Heynick LN. Radiofrequency (RF) effects on blood cells, cardiac, endocrine, and immunological functions. *Bioelectromagnetics* 2003; 24: S187–S195.

199. Wang SG. 5-HT contents change in peripheral blood of workers exposed to microwave and high frequency radiation. *Chung Hua Yu Fang I Hsueh Tsa Chih* 1989; 23: 207–210.

200. Burch JB, Reif JS, Pittrat CA, Keefe TJ, Yost MG. Cellular telephone use and excretion of a urinary melatonin metabolite. In: *Annual Review of Research in Biological Effects of Electric and Magnetic Fields from the Generation, Delivery and Use of Electricity*, Nov. 9–13, P-52, San Diego, CA, 1997.

201. Burch JB, Reif JS, Noonan CW, Ichinose T, Bachand AM, Koleber TL. Melatonin metabolite excretion among cellular telephone users. *Int J Radiat Biol* 2002; 78: 1029–1036.

202. Radon K, Parera D, Rose D-M, Jung D, Volrath L. No effects of pulsed radio frequency electromagnetic fields on melatonin, cortisol, and selected markers of the immune system in man. *Bioelectromagnetics* 2001; 22: 280–287.

203. Bortkiewicz A, Pilacik B, Gadzicka E, Szymczak W. The excretion of 6-hydroxymelatonin sulfate in healthy young men exposed to electromagnetic fields emitted by cellular phone—an experimental study. *Neuroendocrinol Lett* 2002; 23: S88–S91.

204. Brusick D, Albertini R, McRee D, Peterson D, Williams G, Hanawalt P. Genotoxicity of radiofrequency radiation. *Environ Mol Mutagen* 1998; 32: 1–16.

205. Boice JD, McLaughlin JK. *Epidemiologic Studies of Cellular Telephones and Cancer Risk—A Review*. Swedish Radiation Protection Authority, Stockholm, Sweden, 2002.

206. Juutilainen J, de Seze R. Biological effects of amplitude-modulated radiofrequency radiation. *Scand J Environ Health* 1998; 24: 245–254.

207. Cook CM, Thomas AW, Prato FS. Human electrophysiological and cognitive effects of exposure to ELF magnetic and ELF modulated RF and microwave fields: a review of recent studies. *Bioelectromagnetics* 2002; 23: 144–157.

208. Adair RK. Biophysical limits on athermal effects of RF and microwave radiation. *Bioelectromagnetics* 2003; 24: 39–48.

209. Health Council of the Netherlands. *Mobile Telephones: An Evaluation of Health Effects*. The Hague: Health Council of the Netherlands, Publication No. 2002/OIE, 2002.

210. Repacholi M, Saunders R, van Deventer E, Kheifets L. Is EMF a potential environmental risk for children? *Bioelectromagnetics* 2005; 26: S2–S4.

7 Electromagnetic Risk Analysis

7.1 INTRODUCTION

Modern technology offers powerful tools to stimulate a range of benefits for society, in addition to economic development. However, technological progress in the broadest sense has always been associated with hazards and risks [1]. Traditionally, risk has been defined from a technical perspective, namely the product of the probability and consequences of an adverse event. In this case, the adverse event would be exposure to EM fields. These technical assessments are portrayed as representing the actual risks. However, this approach ignores essential social, economic, and cultural dimensions of risk assessment and management. A broader set of criteria must be used to obtain an accurate representation of risk.

EM fields, including both EMF and RFR, have become a driving force of our civilization through their numerous applications in the workplace, home, and external environment. Most public exposure to EM fields comes from electrical power generation, distribution, and use; transportation and telecommunication systems; scientific, medical, and industrial equipment; radar devices; radio and television broadcast facilities; and mobile phones and their base stations [2].

EM fields may have a biological effect on human cells that may disrupt cellular processes, which could in turn lead to adverse health consequences. As the reliance on technologies involving EM fields has increased, so has the public's concern over possible related health risks. This is due to our lack of understanding of the health consequences of increasing levels of exposure of the population to EM fields. However, there are several organizations that have initiated research programs to study this issue and thus improve our understanding of the health risks and our ability to manage them.

Risk analysis is implicitly or explicitly used as the foundation of a large number of standards, including those related to environmental protection, occupational safety and health, food safety, medical devices, drugs, and others [3]. The risk analysis process can be logically divided into three clear and distinct categories: (1) risk assessment, (2) risk management, and (3) risk communication [4].

In recent years it has become widely recognized that a number of determinants (including social and behavioral factors, environmental and occupational exposures, biology and genetic endowment, and health services) affect individual health status and that the health status of individuals and of entire populations is linked. At the same time, risk science has emerged as an important new discipline for the assessment and management of health risks [5].

Concerning the controversial issue of EM health hazard, there exist three main uncertainties: (1) whether EM exposure poses a health hazard or not, (2) what components of the exposure contribute to the health effects (e.g., time-weighted average

179

or exposures above certain thresholds), and (3) how serious the health effects are. Expert opinions regarding these three uncertainties vary widely. They range from a firm belief, based on physical reasoning, that EM exposure cannot possibly pose a health hazard to a conviction, based on epidemiological findings, that they pose a serious health hazard that might double or triple certain cancer rates. Given this broad range of opinions, it seems futile to conduct a formal risk analysis [6].

To effectively address potential health risks associated with EM exposure, it is important to have (1) a clear understanding of the biological and health effects of EM field exposure; (2) a risk management plan highlighting the possible undesirable consequences of EM field exposure, incorporating the key elements of both risk assessment and risk perception; and (3) effective communication of the biological and health effects of EM exposure and the risk management plan to the public.

The goal of this chapter is to provide biomedical researchers with an overview of EM exposure-health risk assessment. The main issue is whether the existing exposure limits, which have been discussed in Chapters 3 and 5, are sufficient to protect public health. An evaluation of the literature has been provided to develop a sound risk assessment and risk perception. Particular attention is paid to measured and perceived risk as part of a thorough risk management agenda.

7.2   RISK ASSESSMENT

Risk assessment is an organized process used to describe and estimate the likelihood of adverse health outcomes. Quantitative risk assessment estimates the hazard for an exposure or situation that cannot be measured directly. This process involves several steps: (1) hazard identification (situations that threaten human health), (2) exposure assessment (exposure to hazard is quantified), (3) dose response analysis (amount of exposure that causes harm), and (4) risk characterization (combination of above). For a particular hazard, exposure is combined with dose response to predict the risk for an individual or population.

Prior to an established interaction mechanism or known effect, health risk assessment studies should start with a null hypothesis, i.e., the objective of the exposure regime and study design is to provide maximized significance for negative findings with respect to the technology. In other words, the likelihood of evoking effects should be maximized. Therefore, worst case values should be applied for various parameters including exposed tissues, exposure strength, and signal characteristics. If positive effects are detected, the parameters causing effects should be subsequently evaluated to assess the actual health risk [7].

7.2.1   SCIENTIFIC EVIDENCE

Risk assessment is a scientific process [8] and, ideally, entirely free of nonscientific parameters. As currently performed, much of the scientific information upon which risk assessment is based falls in the category of scientific extrapolation and scientific judgment [3]. Guidance for EM policy has come primarily from epidemiology studies of health risks associated with power lines in the case of EMF and cell phones in the case of RF. In both frequency ranges, the refining of epidemiological studies over the years has helped to clarify the factors involved in health risk [9].

Laboratory studies have provided the background for all related studies and particularly for realizing the interaction mechanisms that highlight health risk. In this regard, explicit distinctions should be made between the concepts of EM interaction mechanisms, biological effects, and health hazards, consistent with the criteria used by international bodies when making health assessments [10]. Biological effects occur when EM fields interact to produce cellular responses that may or may not be perceived by people. Deciding whether biological changes have health consequences depends, in part, on whether they are reversible, are within the range for which the body has effective compensation mechanisms, or are likely to lead to unfavorable changes in health.

Two major research programs were launched during the 1990s. The NIEHS and the Department of Energy (DOE) were commissioned by the U.S. Congress in 1992 to develop a comprehensive research program and together they formed the Electric and Magnetic Fields Research and Public Information Dissemination (EMF RAPID) program. This five-year program was supported through federal and private funds and focused on health effects, education, and assessment of health risks [11]. In 1996, the WHO established the International EMF project. The mandate of these programs is to conduct targeted research that will permit improved health risk assessments to be made and identify any environmental impacts of EM exposure.

WHO defines health as the state of complete physical, mental, and social well-being, and not merely the absence of disease or infirmity. Not all biological effects are hazardous. Some may be innocuously within the normal range of biological variation and physiological compensation, while others may be beneficial under certain conditions, and the health implications of yet others may be simply indeterminate. Health hazard is generally defined to be a biological effect of EM exposure outside the normal range of physiological compensation and adverse to a person's well-being [12].

A distinction must be made between the biological effects of EM fields and damage to health due to such fields. This distinction is indeed central to risk assessment, since any effect is relevant for risk assessment only insofar as this effect can be considered to be damaging (potentially) to health [13]. While there is a general understanding of the biological effects of EM energy, there is still much to be learned about its long-term health consequences. EMF exposure induces circulating currents inside the human body, while RFR causes thermal effects. Nearly all regular electrical appliances and wireless equipment produce EM fields far weaker than those required for inducing currents or producing heat [14–18].

Studies have shown that weak EM fields can affect a few biological processes. On their own, these effects do not appear to comprise a serious health risk. However, their long-term impact is unknown. The level of association between EM exposure and adverse health effects, although limited, has a considerable public impact. Limitations are partly attributed to a gap in knowledge. Further research is needed in many areas to better assess the health risk. These include laboratory studies of cells and animals, clinical studies of humans, computer simulations, and human population (epidemiological) studies. No single study or class of study provides the entire answer. Often the results of studies are inconsistent or they have not investigated the characteristics of the dose–response relationship (field strength, threshold, and exposure duration), and sometimes have found responses only in exposure "windows," ranges above and below which no effects are seen [12].

Unlike clinical studies, animal studies investigate the response of nonhuman species to EM exposures under laboratory conditions. Animal studies are unable to address many human exposure factors that are sociologically or geographically based, such as personal use of appliances. There is also some uncertainty about the ability to extrapolate evidence from animal studies across species. However, it is widely accepted that the demonstration of an effect in one species increases the plausibility of a similar effect in another species.

Cellular studies provide an understanding of the potential physiological alterations at the basic cellular level and are necessary in the assessment of the human health effects of chronic or long-term EM exposure. In assessing the significant amount of data assembled and wide range of cases studied, the general conclusion seems to be that the current studies indicate no evident pattern of increased health risk associated with EM fields. However, there might be rational grounds for possible suspicion of health risks with long-term exposure to EM fields. To clarify this matter, further research is required. The inconsistency between laboratory data, human data, and interaction mechanisms severely complicates the interpretation of the research outcomes. Given the complexity of living organisms, it is difficult to apply and correlate knowledge from these sources [2].

As progress in technology continues and human beings are enjoying an increased quality of life, it is essential for scientists to ensure that safety is not compromised. Scientists must conduct well-designed studies and report the results in a clear and detailed manner, so other independent investigators can repeat the studies or explore further. Mistakes must be minimized and stopped at the first level of scientific research [19].

7.2.2 SETTING STANDARDS

Standards-setting bodies for safety are faced with conflicting pressures. One is to protect the worker and the public against risks of injury, and health problems. Another is to make useful technology available to the public. How these possibly conflicting requirements are met depends on many factors, including how well the hazards are understood by the public, regulators, the value of the technology, and public view of the kind of potential damage the technology may do to their health and their degree of control over exposure to it [20]. The main issue is whether the existing EM safety standards, which have been discussed in Chapters 3 and 5, are sufficient to protect public health. These standards are based on the scientific evidence about thermal (i.e., heating) effects of EM exposure. Whether exposure below the safety standard levels might cause detrimental health effects is scientifically controversial [13]. The scientific literature suggests that there is no solid evidence for a link between EM fields above these levels and adverse health effects. In addition, a number of recent reports have evaluated the scientific evidence on potential health risks from EM exposure below the exposure limits [11,15–18,21–29]. Most of these reports agree that there is no scientific proof of health risk below the EM exposure limits. However, the reports show differences with regard to the extent and significance of uncertainties in the scientific knowledge about this matter. Importantly, the health consequences may not become apparent until years of exposure have accumulated. With chronic diseases such as cancer, it is impossible to establish any "proof of risk" or "proof of safety," which can be sustained "beyond all reasonable doubt," in just a few years. This reflects the dilemma of risk assessment.

It is evident that the evaluation of the existing evidence leaves space for differing assessments and allows compelling new evidence that challenges any judgments. Under these circumstances, one must consider the subset of possible health risks of EM exposure in our daily life that is subject to scientific uncertainty. The pervasive and complex character of EM fields in our environment makes it impossible to ignore even the most remote suggestion of such a risk.

7.2.3 Structured Risk Assessment

Risk management is a systematic approach to setting the best course of action under uncertainty by identifying, assessing, acting on, and communicating risk issues. A major development in the field of EM health risk would be the introduction of structured risk assessment tools. These tools may be of two main types: (1) structured guidelines, which only specify the relevant risk factors to consider, and (2) implementation measures, which identify items to consider as well as how to combine these items into a comprehensive evaluation agenda. These approaches to risk assessment are far from perfect, but they are more accurate than the unguided judgment used to assess the risk of EM fields. For organizing and structuring the risk assessment process, further investigation should be done to (1) determine whether any health effect can be substantiated and related to EM fields and (2) clarify the relevance of research results. Attention should be paid to the impact of bias (selection, reporting, publication, sponsorship, and pro-industry conclusions) on the existence of health risk. To achieve that, a risk assessment requires the establishment of scientific discussion by different scientific experts related to the field of EM health risk such as biology, epidemiology, biophysics, dosimetry, medicine, environment, etc., to exchange views and facts. However, one problem associated with incorporating a variety of viewpoints into a risk management plan is that it can lead to differences in the evaluation of risk.

In the meantime, standard-setting groups need to decide what to do, taking into account both the results of research showing biological effects at low levels of exposure and the large number of studies that do not. In addition, they need to take into account the benefit of having EM technology services that are used to enhance the standard of living for the public. With these together, the scientific community will be able to develop rules for categorizing scientific evidence, provide more thorough analyses of health risk, and share the information with the public and authorities.

7.3 PERCEPTION OF RISK

In trying to understand people's perception of risk, it is important to distinguish between a health hazard and a health risk. A hazard can be an object or a set of circumstances that could potentially harm a person's health. Risk is the likelihood, or probability, that a person will be harmed by a particular hazard [1].

7.3.1 PUBLIC PERCEPTION OF RISK

The perception of health risk is quite different between scientists and the public. Such divergence is crucial in the debates and controversies about EM fields; it is significant that the International EMF project of WHO (www.who.int/emf) includes, along with traditional research areas, studies on the mechanisms of risk perception and communication [30]. The public will likely consider other factors in addition to the technical ones considered for a scientific assessment. While they may include probability of harm in their view of risk, they will also incorporate the social, political, economic, and cultural consequences. The psychometric approach [31] expands upon the technical approach and attempts to identify the cognitive, emotional, and social–demographic aspects of public perceptions of risk. This broader and more meaningful approach to risk evaluation (termed risk perception) enables an assessment of why public assessment of risk differs from the technical assessment, and can help explain the public outrage often associated with new technologies.

Risk assessment and risk perception both provide valuable insights into risk management. Traditionally, risk assessment has played a greater role in this process because committees established to deal with this issue are made up of scientific experts. However, poor communication of these risks to the general public has led to a call for the development of a new model for risk management. Approaches to risk differ considerably between technical experts and the general public. Technical experts focus on the quantifiable level of risk and view reasonable risk-taking and technological innovation as necessary aspects of social progress. The general public focuses on the safety issues surrounding a particular project and any associated community health risks.

Major causes of different perception are undoubtedly the limited ability of experts to communicate risks to the public, and an attitude of the media to privilege sensationalism rather than a correct transfer of information. However, difficulties in scientific communication have objective causes in the quality of data that are still controversial, sometimes contradictory, and in any case difficult to read and interpret. Therefore, risk assessment faces two main problems: on one side, the correct analysis of scientific data, on the other the understanding of mechanisms of risk communication and perception [30].

Regardless of how much scientific evidence there is, authorities need to consider the degree of public concern, even if low, about possible risk of EM exposure and how that compares with expert assessment. The challenge of risk analysis will not be resolved by scientific knowledge only. Reaching beyond a technical assessment of risk and moving towards a more psychometric approach is necessary if the legitimate concerns of the public are to be recognized.

7.3.2 FACTORS RELEVANT TO ELECTROMAGNETIC FIELDS

There are many factors that shape an individual's perception of risks, including age, sex, and cultural and educational backgrounds. In addition, specific characteristics of the risk such as familiarity with the agent, understanding of the mechanism, voluntary of exposure, fairness, controllability of risk, uncertainty of knowledge, effect on children, effect on future generations, trust in institutions, attention of media, previous accidents, clarity of benefits, and scientific evidence can influence risk perception.

Most of the above factors are of special importance for EM fields. Emotional impact of risks for children is probably the most relevant, but involuntarity, uncertainty in knowledge, and limited understanding of interaction mechanisms are likely to play a significant role. Other factors specific to EM exposure must be added, including imperceptibility, visual impact of power lines and antennas, and use of the term "nonionizing radiation" that may lead to erroneous analogies and extrapolations [30].

Exposure to EM fields can be considered voluntary among cell phone users and involuntary among nonusers. As a result, cell phone users will likely perceive the exposure risk from base stations as lower than nonusers. In addition, the nonusers will consider EM exposure as unfair and this will also alter their perception. The risk will also be perceived as higher by the public if power lines or base stations are installed in their community without prior discussion or consultation. EM technology is new, difficult to understand, and the potential health effects are not well defined. This unfamiliarity of EM technology serves to increase the perceived risk. Consideration of these factors may explain local concerns, possible biases, or assumptions about the technology. Careful attention to the nontechnical risk dimensions of any project allows policy makers and managers to make informed decisions as part of a thorough risk management program [1].

Perceptions of EM fields risk associated with high-voltage transmission lines and other sources of EM fields have been examined in several studies [32–35]. Read and Morgan [34] confirmed an earlier finding that most people believe that any high-voltage power line they can see is exposing them to strong fields. The authors explored a number of strategies that might be used in risk communications to correct this misperception.

7.3.3 HEALTH CONSEQUENCES OF RISK PERCEPTION

One of the most perplexing problems in risk analysis is why some relatively minor risks or risk events, as assessed by technical experts, often elicit strong public concerns and result in substantial impacts upon society and economy. The main reason is that hazards interact with psychological, social, institutional, and cultural processes in ways that may amplify or attenuate public responses to the risk or risk event [36]. A distorted perception of risks is not just a social issue. It strongly affects the psychological attitude of nonexperts toward EM fields. This aspect was made clear in the final report [37] of a study group set up by the European Commission to investigate subjective symptoms (i.e., psychological and neurovegetative disturbances) attributed to EM field exposure. Several medical reports were reviewed for symptoms such as headache, asthenia, weakness, and irritability that patients or physicians attributed to EM fields. The study group concluded that most symptoms, if not all, were of psychosomatic origin. In controlled tests, the symptoms turned out to be statistically correlated to the degree of worry of patients, while no significant association with exposure was found. The suffering of these patients is true and sometimes even intolerable. This confirms a hypothesis put forward by several social scientists and medical doctors: a distorted perception of risk may cause excessive or unjustified worries, which in turn may lead to real health effects [30].

7.4   RISK MANAGEMENT

Today, risk assessment methods are widely applied in industrial and government regulatory applications involving new and existing technologies. These contribute to the development of risk management policies and strategies focusing on technological change [5].

Risk management is fundamentally a societal decision [4]. It includes not only the outcome of risk assessment expressed in characterized risk, but also numerous other parameters, such as cost–benefit and risk–benefit analyses, views of stakeholders, sociopolitical factors, and other nonscientific judgments [38,39].

7.4.1   INVOLVING THE PUBLIC

Love et al. [40] have classified the public, including stakeholders, into several categories: (1) personally impacted, (2) administratively impacted (regulators, permit writers, elected officials), (3) generally concerned (interest based on ideological, philosophical, moral, religious, and other beliefs) stakeholders, (4) process-concerned stakeholders, consisting of those who are concerned over the appropriate role of stakeholders in the decision process, and (5) uninvolved public. The authors recommend an affirmative outreach to ensure the participation of personally impacted stakeholders in the risk management process. They suggest that the next priority should be given to the inclusion of administratively impacted stakeholders. The generally concerned and process-concerned stakeholders should be accommodated after the other two categories have been heard.

Two suggested risk management models stress the importance of involvement in risk management. The NRC 1983 model incorporates analysis (traditional risk assessment) along with deliberation (communication, discussion, and debate) [41]. The advantage of this framework is that it requires input from both scientists and stakeholders. The second framework is the U.S. Presidential/Congressional Commission of Risk Assessment and Risk Management's Framework for Environmental Health Risk Management (FEHRM). It views risk management as a six-stage cycle with stakeholder collaboration at the center, linking and interacting with all the other stages of risk assessment and management [42].

It is important to involve the public in risk management decisions. Experts should listen to the public because in a democratic society these stakeholders have a right to be heard; their views will reflect values about risks. This is currently lacking in the risk assessment approach. Allowing stakeholders to voice their opinion will also enhance communication. While this is initially time consuming, in the long run it will produce a more sound management plan. Finally, incorporating more diverse points of view will only enrich the final discussion and debate [41].

Public risk perception should be taken into account in decisions about risk management. When the public is concerned about a risk, risk managers should address these concerns by invoking additional protective measures. Further, risk management underlines that societal values and public willingness to accept a risk are key factors in determining a society's level of protection [43].

Even if the risk associated with a perceived hazard is low, the affected public will view it as unacceptable if industry officials have not shared information and allowed public involvement in project planning. Public participation in risk management offers many advantages to industry. It will provide an opportunity to defuse public anxiety associated with the technology, enhance public trust, improve industry credibility, create a positive working relationship between industry and the public, facilitate cooperation, and ultimately help the organization acquire regulatory approval. While this seems to be a logical step in project planning, it is not included in many management plans.

7.4.2 Public Meetings

While public meetings can provide a powerful forum for individuals and groups to voice their concerns, they are not encouraged for a number of reasons. For example, the majority of individuals may not have an opportunity to express their views, representation may be biased in terms of demographics, issues are often oversimplified, and there is not always time to properly convey ideas.

Citizen advocacy councils remedy some of these problems. They are a better medium for input of ideas and permit better communication, information exchange, and interaction between individuals. However, they require a large commitment of time and the councils may not represent the prevailing viewpoints. The success of these councils is also contingent upon the offending industry.

It is essential to have the full support of the industry. There are a number of ways that industry can improve the success of the process. They can hold public meetings early on and supplement public meetings with group discussions. Meetings should be held in neutral areas to enhance the comfort of all involved. It is important to evaluate the success of public participation and look for ways to improve the process. Industry representatives can assess the relationship between stakeholders—reviewing cooperation and conflict between the parties and how it was handled. This feedback will be helpful in managing future interactions between stakeholders.

7.4.3 Precautionary Approaches

There has been an increasing movement to consider precautionary approaches within a structured methodology for the management of risk in the face of scientific uncertainty. These approaches include both prudent avoidance and the precautionary principle. Prudent avoidance became an attractive option because it serves to minimize exposure to the perceived problem with minimal costs. For instance, no radical changes to power lines or wireless base stations should be implemented until science shows clear evidence that there is a health risk. By acting prudently, management can embrace a wide range of sensible actions that take into account the research results and community concerns.

The precautionary principle is another process that emerged in the 1970s in response to concerns about the extent to which complex and uncertain risks could be addressed within existing science and policy structures. Under this principle, any claim that an action might pose a risk to the environment or to people's health, however unjustified, seeks the initiator to prove that the action will do no harm before being allowed to act. One form of the principle dictates inaction when action may pose a risk. It can also involve choosing less risky alternatives when they are available and taking responsibility for potential risks.

The precautionary principle alters environmental policy-making by markedly changing the balance in the contest between opposing views on where to set the balance point when science is uncertain and the environment and human health are at stake [44]. This principle is an extremely conservative decision that leads to prudent actions in the face of uncertainty. It reflects the need to take action at reasonable expense and with reasonable consequences for a potentially serious risk without awaiting the results of scientific research. The precautionary principle has been incorporated into numerous international treaties and declarations throughout Europe and several other countries. In fact, Italy, Switzerland, and New Zealand have adopted it to help set precautionary limits for EM exposure.

7.4.4 PUBLIC UNDERSTANDING OF PRECAUTIONARY ACTIONS

There is currently little empirical work that has addressed the question of if, under what circumstances, and how the introduction of precautionary actions and advice affects public appreciations of risks, and of those managing those risks [45]. An extensive exploration of this issue has been provided by Burgess [46], who maintains that precautionary actions and advice do not reduce concern but rather exacerbate it, acting to increase protest activity and intensify media presentation of risk. Burgess argues in relation to mobile telecommunications: "While the data supporting mobile phone risk is illusory, our commitment to risk is quite real. The evidence has only a walk on part in a drama that is being propelled by feelings and beliefs derived from experience of society. Mobile phone risk derives authority not from science, but from the widespread expectation of destruction facing humanity and the wider precautionary climate surrounding human action. The call for additional research, therefore, is naive, at best. No study can ever hope to provide the definitive negative proof, and the necessary qualifications of any future work will only add uncertainty and fuel skepticism that something must be dangerous."

Whether public risk perception should be a stimulus for invoking precautionary measures in risk management is a sensitive question [47]. Opponents of this approach stress the point that risk management should be based on sound science using the best available scientific evidence. They assume that perceived risk differs from assessed risk in that it may more readily be manipulated. In addition, they fear that precautionary measures may undermine the scientific basis for the established exposure limits. In their view, precautionary measures for EMF should be adopted only with great care [43].

7.5 RISK COMMUNICATION

In today's world, technological change and uncertainty are constants. With increased demand by the public for greater transparency, it is essential that any communication involve a comprehensive discussion of the EM health risks as well as the technology itself. Key technological questions that must be answered in a concise manner are (1) How does EM technology function? (2) What power levels are used with EM sources? (3) What is the difference between thermal and nonthermal effects of EM fields? (4) What is the difference between EMF and RFR, and how do they differ with respect to their effects? When answering these questions, the experts should ensure that they classify questions and problems in terms of their importance to the communication partner and provide assistance in understanding.

Clear and effective discussions about EM technology will serve to facilitate further communication about the risks associated with EM fields. The next step involves the planning and organization of the stakeholder discussion. Clarification of the discussion's goals at the outset will enhance the process. These goals could include: (1) fair distribution of risks, (2) legitimizing risk-taking expectations, (3) awareness of the EM issue, and (4) knowledge of the interests, concerns, fears, and attitudes of other group members.

Effective communication demands a clear set of rules. It is essential that all members have the opportunity to express their viewpoint, discuss the views of others, respond to criticisms, and ask questions.

Since communication about EM technology will form an essential part of this process, it is important that the explanations provided are clear and unambiguous. Once this background has been firmly established, it will be easier to discuss the risks associated with EM technology [2].

7.5.1 ROLE OF COMMUNICATION IN RISK ASSESSMENT

When assessing the health risks of EM fields, scientists need to follow certain guidelines. This will ensure that the process is based on solid scientific principles and not influenced by any of the stakeholder groups. An exhaustive review of available data is necessary to ensure an accurate and comprehensive assessment. It would also be useful to document the procedures used to prepare the risk assessment, thereby allowing an evaluation of the entire process. Bailey also recommends a transparent evaluation to permit further scrutiny and evaluation by a broader audience. This will serve to strengthen the risk assessment. To further ease stakeholder apprehension, Bailey suggests that scientists acknowledge the uncertainties surrounding their claims and prepare their assessment using clear and unambiguous language.

7.5.2 ROLE OF COMMUNICATION IN RISK MANAGEMENT

Incorporating risk communication into models of risk management may appear to be more time consuming than simply relying on risk assessment. However, greater emphasis on communication in the long term can simplify matters.

Difficult situations are likely to arise and dealing with these in the early discussion or planning stages will only serve to enhance the overall risk management plan. Properly planned discussions will enhance credibility and provide greater understanding between the individuals within the group. It is essential to evaluate the effectiveness of the communication and note where improvements can be made.

For risk managers and risk communicators who seek to foster a low level of public concern until all answers are in, brochures and similar materials are unlikely to achieve that goal. The EM problem may be with us for a long time before science is able to provide the answers that risk managers and policy makers need to implement technical changes that will alter the public's exposure to EM fields. If the public is to become an effective partner in the future decisions about EM health and safety issues, they will need to become informed and aware of the state of the science. Though initial awareness of the science associated with EM health and safety research may bring an elevation of concern, that concern may leave in its wake a public better prepared to deal with uncertainties about EM exposure and consequences [48].

While society has become increasingly informed and educated about environmental issues and more demanding about consumer information access, people are still anxious about scientific and technological innovation. Genetically modified foods, cloning, bovine somatotrophin, and EM fields represent several of the recent advances that have the potential to create uneasiness amongst the general public simply because of poor communication.

The EM background environment must be carefully assessed. Because of more assertive consumer activism, there is widespread skepticism and uncertainty due to risk mismanagement. For instance, the public has not always been properly informed of the health risks associated with asbestos, tobacco, and silicone breast implants. All of these were initially believed to be safe.

The bovine spongiform encephalopathy (BSE or mad cow disease) scare in Britain has led to uneasiness among the public about things as basic as their own food and food-processing standards. In this milieu, it is easy to see how the alleged health effects of EM fields are equated with tobacco and BSE.

7.5.3 MEDIA COVERAGE

Conflicting safety reports from the experts and the sensationalistic media coverage frequently add to anxiety. Media reports often lack the scientific/industrial knowledge necessary to accurately assess the facts. Also, due to time and space constraints and the fact that sensationalism sells, there is often a biased presentation of the information.

Communicating with media is important. Currently, media reports are rarely reviewed by the source, unlike the peer review process in scientific publication. Media reports are mostly on the spotlight stories instead of those that weigh scientific evidence. In my opinion, accumulated misinformation from the media is the source of electrophobia in the general public. It is the responsibility and moral obligation of scientists to bring "verified" information to the public through the media [49].

Media coverage must also be carefully monitored. It is often irresponsible, using scare tactics to enhance arguments. Sensational headlines such as "my mobile gave me cancer" do little to dispel the myths of EM dangers. They fail to quantify the risks associated with EM fields, and their coverage often focuses on nontechnical issues. Reports often have an anti-industry tone. This is likely due to their information sources, rather than industrial experts. Scientists have an important role in shaping public perception because they are generally viewed as having greater credibility. It is the responsibility of scientists to provide accurate information to the media and balance the information flow between the media and activists [2].

7.5.4   ROLE OF INDUSTRY

A critical issue for industry and government is how to communicate with the public about EM exposure and its potential health risk. What models of risk can be used as a basis for risk communication, and how will the public react to new information about EM exposure [48]. Industry influences public perception, but not always in a positive way. The safety of new technology has not been properly addressed by industry; as a consequence, fears among the public are widespread. Industry is urged to take a more active role in public education to improve its failing credibility and avoid costly commercial consequences.

Industry should think carefully when communicating with the public. It is important to ensure the person or organization is experienced, listens to public concerns, has integrity, and communicates in simple language (not very technical or defensive). The communicator must be more responsible when reporting risks associated with EM technology. There is often uncertainty and disagreement among industry experts concerning the level of risk.

The importance of good risk communication between the industry and concerned residents is essential when one considers the problems encountered with mobile phones, base stations, and power lines. Base stations, for instance, continue to be a public concern even though cellular phones expose users to 1000 times stronger fields than the actual base stations [22]. People who do not use cellular phones will likely oppose the towers because they are exposed to some level of risk without any perceived benefits. While these stations are not constructed in residential areas, the public is still outraged because of poor relations with the service providers. Phone companies as yet do not recognize the merit of a monitoring service to ease public concern, particularly because it is too expensive. As a result, the public continues to protest and the construction of new phone towers has been halted.

The WHO EMF program has been instrumental in bridging the gap between the media, industry, scientists, and the general public. WHO's publications have provided valuable and readily accessible information to the concerned parties.

7.5.5   ROLE OF THE INTERNET

One way to effectively communicate EM risk to the public is through the Internet. The Internet can be used to gather resources, ask questions, and provide an opportunity for the public to become skilled interveners. It facilitates exchanges between experts and the stakeholders and forces industry to be open and accountable. Despite its many advantages, the public must exercise caution when reviewing Internet resources. Not all information is peer reviewed and some may be simply anecdotal in nature. Since activists maintain many of the sites, the information may be biased.

7.5.6   COMMUNICATION WITH CHILDREN

There is a wealth of research on potential health hazards of EM fields, but very little is targeted specifically at children. Not a lot of information is available with regard to specific EM field communication to adolescents and children [50]. Few websites have been identified that are more or less oriented to inform adolescents.

These include three websites from: Belgium [51], Switzerland [52], and Canada [53]. Information on EM fields needs to be converted in material suitable for different age groups. An EM communication strategy and material for children and adolescents are scarce and need to be further developed.

7.6   TRENDS AND FUTURE RESEARCH

In spite of a vast array of studies investigating the association between EM fields and human health, a number of unresolved issues still remain. The unresolved issues continue to raise public concern that there could be some degree of risk from EM exposure. These concerns influence risk management and public acceptance of scientific health risk assessments. Reasonable risk management should build on evidence stemming from both risk assessments and insights from social studies that investigate this concern through well-organized research.

7.6.1   CHALLENGES AND IMPLICATIONS

At the scientific level, characterization of potential adverse health effects associated with exposure to EM fields has been difficult. Science has been under fire for not addressing the key issues surrounding this risk. However, we should learn that scientific research on possible hazards and risk assessment process should start from the very beginning of every new technological development. Following extensive efforts by the scientific community, including well-funded broad-based research programs coordinated by national and international organizations, epidemiological and toxicological studies conducted to date have provided ambiguous evidence of human health hazards.

The management of EM risks is complicated not only by scientific uncertainty about the level of potential risk, but also by public perceptions of risk. Public concern is heightened by a lack of understanding of EM fields, which cannot be seen or sensed, but are ubiquitous in our environment. Public concerns may also be heightened by media reports on EM fields, which are generally not based on a comprehensive evaluation of the weight of scientific evidence in support of a documented population health risk, but rather on reports of individual studies that might attract the attention of the public.

What is needed is greater public involvement in the risk-management decision-making process, including both individuals and stakeholder groups. Participation in the development of an appropriate risk management strategy can go a long way toward the achievement of consensus solutions that enjoy the support of interested and affected parties, even if all participants do not fully understand all of the scientific complexities involved in the evaluation of risk. With technologically based risks, such as those that may be associated with EM fields, industry has a particular responsibility to take a leadership role in open participatory discussions on risk management strategies. As risk management options are debated, consideration will need to be given to the level of risk that might be associated with exposure to EM fields and the attendant scientific uncertainty about EM risks. In addition to considering risk, social values and economic costs and benefits will require consideration [2].

The evaluation and management of potential human health risks from EM fields presents many challenges. When the scientific database is ambiguous, as is the case with EM fields, expert judgment of the overall weight of scientific evidence becomes particularly important. Because of this uncertainty about EM risks, the public is more likely to experience difficulty in evaluating the available information and rely more on perceptions than facts when drawing conclusions. Effective risk communication techniques assume even greater importance in issues such as EM fields than in cases where risks are more clearly delineated and the need for risk mitigation actions more obvious. However, since even the most effective risk communication techniques are not likely to clarify all of the subtleties surrounding EM fields as a population health issue, it is important that all stakeholders in this issue participate in developing consensus solutions.

7.6.2 RESEARCH AND POLICY

Risk assessment research is one of the costs of bringing new technologies into society. The present response of society is ponderous and often features a barely hidden contest involving manufacturers, government, and the public. Manufacturers face conflict in trying to establish the safety of a product but avoid the taint of hazard that can come just by doing the research. Parties in government or the public may be poised to believe there is hazard and to be suspicious of biases introduced by the manufacturer's self-interest. In the present system, these conflicts often produce a protracted tug-of-war before research can begin [44].

The results of Chapters 3, 4, 5, and 6 have revealed that there is no conclusive and consistent evidence to suggest exposure to EM fields at levels below the recommended safe limits can cause cancer and other adverse health effects. However, in recognition of widespread debate and conflicting views—particularly in the contexts of public health and environmental protection—government, scientists, and industry should take effective research and policy actions to address the concerns about potential health risks of EM energy. These actions may include:

- Independent and unbiased research to further our understanding of the potential EM health risks.
- Transparency and full divulgence of data on EM emissions from various sources.
- Public access to the most up-to-date research on biological and health effects associated with EM fields.
- Scientific risk assessment that goes beyond technical issues and identifies a need for psychometric approach—including cognitive, emotional, and social demographic determinants of risk.
- Thorough risk assessment and research projects with a potential to discover even the smallest of health risks with aims and results to be well communicated to all stakeholders.
- Public participation in risk management actions taken in response to concerns about the potential health risks of EM fields.
- Assessment of the impact of precautionary measures on public concern and the adoption of voluntary or mandatory policies.
- Adequate communication with individuals and groups on the various levels of scientific uncertainty.

7.6.3 Concluding Remarks

As the development of science and technology advances and as we are enjoying a better quality of life, it is required from scientists to ensure that safety is not compromised. Scientists must be very careful in reporting their findings. Mistakes must be minimized and stopped at the first level of scientific research.

In closing, I would like to summarize Part I of this book and make a good reason to start Part II with this conclusion made by Chou C-K [49]: "After more than 50 years of studies looking for EMF bioeffects, it is time for the bioelectromagnetics research community to clarify the identified gaps in knowledge on EM bioeffects as listed in the WHO research agenda and move on to study what EM fields can do for people. Dr. d'Arsonval would have been pleased to learn that what he started in the late 19th century on medical applications of EM fields holds promise for much fruit in the 21st Century."

REFERENCES

1. WHO. *WHO Handbook on Establishing a Dialogue on Risks from Electromagnetic Fields*. Geneva: World Health Organization, 2002.
2. Brodsky LM, Habash RWY, Leiss WL, Krewski D, Repacholi M. Electromagnetic fields and possible health risk. Part III: Risk analysis. *Crit Rev Biomed Eng* 2003; 31: 333–354.
3. Moghissi AA, Straja SR, Love BR. The role of scientific consensus organizations in the development of standards. *Health Phys* 2003; 84: 533–537.
4. AAES. Statement on risk analysis: the process and its application. American Association of Engineering Societies. *Technol J Franklin Institute* 1996; 333 (A): 95–106.
5. Krewski D, Hogan V, Birkwood P, McDowell I, Losos J. An integrated framework for risk management and population health, Draft 17, Institute of Population Health, University of Ottawa, Canada, 2003.
6. Von Winterfeldt D, Eppel T, Adams J, Neutra R, DelPizzo V. Managing potential health risk from electric powerlines: a decision analysis caught in controversy. *Risk Anal* 2004; 24: 1487–1502.
7. Kuster N, Schuderer J, Christ A, Futter P, Ebert S. Guidance for exposure design of human studies addressing health risk evaluations of mobile phones. *Bioelectromagnetics* 2004; 25: 524–529.
8. NRC. *A Study of the Isolation System for Geologic Disposal of Radioactive Wastes*. National Research Council. Washington, DC: National Academy Press, 1983.
9. Blank M. The precautionary principle must be guided by EMF research. *Electromag Biol Med* 2006; 25: 203–208.
10. Repacholi MH, Cardis E. Criteria for EMF health risk assessment. *Radiat Prot Dosim* 1997; 72: 305–312.
11. Portier C, Wolfe M, Editors. *Assessment of health effects from exposure to power line frequency electric and magnetic fields*. National Institute of Environmental Health Sciences (NIEHS) Working Group Report of the National Institute of Health, NIH Publication No. 98-3981:50, Research Triangle Park, N.C., 1998.
12. Repacholi MH, Greenebaum B. Interaction of static and extremely low frequency electric and magnetic fields with living systems: health effects and research needs. *Bioelectromagnetics* 1999; 20: 133–160.
13. Schütz H, Wiedemann P. How to deal with dissent among experts? Risk evaluation of EMF in a scientific dialogue. *J Risk Res* 2005; 8: 531–545.

14. Habash RWY. *Electromagnetic Fields and Radiation: Human Bioeffects and Safety.* New York: Marcel Dekker, 2001.

15. Habash RWH, Brodsky LM, Leiss W, Krewski DK, Repacholi M. Health risk of electromagnetic fields. Part II: Evaluation and assessment of electric and magnetic fields. *Crit Rev Biomed Eng* 2003; 31: 141–195.

16. Habash RWH, Brodsky LM, Leiss W, Krewski DK, Repacholi M. Health risk of electromagnetic fields. Part II: Evaluation and assessment of radio frequency radiation. *Crit Rev Biomed Eng* 2003; 31: 197–254.

17. Habash RWY. Electromagnetics—the uncertain health risks. *IEEE Potentials* 2003; 22: 23–236.

18. Habash RWY. Foreseeable health risk of electric and magnetic field residential exposure. *Energy Environ* 2003; 14: 473–487.

19. Chou CK. Basic problems of diversely reported biological effects of radio frequency fields. *Radiats Biol Radioecol* 2003; 43: 512–518.

20. Barnes F. Setting standards in the presence of developing scientific understanding. *Electromag Biol Med* 2006; 25: 209–215.

21. NIEHS. *Report on health effects from exposure to power-line frequency electric and magnetic fields.* National Institute of Environmental Health Sciences (NIEHS) Working Group Report of the National Institute of Health. NIH Publication No. 99-4493, Research Triangle Park, N.C., 1999.

22. Byus CV, Glickman BW, Krewski D, Lotz WG, Mandeville R, McBride ML, Prato FS, Weaver DF. *A Review of the Potential Health Risks of Radiofrequency Fields from Wireless Telecommunication Devices.* Ottawa: Royal Society of Canada, 1999.

23. IEGMP. *Mobile Phones and health. Independent Expert Group on Mobile Phones.* Independent Expert Group on Mobile Phones, National Radiological Protection Board, Chilton, Didcot, Oxon, UK, 2000.

24. Krewski D, Byus CV, Glickman BW, Lotz WG, Mandeville R, McBride ML, Prato FS, Weaver DF. Potential health risks of radiofrequency fields from wireless telecommunication devices. *J Toxicol Environ Health* 2001; 4: 1–143.

25. NRPB. *ELF electromagnetic fields and risk of cancer.* Report of an Advisory Group on Non-Ionising Radiation, National Radiological Protection Board, Doc. NRPB 12(1): 1-179, Chilton, Didcot, Oxon, UK, 2001.

26. Health Council of the Netherlands. Mobile telephones: an evaluation of health effects. The Hague: Health Council of the Netherlands, Publication No. 2002/OIE, 2002.

27. Neutra R, DelPizzo V, Lee GM. *An Evaluation of the Possible Risks from Electric and Magnetic Fields (EMF) from Power Lines, Internal Wiring, Electrical Occupations, and Appliances.* Oakland, CA: California EMF Program, 2002.

28. IARC. Non-ionizing radiation, Part 1: Static and extremely low-frequency (ELF) electric and magnetic fields. International Agency for Research on Cancer. Monographs on the Evaluation of Carcinogenic Risks to Humans. Report No. 80, Lyon, France, 2002.

29. Repacholi M, Saunders R, van Deventer E, Kheifets L. Is EMF a potential environmental risk for children? *Bioelectromag Suppl* 2005; Suppl 7: S2–S4.

30. Vecchia, P. Perception of risks from electromagnetic fields: lessons for the future. *J Biol Phys* 2003; 29: 269–274.

31. Bradbury JA. The policy implications of differing concepts of risk. *Sci Tech Hum Values* 1989; 14: 380–389.

32. Morgan MG, Slovic P, Nair I, Geisler D, MacGregor D, Fischhoff B, Lincoln D, Florig K. Powerline frequency electric and magnetic fields: a pilot study of risk perception. *Risk Anal* 1985; 5: 139–149.

33. Furby L, Slovic P, Fischhoff B, Gregory R. Public perceptions of electric power transmission lines. *J Environ Psychol* 1988; 8: 19–43.

34. Read D, Morgan G. The efficacy of different methods for informing the public about the range dependency of magnetic fields from high voltage power lines. *Risk Anal* 1998; 18: 603–610.
35. Wiedemann PM, Clauberg M, Schutz H. Understanding amplification of complex risk issues: the risk story model applied to EMF case. In: Pidgeon N, Kasperson RE, Slovic P, Editors. *The Social Amplification of Risk*. Cambridge: Cambridge University Press, pp. 286–301, 2003.
36. Kasperson RE, Renn O, Slovic P, Brown HS, Emel J, Goble R, Kasperson JX, Ratick S. The social amplification of risk: a conceptual framework. *Risk Anal* 1988; 8: 177–187.
37. Berqvist U, Vogel E. Possible health implications of subjective symptoms and electromagnetic fields. A report prepared by a European group of experts for the European Commission, DG V. *Arbete Och Halsa* 1997; 19: 1–45.
38. Head G. *Collected Assays in Risk Management*. Malvern, PA: Insurance Institute of America, 1986.
39. Fischhoff B, Lichtenstein S, Slovic P, Derby SL, Keeney R. *Acceptable Risk*. New York: Cambridge University Press, 1983.
40. Love BR, Straja SR, Moghissi AA. *Manual for Stakeholder Participation*. Columbia, MD: Institute for Regulatory Science, 2002.
41. NRC. *Understanding Risk: Informing Decisions in a Democratic Society*. National Research Committee on Risk Characterization. National Research Council. Washington, DC: National Academy Press, 1996.
42. Presidential/Congressional Commission on Risk Assessment and Risk Management. Framework for Environment Health Risk Management. Final Report 1. Washington, DC, 1997.
43. Wiedemann PM, Schutz H. The precautionary principle and risk perception: experimental studies in the EMF area. *Environ Health Perspec* 2005; 4: 402–405.
44. Balzano Q, Sheppard AR. The influence of the precautionary principle on science-based decision-making: questionable applications to risks of radiofrequency fields. *J Risk Res* 2003; 5: 351–569.
45. Timotijevic L, Barnett J. Managing the possible health risk of mobile telecommunications: public understanding of precautionary action and advice. *Health Risk Soc* 2006; 8: 143–164.
46. Burgess A. *Cellular Phones, Public Fears, and a Culture of Precaution*. Cambridge: Cambridge University Press, 2006.
47. Goldstein B, Carruth RS. The precautionary principle and/or risk assessment in World Trade Organization decisions: a possible role for risk perception. *Risk Anal* 2004; 24: 491–499.
48. MacGregor DG, Slovic P, Morgan G. Perception of risks from electromagnetic fields: a psychometric evaluation of a risk-communication approach. *Risk Anal* 1994; 14: 815–828.
49. Chou C-K. Thirty-five years in bioelectromagnetics research. *Bioelectromagnetics* 2007; 28: 3–15.
50. Martens L. Electromagnetic safety of children using wireless phones: a literature review. *Bioelectromagnetics* 2005; 27: S133–S137.
51. Belgian Government, 2007. http://www.infogsm.be.
52. Research Foundation Mobile Communication, 2007. http://www.emf-info.ch.
53. McLaughlin Centre for Population Health Risk Assessment, Institute for Population Health, University of Ottawa, 2007. http://www.wirc.org.

Part II

Therapeutic Applications of Electromagnetic Energy

8 Electromagnetic Therapy

8.1 INTRODUCTION

Advances in electronics and electromagnetic theory have set the stage for an unprecedented drive towards the development of medical devices with various diagnostic and therapeutic applications. RF (hundreds of kilohertz to a few megahertz) and microwaves (hundreds of megahertz to approximately 10 gigahertz) are forms of nonionizing radiation, unlike much higher frequencies (above visible light) in the EM spectrum, which are ionizing. Therapies using EM sources at RF and microwave frequencies have been called thermal therapy. These therapies have been applied in a number of frequency regions along the EM spectrum, as shown in Figure 8.1. Included among these thermotherapies are hyperthermia and thermal ablation.

Thermotherapy, or thermal therapy, encompasses all therapeutic treatments based on the transfer of thermal energy into or out of the body. In clinical settings, the major objective of thermal therapy is to achieve efficacious treatment outcome without damaging normal tissues. The extent of initial tissue necrosis is predominantly determined by the thermal power and energy applied to the tissue before charring [1]. The use of heat alone or in combination with radiotherapy or chemotherapy to increase direct ablation of tumors is the subject of Part II of this book.

In recent years, a range of medical applications based on various sources of energy, especially EM power, have been widely investigated [2–4]. Owing to the wide range of possible therapeutic effects, thermal therapy is practiced with considerably large variations in methodology based on geography as well as subdisciplines within the medical community [5]. Several books, handbooks, and review papers providing good background information on thermal therapy have been published over the years. Michaelson and Lin [6] reviewed biological effects and health implications of RF radiation. Thuery [7] described the ISM applications of microwaves. Rosen and Rosen [8] discussed a number of topics related to microwave therapeutic medicine. Polk and Postow [9] reviewed biological effects of EM fields. Habash [10] discussed human bioeffects and safety consideration related to EM fields. Rosen et al. [3] highlighted medical applications of RF/microwaves with emphasis on emerging diagnostic and therapeutic applications, such as microwave breast cancer detection and treatment with localized high power used in ablation of the heart and liver, benign prostate hypertrophy, angioplasty, and others. Habash et al. [11] reviewed and evaluated the literature on acute and long-term health risks associated with RF radiation. Dewhirst et al. [12] presented an overview on the carcinogenic effects of hyperthermia alone or combined with known carcinogens, such as ionizing radiation and chemical carcinogens. Stauffer and Goldberg [5] introduced thermal ablation therapy, covering a range of ablation articles included in a special issue on the same subject published by the *International Journal of Hyperthermia*.

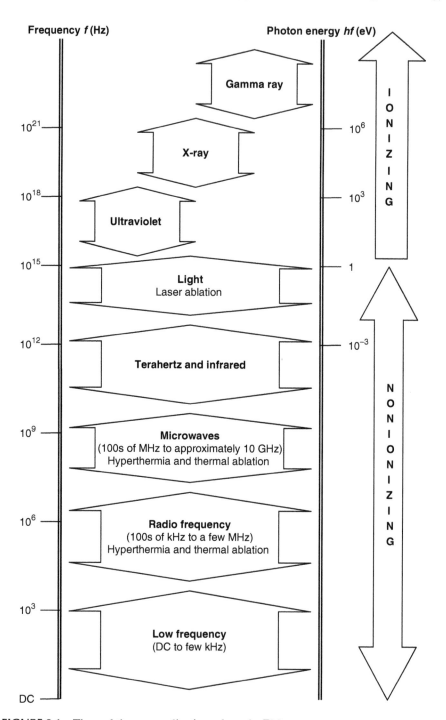

FIGURE 8.1   Thermal therapy applications along the EM spectrum.

Haveman et al. [13] overviewed the current knowledge about effects of hyperthermia at temperatures used in clinical oncology on the peripheral nervous system. Stauffer [14] reviewed the technology used for thermal therapy of cancer, with emphasis on the evolution of equipment from basic single-element devices of the early 1980s to adjustable multielement heating devices in use or in the final stage of development. Vander Vorst et al. [4] addressed the needs of today's engineering community with an interest in the use of RF and microwave energy in public health and in medicine. The authors devoted one chapter of their book to thermal therapy and another chapter to delivery systems for therapeutic applications. Ayrapetyan and Markov [15] edited a book covering a very broad range of frequencies and amplitudes in 24 articles arranged in four chapters: Mechanisms of EM Interactions with Biological Systems, EM Therapy, EM Dosimetry, and Epidemiology and Policy.

In general, thermal therapy is categorized into three different modalities according to the temperature level and time duration.

1. Diathermia. Heating up to 41°C with applications in physiotherapy for the treatment of rheumatic diseases.
2. Hyperthermia. The temperature of a part of the body or of the whole body can be raised to a higher than normal level (41–45°C), which may allow other types of cancer treatments (radiation therapy or chemotherapy) to work better. This type of hyperthermia has applications in oncology for cancer treatment and will be investigated in Chapter 9.
3. Thermal ablation. Very high temperature (above 45°C) can be used to destroy cells within a localized section of a tumor. This is commonly used in oncology for cancer treatment, in urology for benign prostatic hyperplasia (BPH) treatment, and in cardiology for heart stimulations and other areas. Thermal ablation using RF and microwave techniques are discussed in Chapter 10.

8.2   HISTORY OF ELECTROMAGNETIC THERAPY

The use of thermal energy for a therapeutic purpose dates back thousands of years. In the splendor of the Roman Empire, thermal baths constituted a habit, often with complete facilities for the treatment of diseases involving the use of humid and dry heat in local or general applications. Probably the oldest report related to thermal therapy was found in the Egyptian Edwin Smith surgical papyrus, dated around 3000 BC. Researchers like to cite Hippocrates (460–370 BC) in particular, although the method he describes in one of his aphorisms, i.e., hot irons, involves higher temperatures, such as those used in cauterization. In the nineteenth and twentieth centuries, fever therapy has been used as a method to increase temperature, while other investigators started to apply RF techniques in medicine [16].

The modern discipline of thermal therapy emerged from a number of radiation-biology-oriented laboratories in the mid-to-late 1970s [17]. Studies on cell cultures and experimentally induced tumors *in vivo* provided convincing justification for the clinical application of heat. The rationale is based on a direct cell-killing effect at temperatures above 41–42°C [18]. At higher temperatures, equivalent levels of killing can be achieved with shorter exposure times.

Two key papers, published in the mid-1980s, attracted attention to the opportunity to assess the efficacy of cell killing with heat [19,20]. These papers established the first concepts for thermal dosimetry and indicated that significant cell killing could occur if cells or tissues were heated to more than 42°C for 1 h or more. The application of heat has continued to increase in sophistication. Initially, treatments were limited to very cold (ice) or very hot (cautery) temperatures that could not be controlled but were maintained for a sufficient time to obtain visually obvious effects on surface tissues. Over time, there has been renewed interest in therapeutic applications of hot and cold temperature, primarily due to limitations of conventional therapeutic modalities (surgery, chemotherapy, and radiotherapy) and improvements in devices and techniques used to deliver and monitor the effect of energy [5,21,22].

Overall, enthusiasm for thermal therapy waned significantly in the mid-to-late 1990s, partly as a result of the perceived difficulties in achieving adequate treatment as defined by the need to kill cells directly by heating [23]. The problem that was faced by the thermal therapy community at that juncture was unrealistic thermal goals because of the lack of adequate equipment for delivering thermal treatment and inability to measure the treatment delivered. A combination of the above difficulties is still a challenge to the design and implementation of successful clinical trials [24].

8.3   MECHANISM OF THERMAL INJURY

Tissue injury caused by heat occurs in two distinct phases. The initial phase is direct heat injury that is predominantly determined by the total energy applied to the tumor, tumor biology, and tumor microenvironment [1]. The mechanisms of direct thermal injury and thermosensitivity involve complex interactions within tumor tissue at cellular and subcellular levels. The cell membrane appears to be the cellular component most vulnerable to heat injury.

The significance of Joule heating as a mode of injury can be estimated by first determining the tissue temperature as a function of time. Tropea and Lee [25] simulated the Joule heating dynamics using a numerical method to solve the bioheat equation [26]. Joule heating density is the product of the electrical conductivity and the time average square of the electric field. *In vitro* [27] and *in vivo* [28] studies demonstrate that tumor cells are destroyed at lower temperatures than normal cells.

The second phase is indirect injury after focal hyperthermia application that produces a progression in tissue damage. This progressive injury may involve a balance of several factors including microvascular damage, ischemia-reperfusion injury, induction of apoptosis, Kupffer cell activation, altered cytokine expression, and modulation of the immune response [29]. The effects of heat depend on the tissue temperatures attained, determined by the total thermal energy applied, rate of removal of heat, and the specific thermal sensitivity of the tissue (Table 8.1) [29].

Classical hyperthermia relies on a temperature of 42–45°C for periods of 30–60 min to cause irreversible cellular damage [30]. As the tissue temperature rises to 60°C the time required to achieve irreversible cellular damage decreases exponentially. Protein denaturation occurs between 60 and 140°C and leads to immediate cell

TABLE 8.1
Effect of Temperature on Biological Tissues

Temperature Range (°C)	Time Requirements	Physical Effects	Biological Effects
<-50	>10 min	Freezing	Complete cellular destruction
0–25		Decreased permeability	Decreased blood perfusion; decreased cellular metabolism; hypothermic killing
30–39	No time limit	No change	Growth
40–46	30–60 min	Changes in the optical properties of tissue	Increased perfusion; thermotolerance induction; hyperthermic killing
47–50	>10 min	Necrosis, coagulation	Protein denaturation; no subtle effects
<50	After ~2 min	Necrosis, coagulation	Cell death
60–140	Seconds	Coagulation, ablation	Protein denaturation; membrane rupture; cell shrinkage
100–300	Seconds	Vaporization	Cell shrinkage and extracellular steam vacuole
<300	Fraction of a second	Carbonization, smoke generation	Carbonization

death. Vaporization of tissue water is superimposed on this process between 100 and 300°C. In addition, carbonization, charring, and smoke generation occurs at 300–1000°C [31].

The underlying physical principles and engineering aspects of heating mechanisms have been described in a number of review articles [1,12,22,32–39] and books [1,4,16,29,40–42]. In a comprehensive review of the literature, Dewhirst et al. [38] summarized the basic principles that govern the relationships between thermal exposure (temperature and time of exposure) and thermal damage, with an emphasis on normal tissue effects. Methods for converting one time–temperature combination to a time at a standardized temperature are provided as well as a detailed discussion about the underlying assumptions that go into these calculations. This review makes it clear that much more work needs to be done to clarify what the thresholds for thermal damage are in humans.

8.4 THERMAL THERAPY TREATMENT PROTOCOL

Thermal therapy is currently implemented as a minimally invasive alternative to traditional surgery in the treatment of benign disease and cancer, as well as repair of sport injuries and tissue reshaping or modification [17]. Thermal ablation, thermal coagulation, hyperthermia, and thermotherapy are terms often used to describe the use of heat to directly modify or destroy tissues [14]. Figure 8.2 shows the schematic range for thermal therapies.

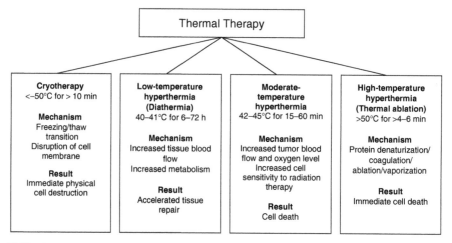

FIGURE 8.2 Schematic range of thermal therapies.

Throughout Part II, we will use the following protocols that describe thermal therapy:

1. Cryoablation [temperature (T) $<-50°C$ for time (t) >10 min]
2. Hyperthermia:
   a. Long-term low-temperature hyperthermia ($40–41°C$ for 6–72 h)
   b. Moderate-temperature hyperthermia ($42–45°C$ for 15–60 min)
3. High-temperature hyperthermia or thermal ablation ($>50°C$ for $>4–6$ min)

It is important to stress that thermal ablation and moderate-temperature hyperthermia should be viewed as complementary forms of thermal therapy. Based on realistic limitations of each approach, neither form of therapy is likely to replace the other. The uniqueness of thermal ablation is the ability to treat a tumor with a defined volume in sites where surgery itself is difficult (e.g., liver) or where organ function preservation is needed or desired (e.g., prostate, uterus). However, this form of therapy will find little use for large bulky tumors such as colorectal cancer primaries, soft tissue sarcomas, head and neck nodules, and superficial disease involving the skin. Whether a consequence of tumor size or infiltrative disease with borders that are difficult to define, there are applications that require more subtle moderate-temperature hyperthermia as opposed to complete ablation to preserve surrounding critical normal tissue structures [5]. Figure 8.3 shows the challenges to the development of thermal therapy.

8.5 POSSIBLE SIDE EFFECTS OF ELECTROMAGNETIC ENERGY AND HEAT

It has been known for some time that high intensities of nonionizing radiation can be harmful due to the ability of its energy to heat biological tissue rapidly. This is the principle by which microwave ovens cook food, and exposure to high EM power densities, i.e., on the order of 100 mW/cm² or more, can result in heating of

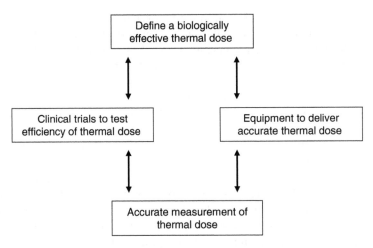

FIGURE 8.3 Challenges to the development of thermal therapy.

the human body. Tissue damage can result primarily because of the body's inability to cope with or dissipate the excessive heat. The amount of damage in tissue as a result of heating is dependent upon both temperature and time. On a different note, Osepchuk and Petersen [43] have noted that millions of people experienced strong EM exposures via clinical diathermy during the last century with only beneficial consequences.

8.5.1 TISSUE PHYSIOLOGY AND RESPONSE TO HEAT

Heat causes numerous subtle changes in tissue physiology, such as increased blood perfusion, vascular permeability, and metabolic activity. The most important physiological parameter in this context is blood flow. When any tissue is heated, various physiological changes occur—the majority of which are secondary to changes in blood flow [44–46]. Blood flow is also one of the major vehicles by which heat is dissipated from tissues; thus the tissue blood supply will have a significant influence on the ability to heat tissues [47]. The lower the rate of blood flow, the easier it is to heat. Although solid tumors can have blood flow values that can be greater than those of certain normal tissues, when compared to normal tissues the tumor blood supply is generally primitive and chaotic in nature, which can result in areas that are nutrient-deprived, low in oxygen, and highly acidic; cells that exist in these adverse conditions are generally more sensitive to the cytotoxic effect of heat [46].

Toxicity of heat generated during thermal therapy in general is low. Burns represent typical thermal therapy associated toxicity with low incidence [48], which can be avoided via correct heating techniques. The primary hazards of thermal therapy are due to either increased body core temperature or increased temperature in specific organs. Regulation of body core is critical in humans because numerous cellular structures and metabolic pathways are affected by changes in temperature. Body core temperatures range from 36 to 38°C, but may increase during, for example, exercise or humid weather. Normally, in healthy persons such excursions seldom exceed 39°C. Compared with other species, humans are especially adept at dissipating heat through increased blood flow and increased sweating over most of the body surface [49]. Most healthy people can tolerate body core temperature excursions up to 40°C when adequately hydrated. At higher temperatures (42–43°C), cellular death begins.

The molecular-biological mechanisms of health effects are still under investigation. Increases in temperature result in increases in molecular motion in cells, tissues, and organs. The increased molecular motion in turn increases chemical reaction rates. If reaction rates within steps of a metabolic process become unbalanced, metabolism may be altered. The activation energies of metabolic reactions are low, of the order of 3–20 kcal/mol. For short duration heat exposures, it was thought that unbalanced metabolism would be transitory and, therefore, unlikely to cause permanent damage. Long periods of unbalanced metabolism could cause permanent, irreversible damage, but there is currently no scientific evidence for this hypothesis [49]. Because EM exposure may produce hyperthermia, it is necessary to delineate whether any observed effects are specific to EM exposure or if they were simply a result of the hyperthermia attendant on EM exposure [50].

8.5.2   Cellular Responses

Various targets in the cell affected by rises in temperature have been found, such as cell activity, growth rate, membranes, the cytoskeleton, synthesis of macromolecules, the cell cycle, regulating molecular functions such as apoptosis, and DNA repair [51–54].

The cell growth rate increases with increasing temperature to some maximum temperature above which growth is sharply inhibited [55–57]. In the hyperthermic region above the maximum growth temperature, there are three significant cellular responses for thermal therapy: cytotoxicity, radiosensitization, and thermotolerance [58,59]. These changes at the cellular level must be due to temperature-induced alterations in molecular pathways. These usually involve inhibition of DNA, RNA, and protein synthesis [58]. While protein synthesis is inhibited during heating at higher temperatures, at milder temperatures and after return to normal growth temperature the induction of heat-shock protein (HSP) occurs [60]. This is an inducing event and closely associated with the induction of thermotolerance. The role of these proteins in neurodegenerative disease and in suppression of neuronal apoptosis led to a strongly enhanced interest in these proteins [61,62].

Hyperthermia may induce both regional and systemic production of cytokines through activation of inflammatory cells. The release of tumor necrosis factor (TNF) is well described after whole-body hyperthermia (WBH) [63]. Increased levels of TNF have direct cytotoxic effects, can induce tumor endothelial injury, and sensitize tumor cells to heat-induced damage [64,65].

A number of studies have documented the adverse effects of hyperthermia on the normal adult testis in several species, including mouse [66], rat [67], and human [68,69]. The reported effects include a temporary reduction in relative testis weight accompanied by a temporary period of partial or complete infertility [70,71]. Sperm quality has also been shown to suffer, with a reduction in progressive sperm motility and a significantly lower *in vitro* fertilization rate of oocytes by sperm from heat-shocked males [70,72].

Studies have shown heat-dependent immunological reactions of human leukocytes [73] and effects on natural killer cells and cytokine depletion [74].

8.5.3 Immunological Effects

The possibility of hyperthermia-induced inhibition of the host immune system must be considered when heat is used clinically for cancer treatment [75]. WBH appears to enhance the synergistic and antiproliferative activities of gamma-interferon, leading to an upgrading of immune surveillance [76,77]. However, this effect is reversed at temperatures greater than 42°C [78]. Whether some of the changes described in WBH occur with focal hyperthermia remains unknown [1].

Heat-shock proteins are the most abundant and ubiquitous soluble intracellular proteins. They are recognized as significant participants in immune reactions. Hyperthermia induces overexpression of HSP at the expense of inhibiting the synthesis of many other proteins, including cytosketetal and regulatory proteins that may be crucial for normal cellular functions. For example, heat may alter the normal body immuno-response by altering thymocyte [79] and leukocyte [76] production as well as inducing T-lymphocyte propagation [80]. Ito et al. [81] suggested that HSP70 is an important modulator of tumor cell immunogenicity and that hyperthermic treatment of tumor cells can induce the host antitumor immunity via the expression of HSP70. These results may benefit further efforts on developing novel cancer immunotherapies based on hyperthermia. Other studies demonstrated a dual role of thermotolerance and immune stimulation of HSPs [82,83]. Ivarsson et al. [84] used an implantation model of colorectal liver metastases to identify increased expression and change in the localization of HSP70 at 10–15 h after laser ablation. It is postulated that increased HSP tumor petite complexes following focal hyperthermia are involved in tumor antigen presentation to macrophages and other antigen presenting cells. The immunological properties of HSPs enable them to be used in new immunotherapies of cancers and infections [85,86].

Milani and Noessner [87] reviewed the topic and concluded: "We emphasize that the response to thermal stress is not a one-time point event, but rather a time period starting with the heat exposure and extending over several days of recovery. In addition, the response of tumor cells and their susceptibility to immune effector cells is strongly dependent on the model system, the magnitude and duration of the thermal stress, and the time of recovery after heat exposure. Consideration of these aspects might help to explain some of the conflicting results that are reported in the field of thermal stress response."

8.5.4 Cardiovascular Responses

Cardiovascular strain and heat-related disorders are quite common, especially in people unaccustomed to heat. Some people are particularly susceptible to the adverse effects of heat, especially the elderly, who are at increased risk of coronary thrombosis in these circumstances, and infants and people with certain medical conditions or taking certain medications [49].

When body temperature rises, heat balance of the body is normally restored by increased blood flow to the skin and by sweating. These responses increase the work of the heart and cause loss of salt and water from the body. They impair working efficiency and can overload the heart and cause hemoconcentration, which can lead to coronary and cerebral thrombosis, particularly in elderly people with atheromatous arteries. These adverse effects of thermoregulatory adjustments occur with even mild heat loads and account for the great majority of heat-related illness and death. Donaldson et al. [88] reviewed the basic thermoregulatory physiology of healthy people in relation to hazards from external heat stress and internal heat loads generated by physical exercise or RF radiation. The authors concluded that exposure to RF exposure levels currently recommended as safe for the general population, equivalent to heat loads of about one-tenth basal metabolic rate, could continue to be regarded as trivial in this context, but that prolonged exposures of the general population to RF exposure levels higher than that could not be regarded as safe in all circumstances.

Gong et al. [89] found that WBH promotes cardiac protection against ischemia/reperfusion injury, in part by up-regulation of HSP. Their experiments on rats subject to WBH at 42°C for 15 min showed that sublethal heat stress can lead to up-regulation of both vascular endothelial growth factor (VEGF) and HSP70 in cardiac tissue, and promote focal endothelial proliferation in the heart. The above finding is supported by a previous study [90].

Compared with animals, humans are exceptionally well adapted to dissipate excess heat; in addition to a well-developed ability to sweat, which in humans can be produced over most of the body surface, the dynamic range of blood flow rates in the skin is much higher than in other species [91]. Most deaths caused by heat are not due to hyperthermia, but to loss of water and salt in sweat, leading to hemoconcentration. This makes the blood more prone to clot and so leads to increased incidence of coronary and cerebral artery thrombosis in elderly people. The importance of this is that any degree of heat exposure sufficient to cause sweating, from any source, will carry a risk to humans [49].

8.5.5 Nervous System Responses

The nervous tissues appear critically sensitive to heat, with a possibility of damage and changes in nerve morphology for nerve conduction and nerve function [13]. Most studies on the effects of hyperthermia on nervous system have focused on the heat-shock response, characterized by the transient induction of HSPs, which play a role in repair and protective mechanisms [92]. Although interspecies variations may play a role, the data indicate that the maximum heat dose without obvious complications after localized hyperthermia in regions of the CNS lies in the range of 40–60 min at 42–42.5°C or 10–30 min at 43°C [93].

A review of the literature on the effects of intermediate- and low-level EM radiation shows that exposure at relatively low SAR (less than 2 W/kg) under certain conditions could affect the nervous system [94–97]. This includes effects on BBB, morphology, electrophysiology, neurotransmitter activity, and metabolism.

Takahashi et al. [98] induced WBH in dogs by extracorporeal heating of blood, to determine the effects 7 days after hyperthermia on the canine brain and spinal cord. The thermal dose resulted in neither microscopic damage to the CNS nor neurological symptoms, as determined by comparison of microscopic and neurological findings with those of dogs whose brain and spinal cord temperatures were maintained at 37°C for 60 min. The findings suggest that, for medical purposes, WBH appears promising for application at a thermal dose of up to 42°C for 60 min.

Histopathological data show that the myelin sheath, which is important for nerve conduction, is the most vulnerable part of the nerve fiber. Hoogenveen et al. [99] observed many demyelinated axons 1 week after heat treatment for 30 min at 44°C. Sasaki and Ide [100] observed demyelinated axons after heating a part of the rat spinal cord.

Studies on nerve conduction 1 h after 30-min [101] or 60-min [102] treatment at 45°C showed a significant decrease in amplitudes and conduction velocities, possibly because of edema and early demyelination. Hogenveen et al. [103] showed that nerve function remained normal for the first few hours after treatment for 30 min at 45°C.

For the CNS, irreversible damage was found after treatment at 42–42.5°C for longer than 40–60 min [104]. Exposure of rats at 38°C for 4 h results in cellular damage in several parts of the brain [49]. Effects of whole-body and localized heating on the CNS are discussed by Sharma and Hoopes [105].

Clinically, Bull et al. [106] studied nerve conduction in four patients with neuropathy after WBH and observed a pattern of scattered demyelination. Haveman et al. [93] indicated in an overview that there are no clear experimental data pointing out an increase in adverse effects specific to the CNS after localized or WBH as a result of combined treatment with chemotherapy.

8.5.6 CARCINOGENIC EFFECTS

With respect to the behavioral effects of heat in humans, it has been shown that cognitive performance is affected well before the physiological tolerance limits are reached. Data from laboratory animals describe the disruption of ongoing vigilance behavior by imposed EM fields [49]. D'Andrea et al. [107] reviewed the literature concerning EM exposure and behavioral and cognitive effects. They conclude: "Reports of change of cognitive function (memory and learning) in humans and laboratory animals are in the scientific literature. Mostly, these are thermally mediated effects, but other low-level effects are not so easily explained by thermal mechanisms. The phenomenon of behavioral disruption by microwave exposure, an operationally defined rate decrease (or rate increase), has served as the basis for human exposure guidelines since the early 1980s and still appears to be a very sensitive EM bioeffect."

Prior to discussing the problems associated with thermal therapy, it should be pointed out that unlike ionizing radiation and toxic drug therapy, nonionizing radiation such as EM fields has not been found to have a mutagenic effect [108,109]. It is now widely agreed that cancer is initiated by alterations in the genetic material (DNA) in the cell (geotaxis effects), although some nongeotaxis chemicals and processes (called epigamic carcinogens) have been recognized. Alterations in genetic material can occur if there is breakage in the DNA, leading to a single- or double-stranded breaks. Studies to investigate whether EM radiation produce genetic effects have been performed on various animal cells and tissue cultures. The results of the studies did not yield any reliable or systematic evidence that RF or microwaves can induce any mutation in living systems other than through induction of heat; it is known that the rate of induction of mutations increases with increasing temperature.

Carcinogenesis is known to follow a multistep process that can be categorized into four main steps: initiation, promotion, malignant conversion, and tumor progression [12,110]. Although hyperthermia alone is not carcinogenic, it may enhance the development of tumors induced by ionizing radiation [111–113]. However, several investigators have examined whether or not hyperthermia alone can cause cancer by causing chromosomal aberrations [114–117], DNA double-strand breaks [118–120], and mutation [121–124].

The controversy over whether EM radiation might initiate or promote cancer continues to receive a great deal of attention, both in the popular press and in the biomedical literature [125] Conflicting reports appear in the literature, suggesting that hyperthermia treatment (via a water bath) can either serve as an antipromoter [126,127] or as a promoter [128], depending on the treatment regimen.

Studies of possible genotoxic effects of EM exposure, enhanced cell proliferation, and inappropriate gene expression have been carried out at the cellular level. In addition, there have been a number of long-term studies of cancer induction in animals, including tests of epigenetic interaction with known carcinogens [129]. Along the years, several studies have investigated potential carcinogenic effects of EM exposure on mammary cancer [130,131], liver cancer [132], lymphoma [133], and brain cancer [134].

8.6   CONCLUDING REMARKS

The primary goal of this chapter was to introduce current concepts of thermal therapy as generally as possible, with a collection of topics that will further expand the usefulness of this therapy and translate thermal technology into clinical practice. It is necessary, however, to provide a superficial covering for the topics while leaving in-depth discussions to subsequent chapters.

8.6.1   Risk Assessment

Thermal therapy techniques are becoming more acceptable as a minimally invasive alternative for the treatment of some cancers and other forms of benign diseases [17]. However, evaluation of human exposure risk to EM sources or the corresponding heat, especially in patients and personnel working in this field, is a difficult task because it involves many physical, biological, and chemical variables. In this chapter, we were largely concerned with the thermal effects of EM exposure. Thermal effects are produced by energy transfer from radiation to tissues, varying with frequency of operation, mostly governed by dielectric loss—the loss that is proportional to the intensity of radiation. In general, elevated temperatures have obvious effects on humans such as cataracts (opacity), increased blood pressure, dizziness, weakness, disorientation, nausea, or a faint pain. Heating the human body, either the whole or part of the body, may affect physiology, particularly the heart and circulatory system. It may induce other thermoregulatory responses, such as sweating, or various heat-related disorders, such as heat stroke.

It should be mentioned that based on the long history of EM exposure in humans, it is reasonably certain that exposures below MPE values have no credible reported adverse health effects and are medically safe [11,135]. Some epidemiological studies addressing possible links between EM exposure and excess risk of cancer have reported positive findings for leukemia and brain tumors. However, in some of these studies there are significant difficulties in assessing the relationship between disease incidence and EM exposure, and with potential confounding factors such as ELF fields and chemical exposure [12].

When considering the impact of EM-induced heating on carcinogenesis, the problem is that there are few or no data from studies using high EM exposures to produce thermal responses, particularly with respect to the initiation, promotion or copromotion of cancer. Studies involving higher thermal exposures from heat alone do suggest modulation of both initiating and promoting events in carcinogenesis. However, the issue is complex [128]. How such data affect the establishment of standards for EM exposure is a challenge [12]. The thermogenic effects of EM energy have been well documented and summarized as follows [136,137]:

1. Biological effects due to thermoregulatory response occur when a living body is thermally loaded at a rate equal to its basal metabolic rate (BMR).
2. Numerous behavioral and endocrine effects, and cardiac and respiratory changes for SARs below the BMR, are manifestations of physiological responses to mild thermal stress.
3. Thermal stress resulting from about twice the BMR, when maintained over long periods of time, leads to significant physiological effects.
4. Responses to thermal load from pulsed fields appear to be the same as the responses to continuous fields of the same average power.
5. It is also important to mention that heat may cause a positive as well as negative effect in the integrated body system.

8.6.2 Trends in Equipment Development

While thermal therapy requires investment in equipment and personnel training, the same is true for other types of therapies. In spite of the required investments, the economic evaluation of thermal therapy can be within an acceptable range. The most important technical areas of thermal therapy development can be specified as follows [137]:

1. Optimization of new heating devices for more effective local, intracavitary, and regional treatment.
2. Integration of noninvasive monitoring capabilities and treatment planning for thermal therapy with the evolving heating systems to dramatically improve clinical efficacy.
3. Utilization of existing technology in clinical settings and encouragement of equipment developers to produce devices for new clinical applications.

4. Acceleration of training programs for physicians and physics staff to make efficient use of the available technology.
5. Further development of fast and dynamic imaging techniques for guidance and monitoring in clinical treatment.

8.6.3 FUTURE RESEARCH DIRECTIONS

Future research should examine, in addition to the above technical advancements, various efforts, including among others [5,12,49,137]:

1. Mechanisms of how cells react to changes in their thermal environment and clarification of thresholds for thermal damage in humans.
2. Accurate EM and thermal dosimetry including further investigations in the following fields: (a) modeling power deposition and estimation of EM energy absorbed by tissues exposed to EM radiation, (b) electrical-thermal modeling for thermal therapy with various models of heat transfer in living tissues, and (c) models of EM energy deposition in humans combined with appropriate models of the human thermoregulatory responses to predict the potential hazards associated with specific EM exposure conditions.
3. Human and animal studies on (a) CNS changes in heat-related illnesses using quantitative immunopathological techniques at the cellular and ultrastructural levels, (b) effect of EM exposure on cognitive performance, (c) effect of prolonged or chronic exposure at ambient temperatures ($<41°C$), and (d) carcinogenic risk of heat, especially for low-temperature hyperthermia.

REFERENCES

1. Nikfarjam M, Muralidharan V, Christophi C. Mechanisms of focal heat destruction of liver tumors. *J Surg Res* 2005; 127: 208–223.
2. Strezer F. Microwave medical devices. *IEEE Microwave Mag* 2002; 3: 65–70.
3. Rosen A, Stuchly MA, Vander Vorst A. Applications of RF/microwaves in medicine. *IEEE Trans Microw Theory Tech* 2002; 50: 963–974.
4. Vander Vorst A, Rosen A, Kotsuka Y. *RF/Microwave Interaction with Biological Tissues*. New York: Wiley-IEEE Press, 2006.
5. Stauffer PR, Goldberg SN. Introduction: thermal ablation therapy. *Int J Hyperthermia* 2004; 7: 671–677.
6. Michaelson S, Lin, JC. *Biological Effects and Health Implications of Radio Frequency Radiation*. New York: Plenum, 1987.
7. Thuery J. *Microwaves—Industrial, Scientific and Medical Applications*. Norwood, MA: Artech House, 1992.
8. Rosen A, Rosen HD. *New Frontiers in Medical Device Technology*. New York: Wiley, 1995.
9. Polk C, Postow E. *Handbook of Biological Effects of Electromagnetic Fields*. Boca Raton, FL: CRC Press, 1996.
10. Habash RWY. *Electromagnetic Fields and Radiation: Human Bioeffects and Safety*. New York: Marcel Dekker, 2001.
11. Habash RWH, Brodsky LM, Leiss W, Krewski DK, Repacholi M. Health risk of electromagnetic fields. Part II: Evaluation and assessment of radio frequency radiation. *Crit Rev Biomed Eng* 2003; 31: 197–254.

12. Dewhirst MW, Lora-Michiels M, Viglianti BL, Dewey WC, Repacholi M. Carcinogenic effects of hyperthermia. *Int J Hyperthermia* 2003; 19: 236–251.

13. Haveman J, Van der Zee J, Wondergem J, Hoogeveen JF, Mulshof MC. Effects of hyperthermia on the peripheral nervous system: a review. *Int J Hyperthermia* 2004; 20: 371–391.

14. Stauffer PR. Evolving technology for thermal therapy of cancer. *Int J Hyperthermia* 2005; 21: 731–744.

15. Ayrapetyan S, Markov M. *Bioelectromagnetics: Current Concepts.* Dordrecht: Springer-Verlag, 2006.

16. Seegenschmiedt MH, Vernon CC. A historical perspective on hyperthermia in oncology. In: Seegenschmiedt MH, Fessenden P, Vernon CC, Editors. *Thermoradiotherapy and Thermochemotherapy*, Vol. 1. Berlin: Springer-Verlag, pp. 3–44, 1995.

17. Diederich CJ. Thermal ablation and high-temperature thermal therapy: overview of technology and clinical implementation. *Int J Hyperthermia* 2005; 21: 745–753.

18. Dewey WC. Arrhenius relationships from the molecule and cell to the clinic. *Int J Hyperthermia* 1994; 10: 457–483.

19. Field SB, Morris CC. The relationship between heating time and temperature: its relevance to clinical hyperthermia. *Radiother Oncol* 1983; 1: 179–186.

20. Sapareto SA, Dewey WC. Thermal dose determination in cancer therapy. *Int J Radiat Oncol Biol Phys* 1984; 10: 787–800.

21. Short JG, Turner PF. Physical hyperthermia and cancer therapy. *Proc IEEE* 1980; 68: 133–142.

22. Cheung AY. Microwave hyperthermia for cancer therapy. *IEEE Proc* 1987; 34: 493–522.

23. Dewhirst MW, Griffin TW, Smith AR, Parker RG, Hanks GE, Brady LW. Intersociety Council on Radiation Oncology essay on the introduction of new medical treatments into practice. *J Natl Cancer Inst* 1993; 85: 951–957.

24. Dewhirst MW, Vujaskovic Z, Jones E, Thrall D. Re-setting the biologic rationale for thermal therapy. *Int J Hyperthermia* 2005; 21: 779–790.

25. Tropea BI, Lee RC. Thermal injury kinetics in electrical trauma. *J Biomech Eng* 1992; 114: 241–250.

26. Pennes HH. Analysis of tissue and arterial blood temperatures in the resting human arm. *J Appl Physiol* 1948; 1: 93–122.

27. Dickson JA, Calderwood SK. Temperature range and selective sensitivity of tumors to hyperthermia: a critical review. *Ann N Y Acad Sci* 1980; 335: 180–205.

28. Overgaard K, Overgaard J. Investigations on the possibility of a thermic tumor therapy. I. Short-wave treatment of a transplanted isologous mouse mammary carcinoma. *Eur J Cancer* 1972; 8: 65–78.

29. Nikfarjam M, Muralidharan V, Christophi C. Focal hyperthermia produces progressive tumor necrosis independent of the initial thermal effects. *J Gastrointest Surg* 2005; 9: 410–417.

30. Welch AJ, Motamedi M, Rastegar S, Le Carpentier GL, Jansen D. Laser thermal ablation. *Photochem Photobiol* 1991; 53: 815–823.

31. Germer CT, Roggan A, Ritz JP, Isbert C, Albrecht D, Muller G, Buhr HJ. Optical properties of native and coagulated human liver tissue and liver metastases in the near infrared range. *Lasers Surg Med* 1998; 23: 194–203.

32. Guy AW, Lehmann J, Stonebridge JB. Therapeutic applications of electromagnetic power. *IEEE Proc* 1974; 62: 55–75.

33. Christensen DA, Durney CH. Hyperthermia production for cancer therapy: a review of fundamentals and methods. *J Microw Power* 1981; 16: 89–105.

34. Fessenden P, Hand JW. Hyperthermia therapy physics. In: Smith AR, Editor. *Medical Radiology: Radiation Therapy Physics.* Berlin: Springer-Verlag, pp. 315–363, 1995.

35. Roemer RB. Engineering aspects of hyperthermia therapy. *Ann Rev Biomed Eng* 1999; 1: 347–376.

36. Gel'vich EA, Mazokhin VN. Technical aspects of electromagnetic hyperthermia in medicine. *Crit Rev Biomed Eng* 2001; 29: 77–97.

37. Moroz P, Jones SK, Gray BN. Magnetically mediated hyperthermia: current status and future directions. *Int J Hyperthermia* 2002; 18: 267–284.

38. Dewhirst MW, Viglianti BL, Lora-Michiels M, Hanson M, Hoopes PJ. Basic principles of thermal dosimetry and thermal thresholds for tissue damage from hyperthermia. *Int J Hyperthermia* 2003; 19: 267–294.

39. Haemmerich D, Laeseke PF. Thermal tumour ablation: devices, clinical applications and future directions. *Int J Hyperthermia* 2005; 21: 755–760.

40. Nussbaum GH, Editor. *Physical Aspects of Hyperthermia*. New York: American Association of Physicists in Medicine, 1982.

41. Field SB, Hand JW, Editors. *An Introduction to the Practical Aspects of Clinical Hyperthermia*. London: Taylor & Francis, 1990.

42. Gautherie M, Editor. *Methods of External Hyperthermia Heating*. Berlin: Springer-Verlag, 1990.

43. Osepchuk JM, Petersen RC. Safety and environmental issues. In: Golio M, Editor. *Modern Microwave and RF Handbook*. Boca Raton, FL: CRC Press, pp. 3.28–3.43, 2001.

44. Song CW. Effect of hyperthermia on vascular functions of normal tissues and experimental tumors. Brief communication. *J Natl Cancer Inst* 1978; 60: 711–713.

45. Vaupel P, Kallinowski F. Physiological effects of hyperthermia. In: Streffer C, Editor. *Recent Results in Cancer Research*. Vol. 104. Heidelberg: Springer-Verlag, pp. 71–109, 1987.

46. Horsman MR. Tissue physiology and the response to heat. *Int J Hyperthermia* 2006; 22: 197–203.

47. Patterson J, Strang R. The role of blood flow in hyperthermia. *Int J Radiat Oncol Biol Phys* 1979; 5: 235–241.

48. Vernon CC, Hand JW, Field SB, Machin D, Whaley JB, Van der Zee J, van Putten WL, van Rhoon GC, van Dijk JD, Gonzalez Gonzalez D, Liu FF, Goodman P, Sherar M. Radiotherapy with or without hyperthermia in the treatment of superficial localized breast cancer: results from five randomized controlled trials. International Collaborative Hyperthermia Group. *Int J Radiat Oncol Biol Phys* 1996; 35: 731–744.

49. Goldstein LS, Dewhirst MW, Repacholi M, Kheifets L. Summary, conclusions and recommendations: adverse temperature levels in the human body. *Int J Hyperthermia* 2003; 19: 373–384.

50. Nelson DA, Nelson MT, Walters TJ, Mason PA. Skin heating effects of millimeter-wave irradiation—thermal modeling results. *IEEE Trans Microw Theory Tech* 2000; 48: 2111–2120.

51. Fajardo LE, Egbert B, Marmor J, Hahn GM. Effects of hyperthermia in the malignant tumor. *Cancer* 1980; 45: 613–623.

52. Dikomy E, Franzke J. Effect of heat on induction and repair of DNA strand breaks in X-irradiated CHO cells. *Int J Radiat Biol* 1992; 61: 221–234.

53. Sakaguchi Y, Stephens LC, Makino M, Kaneko T, Strebel FR, Danhauser LL, Jenkins GN, Bull JM. Apoptosis in tumors and normal tissues induced by whole body hyperthermia in rats. *Cancer Res* 1995; 55: 5459–5464.

54. Roti Roti JL, Kampinga HH, Malyapa RS, Wright WD, van der Waal RP, Xu M. Nuclear matrix as a target for hyperthermic killing of cancer cells. *Cell Stress Chaperones* 1998; 3: 245–255.

55. Sawaji Y, Sato T, Takeuchi A, Hirata M, Ito A. Anti-angiogenic action of hyperthermia by suppressing gene expression and production of tumour-derived vascular endothelial growth factor *in vivo* and *in vitro*. *Br J Cancer* 2002; 86: 1597–1603.

56. Lepock JR. How do cells respond to their thermal environment? *Int J Hyperthermia* 2005; 21: 681–687.

57. Lepock JR. Cellular effects of hyperthermia: relevance to the minimum dose for thermal damage. *Int J Hyperthermia* 2003; 19: 252–266.

58. Laszlo A. The effects of hyperthermia on mammalian cell structure and function. *Cel Prolif* 1992; 25: 59–87.

59. Kampinga HH, Dynlacht JR, Dikoney E. Mechanism of radiosensitization by hyperthermia ($\geq 43°C$) as derived from studies with DNA repair defective mutant cell lines. *Int J Hyperthermia* 2004; 20: 131–139.

60. Kregel KC. Heat shock proteins: modifying factors in physiological stress responses and acquired thermotolerance. *J Appl Physiol* 2002; 92: 2177–2186.

61. Sharp FR, Massa SM, Swanson RA. Heat-shock protein protection. *Trends Neurosci* 1999; 22: 97–99.

62. Sherman MY, Goldberg AL. Cellular defenses against unfolded proteins: a cell biologist thinks about neurodegenerative diseases. *Neuron* 2001; 29: 15–32.

63. Klostergaard J, Barta M, Tomasovic SP. Hyperthermic modulation of tumor necrosis factor-dependent monocyte/macrophage tumor cytotoxicity in vitro. *J Biol Response Mod* 1989; 8: 262–277.

64. Tomasovic SP, Klostergaard J. Hyperthermic modulation of macrophage-tumor cell interactions. *Cancer Metastasis Rev* 1989: 8: 215–229.

65. Isbert C, Ritz JP, Roggan A, Schuppan D, Ruhl M, Buhr HJ, Germer CT. Enhancement of the immune response to residual intrahepatic tumor tissue by laser-induced thermotherapy (LITT) compared to hepatic resection. *Lasers Surg Med* 2004; 35: 284–292.

66. Hand JW, Walker H, Hornsey S, Field SB. Effects of hyperthermia on the mouse testis and its response to X-rays, as assayed by weight loss. *Int J Radiat Biol* 1979; 35: 521–528.

67. Collins P, Lacy D. Studies on the structure and function of the mammalian testis. II. Cytological and histochemical observations on the testis of the rat after a single exposure to heat applied for different lengths of time. *Proc R Soc Lond B Biol Sci* 1969; 172: 17–38.

68. Baranski B. Effects of the workplace on fertility and related reproductive outcomes. *Environ Health Perspect* 1993; 1019 (suppl 2): 81–90.

69. Mieusset R, Bujan L. Testicular heating and its possible contributions to male infertility: a review. *Int J Androl* 1995; 18: 169–184.

70. Jannes P, Spiessens C, Van der Auwera I, D'Hooghe T, Verhoeven G, Vanderschueren D. Male subfertility induced by acute scrotal heating affects embryo quality in normal female mice. *Hum Reprod* 1998; 13: 372–375.

71. Setchell BP, D'Occhio MJ, Hall MJ, Laurie MS, Tucker MJ, Zupp JL. Is embryonic mortality increased in normal female rats mated to subfertile males? *J Reprod Fertil* 1998; 82: 567–574.

72. Rockett JC, Mapp FL, Garges JB, Christopher Luft J, Mori C, Dix DJ. Effects of hyperthermia on spermatogenesis, apoptosis, gene expression, and fertility in adult male mice. *Biol Reprod* 2001; 65: 229–239.

73. Shen RN, Lu L, Shidnia H, Hornback NB, Broxmeyer HE. Influence of elevated temperature on natural killer cell activity and lectin-dependent cytotoxicity of human umbilical cord blood and adult blood cells. *Int J Radiat Oncol Biol Phys* 1994; 29: 821–826.

74. Multhoff G, Botzler C, Jennen L, Schmidt J, Ellwart J, Issels R. Heat shock protein 72 on tumor cells: a recognition structure for natural killer cells. *J Immunol* 1997; 158: 4341–4350.

75. Yoshioka A, Miyachi Y, Imamura S. Immunological effects of in vitro hyperthermia. *J Clin Lab Immunol* 1989; 29: 95–97.

76. Roberts NJ Jr. Differential effects of hyperthermia on human leukocyte production of interferon-alpha and interferon-gamma. *Proc Soc Exp Biol Med* 1986; 183: 42–47.

77. Downing JF, Taylor MW, Wei KM, Elizondo RS. In vivo hyperthermia enhances plasma antiviral activity and stimulates peripheral lymphocytes for increased synthesis of interferon-gamma. *J Interferon Res* 1987; 7: 185–193.

78. Alfieri AA, Hahn EW, Kim JH. Role of cell-mediated immunity in tumor eradication by hyperthermia. *Cancer Res* 1981; 41: 1301–1305.

79. Mansoor S, Spano M, Baschieri S, Cividalli A, Mosiello L, Doria G. Effect of in vivo hyperthermia on thymocyte maturation and selection. *Int Immunol* 1992; 4: 227–232.

80. Moliterno R, Woan M, Bentlejewski C, Qian J, Zeevi A, Pham S, Griffith BP, Duquesnoy RJ. Heat shock protein-induced T-lymphocyte propagation from endomyo-cardial biopsies in heart transplantation. *J Heart Lung Transplant* 1995; 14: 329–337.

81. Ito A, Shinkai M, Honda H, Wakabayashi T, Yoshida J, Kobayashi T. Augmentation of MHC class I antigen presentation via heat shock protein expression by hyperthermia. *Cancer Immunol Immunother* 2001; 50: 515–522.

82. Asea A, Kraeft SK, Kurt-Jones EA, Stevenson MA, Chen LB, Finberg RW, Koo GC, Calderwood SK. HSP70 stimulates cytokine production through a CD14-dependent pathway, demonstrating its dual role as a chaperone and cytokine. *Nat Med* 2000; 6: 435–442.

83. Calderwood SK, Asea A. Targeting HSP70-induced thermotolerance for design of thermal sensitizers. *Int J Hyperthermia* 2002; 18: 597–608.

84. Ivarsson K, Myllymaki L, Jansner K, Bruun A, Stenram U, Tranberg KG. Heat shock protein 70 (HSP70) after laser thermotherapy of an adenocarcinoma transplanted into rat liver. *Anticancer Res* 2003; 23: 3703–3712.

85. Srivastava P. Roles of heat-shock proteins in innate and adaptive immunity. *Nat Rev Immunol* 2002; 2: 185–194.

86. Li Z, Menoret A, Srivastava P. Roles of heat-shock proteins in antigen presentation and cross-presentation. *Curr Opin Immunol* 2002; 14: 45–51.

87. Milani V, Noessner E. Effects of thermal stress on tumor antigenicity and recognition by immune effector cells. *Cancer Immunol Immunother* 2006; 55: 312–319.

88. Donaldson GC, Keating WR, Saunders RD. Cardiovascular responses to heat stress and their adverse consequences in healthy and vulnerable human populations. *Int J Hyperthermia* 2003; 19: 225–235.

89. Gong B, Asimakis GK, Chen Z, Albrecht TB, Boor PJ, Pappas TC, Bell B, Mota-medi M. Whole-body hyperthermia induces up-regulation of vascular endothelial growth factor accompanied by neovascularization in cardiac tissue. *Life Sci* 2006; 79: 1781–1788.

90. Gowda A, Yang CJ, Asimakis GK, Ruef J, Rastegar S, Runge MS, Motamedi M. Cardioprotection by local heating: improved myocardial salvage after ischemia and reperfusion. *Ann Thorac Surg* 1998; 65: 1241–1247.

91. Kheifets L, Repacholi A, Saunders R. Thermal stress and radiation protection principles. *Int J Hyperthermia* 2003; 19: 215–224.

92. Khan VR, Brown IR. The effect of hyperthermia on the induction of cell death in brain, testis, and thymus of the adult and developing rat. *Cell Stress Chaperones* 2002; 7: 73–90.

93. Haveman J, Smina P, Wondergem J, Van der zee J, Mulshof MCCM. Effects of hyper-thermia on the central nervous system: what was learnt from animal studies? *Int J Hyperthermia* 2005; 21: 473–487.

94. Lai H. Research on the neurological effects of nonionizing radiation at the University of Washington. *Bioelectromagnetics* 1992; 13: 513–526.

95. Dimbylow PJ. FDTD calculations of SAR for a dipole closely coupled to the head at 900 MHz and 1.9 GHz. *Phys Med Biol* 1993; 38: 361–368.

96. Dimbylow PJ, Mann JM. SAR calculations in an anatomically realistic model of the head for mobile communication transceivers at 900 MHz and 1.8 GHz. *Phys Med Biol* 1994; 39: 1527–1553.

97. Martens LJ, DeMoerloose C, DeWagter, DeZutter D. Calculation of the electromagnetic fields induced in the head of an operator of a cordless telephone. *Radio Sci* 1995; 30: 415–420.

98. Takahashi S, Tanaka R, Watanabe M, Takahashi H, Kakinuma K, Suda T, Yamada M, Takahashi H. Effects of whole-body hyperthermia on the canine central nervous system. *Int J Hyperthermia* 1999; 15: 203–216.

99. Hoogenveen JF, Troost D, Wondergem J, van der Krachi AH, Haveman J. Hyperthermic injury versus crush injury in the rat sciatic nerve: a comparative functional, histopathological and morphometrical study. *J Neurol Sci* 1992; 108: 55–64.

100. Sasaki M, Ide C. Demyelination and remyelination in the dorsal funiculus of the rat spinal cord after heat injury. *J Neurocytol* 1989; 18: 225–239.

101. De Vrind HH, Wondergem J, Haveman J. Hyperthermia-induced damage to rat sciatic nerve assessed in vivo with functional methods and with electrophysiology. *J Neurosci Methods* 1992; 45: 165–174.

102. Vujaskovic Z, Gillette SM, Powers BE, Larue SM, Gillete EL, Borak TB, Scott RJ, Ryan TB, Colacchio TA. Effects of intraoperative hyperthermia on peripheral nerves: neurological and electrophysiological studies. *Int J Hyperthermia* 1994; 10: 41–49.

103. Hogenveen JF, Troost D, van der Kracht AH. Wondergen J, Haveman J, Gonzalez Gonzalez D. Ultrastructural changes in the rat sciatic nerve after local hyperthermia. *Int J Hyperthermia* 1993; 9: 723–730.

104. Sminia P, Van der Zee J, Wondergem J, Haveman J. Effect of hyperthermia on the central nervous system: a review. *Int J Hyperthermia* 1994; 10: 1–130.

105. Sharma HS, Hoopes PJ. Hyperthermia induced pathophysiology of the central nervous system. *Int J Hyperthermia* 2003; 19: 325–354.

106. Bull JM, Lees D, Schuette W, Whang-Peng J, Smith R, Bynum G, Atkinson ER, Gottdiener JS, Gralnick HR, Shawker TH, DeVita VT, Jr. Whole body hyperthermia: a phase-I trial of a potential adjuvant to chemotherapy. *Ann Intern Med* 1979; 90: 317–323.

107. D'Andrea JA, Adair ER, de Lorge JO. Behavioral and cognitive effects of microwave exposure. *Bioelectromagnetics* 2003; 24: S39–S62.

108. Dhahi SJ, Habash RWY, Alhafid HT. Lack of mutagenic effects on conidia of aspergillus amstelodami irradiated by 8.7175 GHz microwaves. *J Microw Power* 1982; 17: 346–351.

109. Ned B, Hornback MD. Is the community radiation oncologist ready for clinical hyperthermia? *Radiographics* 1987; 7: 139–149.

110. Weston A, Harris CC. Chemical carcinogenesis. In: Bast RC, Kufe DW, Pollock RE, Weichselbaum RR, Holland JF, Frei E, Editors. *Cancer Medicine-5*. Hamilton: B.C. Decker, Inc., pp. 189–94, 2000.

111. Baker DG, Constable WC, Sager H. The effect of hyperthermia on radiation-induced carcinogenesis. *Radiat Res* 1988; 115: 448–460.

112. Sminia P, Haveman J, Jansen W, Hendriks JJ, van Dijk JD. Hyperthermia promotes the incidence of tumours following X-irradiation of the rat cervical cord region. *Int J Radiat Biol* 1991; 60: 833–845.

113. Sminia P, van der Kracht AHW, Frederiks WM, Jansen W. Hyperthermia, radiation carcinogenesis and the protective potential of vitamin A and N-acetylcysteine. *J Cancer Res Clin Oncol* 1996; 122: 343–350.

114. Eki T, Enomoto T, Murakami Y, Hanaoka F, Yamada M. Characterization of chromosome aberrations induced by incubation at a restrictive temperature in the mouse temperature-sensitive mutant tsFT20 strain containing heat-labile DNA polymerase alpha. *Cancer Res* 1987; 47: 5162–5170.

115. Mackey MA, Dewey WC. Time-temperature analysis of cell killing of synchronous G1 and S phase Chinese hamster cells in vitro. *Radiat Res* 1988; 113: 318–333.

116. Dewey WC, Li XL, Wong RS. Cell killing, chromosomal aberrations, and division delay as thermal sensitivity is modified during the cell cycle. *Radiat Res* 1990; 122: 268–274.

117. Li XL, Wong RS, Dewey WC. Thermal tolerance during S phase for cell killing and chromosomal aberrations. *Radiat Res* 1990; 122: 193–196.

118. Nevaldine B, Longo JA, Hahn PJ. Hyperthermia inhibits the repair of DNA double-strand breaks induced by ionizing radiation as determined by pulsed-field gel electrophoresis. *Int J Hyperthermia* 1994; 10: 381–388.

119. Wong RS, Dynlacht JR, Cedervall B, Dewey WC. Analysis by pulsed-field gel electrophoresis of DNA double-strand breaks induced by heat and/or X-irradiation in bulk and replicating DNA of CHO cells. *Int J Radiat Biol* 1995; 68: 141–152.

120. Wachsberger PR, Iliakis G. Hyperthermia does not affect rejoining of DNA double-strand breaks in a cell-free assay. *Int J Radiat Biol* 2000; 76: 313–326.

121. Lindquist S. Heat-shock proteins and stress tolerances in microorganisms. *Curr Opin Genet Dev* 1992; 2: 748–755.

122. Waters ER, Schaal BA. Heat shock induces a loss of rRNA-encoding DNA repeats in Brassica nigra. *Proc Natl Acad Sci USA* 1996; 93: 1449–1452.

123. Leonhardt EA, Trinh M, Forrester HB, Johnson RT, Dewey WC. Comparisons of the frequencies and molecular spectra of HPRT mutants when human cancer cells were X-irradiated during G1 or S phase. *Radiat Res* 1997; 148: 548–560.

124. Davidson JF, Schiestl RH. Cytotoxic and genotoxic consequences of heat stress are dependent on the presence of oxygen in *Saccharomyces cerevisiae*. *J Bacteriol* 2001; 83: 4580–4587.

125. Mason PA, Walters TH, DiGiovanni J, Beason CW, Jauchem JR, Dick EJ Jr, Mahajan K, Dusch SJ, Shields BA, Merritt JH, Murphy MR, Ryan KL. Lack of effect of 94 GHz radio frequency radiation exposure in an animal model of skin carcinogenesis. *Carcinogenesis* 2001; 22: 1701–1708.

126. Mitchel REJ, Morrison DP, Gragtmans NJ, Jevcak JJ. Hyperthermia and phorbol ester tumor promotion in mouse skin. *Carcinogenesis* 1986; 7: 1505–1510.

127. Mitchel REJ, Morrison DP, Gragtmans NJ. Tumorigenesis and carcinogenesis in mouse skin treated with hyperthermia during stage I or stage II of tumor promotion. *Carcinogenesis* 1987; 8: 1875–1879.

128. Mitchel RE, Morrison DP, Gragtmans NJ. The influence of a hyperthermia treatment on chemically induced tumor initiation and progression in mouse skin. *Carcinogenesis* 1988; 9: 379–385.

129. IEGMP. Mobile phones and health. National Radiological Protection Board. Chilton, Didcot, Oxon, UK, 2000.

130. Toler JC, Shelton WW, Frei MR, Merritt JH, Stedham MA. Long-term, low-level exposure of mice prone to mammary tumors to 435 MHz radiofrequency radiation. *Radiat Res* 1997; 148: 227–234.

131. Frei MR, Berger RE, Dusch SJ, Guel V, Jauchem JR, Merritt JH, Stedham MA. Chronic exposure of cancer-prone mice to low-level 2450 MHz radiofrequency radiation. *Bioelectromagnetics* 1998; 19: 20–31.

132. Imaida K, Taki M, Watanabe S, Kamimura Y, Ito T, Yamaguchi T, Ito N, Shirai T. The 1.5 GHz electromagnetic near-field used for cellular phones does not promote rat liver carcinogenesis in a medium-term liver bioassay. *Jpn J Cancer Res* 1998; 89: 995–1002.

133. Repacholi MH, Basten A, Gebski V, Noonan D, Finnie J, Harris AW. Lymphomas in Eμ-*Pim 1* transgenic mice exposed to pulsed 900 MHz electromagnetic fields. *Radiat Res* 1997; 147: 631–640.

134. Adey WR, Byus CV, Cain CD, Higgins RJ, Jones RA, Kean CJ, Kuster N, MacMurray A, Stagg RB, Zimmerman G. Spontaneous and nitrosourea-induced primary tumors of the central nervous system in Fischer 344 rats exposed to frequency-modulated microwave fields. *Cancer Res* 2000; 60: 1857–1863.

135. Feychting M, Ahlbom A, Kheifets L. EMF and health. *Ann Rev Public Health* 2005; 26: 165–189.

136. Tell RA, Harlen F. A preview of selected biological effects and dosimetric data useful for development of radiofrequency safety standards for human exposure. *J Microw Power* 1979; 14: 405–424.

137. Habash RWY, Bansal R, Krewski D, Alhafid HT. Thermal therapy, Part 1: An introduction to thermal therapy. *Crit Rev Biomed Eng* 2006; 34: 459–489.

9 Electromagnetic Hyperthermia

9.1 INTRODUCTION

The term hyperthermia broadly refers to either an abnormally high fever or the treatment of a disease by the induction of fever, as by the injection of a foreign protein or the application of heat [1]. Hyperthermia as a method of treating cancer has a long history. Many Greek and Roman physicians thought that if they could simply control body temperature they could cure all diseases. This included cancer, because the pathology of tumor development had been described in the Greek literature [2].

Hyperthermia may be defined more precisely as raising the temperature of a part of or the whole body above normal for a defined period of time. The amount of temperature elevation is on the order of a few degrees above normal temperature (41–45°C). The effect of hyperthermia depends on the temperature and exposure time. First, there is the curative, physiologically based therapy (physiological hyperthermia), which treats aches, pains, strains, and sprains. This is applied in multiple sessions, uses low temperature (e.g., below 41°C) for approximately an hour, has a reparative goal of accelerated tissue healing, and uses physiological mechanisms of increasing blood flow and metabolic rates [3]. At temperatures above 42.5–43°C, the exposure time can be halved with each 1°C temperature increase to give an equivalent cell kill [4]. Most normal tissues are undamaged by treatment for 1 h at a temperature of up to 44°C [5]. The main mechanism for cell death is probably protein denaturation, observed at temperatures >40°C, which leads to, among other things, alterations in multimolecular structures like cytoskeleton and membranes, and changes in enzyme complexes for DNA synthesis and repair [6].

The first paper on hyperthermia was published in 1886 [7]. According to the author, the sarcoma that occurred on the face of a 43-year-old lady was cured when fever was caused by erysipelas. Westermark [8] tried to circulate high-temperature water for the treatment of an inoperable cancer of the uterine cervix and the effectiveness was confirmed. In the early twentieth century, applied research was carried out together with basic research; however, since the heating method and temperature-measuring technology, for example, had not developed sufficiently at that time, the positive clinical application of hyperthermia treatment was not carried out. Therefore, surgeries, radiotherapy, chemotherapy, and so on, were dominant as therapy of tumors [9]. Worldwide interest in hyperthermia was initiated by the first international congress on hyperthermic oncology in Washington in 1975. In the United States, a hyperthermia group was formed in 1981, while the European Hyperthermia Institute was formed in 1983. In Japan, hyperthermia research started in 1978 and the Japanese Society of Hyperthermia Oncology was established in 1984.

This interest has followed a course that is usual for a new type of treatment. In the first decade there was a growing enthusiasm, reflected by an exponential increase in the number of papers and participants at meetings. Thereafter, the interest waned, due to disappointing clinical results from some of the first randomized studies, accompanied by reluctance among sponsoring authorities and hospital boards to support further research. Nowadays, there appears to be a renewed interest, thanks to several investigations demonstrating that the improvements in treatment outcome by adjuvant hyperthermia can be very substantial, provided that adequate heating procedures are used [10].

In the past decade, extensive studies have been performed in the field of hyperthermia, ranging from the mechanisms of thermal cell kill to clinical trials and treatments. A book series was initiated to summarize and pass on the many experimental and clinical studies in the field of hyperthermia [11–14]. Other books describing hyperthermia and its clinical applications have been authored or edited [9,15–20]. Several book chapters also focused on hyperthermia [21–25]. There is an increasing number of relevant published periodicals as well as a large number of scientific articles published in high-ranked journals that review physical background and technical realization of hyperthermia [26–49]. A large body of scientific and clinical literature demonstrating the effectiveness of hyperthermia, either alone or combined with radiotherapy or chemotherapy has been published during the past few years [50–68]. The increasing number of applications and clinical trials at universities, clinics, hospitals, and institutes prove the feasibility and applicability of clinical hyperthermia in cancer therapies [49].

The objective of this chapter is to outline and discuss the means by which electromagnetic (EM) energy and other techniques can provide elevation of temperature within the human body. Clinical hyperthermia falls under three major categories: localized, regional, and WBH. Because of the individual characteristic of each type of treatment, different types of heating systems have evolved. Hyperthermia may be applied alone or jointly with other modalities such as radiotherapy, chemotherapy, surgical treatment, immunotherapy, and so on. The chapter concludes with a discussion of challenges and opportunities for the future.

9.2 BIOLOGICAL RATIONALE

The clinical exploitation of hyperthermia was and still is hampered by technical limitations and the high degree of interdependency between technology, physiology, and biology [69,70]. Extensive biologic research has shown that there are sound biological reasons for using hyperthermia in the treatment of malignant diseases [35]. The biological rationale for the treatment of malignant disease by heat is mediated by various specific facts, including:

1. The survival of cells depends on the temperature and duration of heating in a predictable and repeatable way. For example, when the temperature increases, the survival rate of the cell becomes lower.
2. Tumor cell environment, such as hypoxia, poor nutrition, and low pH, while detrimental to cell kill by ionizing radiation, is beneficial to heat therapy.

3. Cells may develop resistance to subsequent heat following previous heat treatment. This condition is known as thermotolerance.
4. The differential sensitivity of normal and tumor cells to heat is dependent on cell type and environmental conditions.
5. Heat treatment enhances biological effect of both radiation and chemotherapy agents [9,34].

9.2.1 HEAT ALONE

The biological rationale is based on a direct cell-killing effect at temperatures above 41–42°C [6]. However, the thermal-dose response relation varies among cell lines and depends, furthermore, on microenvironmental factors such as pH [71]. Protein damage is the main molecular event underlying the biological effects of hyperthermia in the clinically relevant temperature range (39–45°C). The activation energies for protein denaturation and heat-induced cell death are within the same range [6]. Cellular and tissue level studies, both *in vitro* and *in vivo*, indicate that protein denaturation is the most likely thermal effect causing permanent irreversible damage [72]. Biophysical approaches [73–75] as well as work with model proteins [76,77] have directly shown that substantial protein denaturation occurs in the clinically relevant temperature range. As a result of denaturation, proteins are prone to aggregation. Without chaperones, these aggregates can have destructive consequences for many macromolecular structures and their functions [66].

The responses of tumors to hyperthermia involve both cellular and host-related factors. Experimentally, frequently it is not easy to separate these. When cells are exposed to elevated temperatures, they are inactivated in a time- and temperature-dependent fashion. Inactivation starts at 40–41°C, at least, for murine cells and tumors. At these low temperatures, cell inactivation continues for only a few hours; beyond that time, the surviving cells appear resistant to further exposure to such temperatures. Studies have shown that this is not a selection of heat-resistant subpopulations but that it results from the induction of a temporary resistance to heat. This transient phenomenon is referred to as thermotolerance. However, very prolonged heating at mild temperatures (41–42°C) overcomes this transient thermotolerance [78]. Above 43°C, for most rodent lines, inactivation is exponential with time and thus resembles cell inactivation by ionizing radiation. Human cells tend to be more resistant, and in some human tumor cell lines this temperature threshold is as high as 44.5°C. Hence, thermotolerance can develop during treatment of human lesions, since tumor temperatures only rarely exceed 44°C. At even higher temperatures, thermotolerance does not develop, but if the cells are returned to 37°C, within a few hours the surviving cells do become resistant. At temperatures between 41 and 42°C, human tumor cell lines may be more sensitive than rodent tumor cells, and a potential therapeutic advantage may be achieved with prolonged heating at these milder temperatures [79].

The development of thermotolerance is accompanied by the preferential synthesis (or *de novo* synthesis) of a series of proteins referred to as HSP. These molecules are the subject of intense study because of their importance in normal cell function and in various disease states [80]. Thermotolerance can also greatly modify the cells' response to some drugs, heat, and x-irradiation, but it does not seem to have much effect on the cells' response to x-irradiation alone [81].

In addition to thermotolerance, there is great variability in genetically deter-mined heat sensitivity of tumor cells. Heat-resistant variants of B16 melanoma cells and of a radiation-induced fibrosarcoma (RIF-1) have been isolated and character-ized. Very likely, many human neoplasms also contain subpopulations of resistant cells. The frequency of occurrence of such cells appears to be very low; however, there is no evidence of cross-resistance between heat sensitivity and x-irradiation or most anticancer drugs. Hence, genetically heat-resistant cells may be of little impor-tance during combination treatments with heat and radiation or chemotherapy.

9.2.2 HEAT AND RADIATION

Aggregation of nuclear protein damage is thought to be the central event by which heat makes cells more sensitive to radiation [74,82]. The synergy between heat and radiation, often expressed as thermal enhancement ratios (TER), is highest when the two modalities are given simultaneously. When heat precedes radiation, the synergy is lost when the time interval between the two modalities increases and this loss of TER nicely parallels the decline in protein aggregation [83].

Heat enhances the cytotoxicity of x-rays, in both a super additive and a comple-mentary fashion. Super additivity means an increased cytotoxicity observed over what would be expected on the basis of additivity of the two treatments and it is maximum when these are given simultaneously. It decays with time when the treat-ments are separated by more than 1–2 h, even less in some systems [15,35].

9.2.3 HEAT AND DRUGS

A lot of physiology-related features make a combination of heat and drugs very attractive. Moreover, heat can cause more than additive killing when combined with alkylating agents, nitrosureas, platinum drugs, and some antibiotics [84], although for some drugs only additive effects or even less than additive effects on cell death are found [66]. Most impressive are data for heat and cisplatin treatments. Synergistic cell killing has already been found at rather mild heat treatments [85].

When cells are exposed at elevated temperatures to drugs, their response is fre-quently very different from that seen at 37°C. Drugs whose rate-limiting reaction is primarily chemical (i.e., not involving enzymes) would, on thermodynamic grounds, be expected to be more efficient at higher temperatures. The rates of alkylation of DNA, or of conversion of a nonreactive species to a reactive one, can be expected to increase as the temperature increases. Tissue culture studies have shown this to be true for the nitrosoureas and cisplatin. For other drugs, there appears to be a threshold at or near 43°C. Below that temperature, drug activity is only mildly enhanced. At higher tem-peratures, however, cell killing proceeds at a greatly enhanced rate. The combination of chemotherapy with hyperthermia still deserves attention and has high potential [66].

9.3 TYPES OF HYPERTHERMIA

Hyperthermia is mostly applied within a department of radiation oncology under the authority of a radiation oncologist and a medical physicist. Hyperthermia is always implemented as part of a multimodal, oncological strategy, i.e., in combination with radiotherapy or chemotherapy [69]. The effectiveness of hyperthermia treatment is related to the temperature achieved during the treatment, as well as the length of treatment and cell and tissue characteristics [10,86]. To ensure that the desired temperature is reached, but not exceeded, the temperature of the tumor and surrounding tissues is monitored throughout the hyperthermia procedure [59,60]. The majority of the hyperthermia treatments are applied using external devices, employing energy transfer to tissues by EM technologies [87,88].

9.3.1 LOCAL HYPERTHERMIA

The success of hyperthermia as a treatment modality lies in the localization of the heat inside the cancerous tumor without causing thermal damage to surrounding normal tissues. In local hyperthermia, the aim is to increase mainly the tumor temperature while sparing surrounding normal tissue, using either external or interstitial modalities. Heat is applied to a small area, such as a tumor, using various techniques that can deliver energy to heat the tumor. Local hyperthermia treatment is a well-established cancer treatment method with a simple basic principle: If a rise in temperature to 42°C can be obtained for 1 h within a cancer tumor, the cancer cells will be destroyed. Primary malignant tumors have poor blood circulation, which makes them more sensitive to changes in temperature.

Local hyperthermia is performed with superficial applicators (RF, microwave, or ultrasound) of different kinds (waveguide, spiral, current sheet, etc.) placed on the surface of superficial tumors with a contacting medium (bolus). The resulting SAR distribution is subject to strong physical curtailment resulting in a therapeutic depth of only a few centimeters. The penetration depth depends on the frequency and size of the applicator, and typically the clinical range is not more than 3–4 cm. A system for local hyperthermia consisting of a generator, control computer applicator, and a scheme to measure temperature in the tumor is shown in Figure 9.1. The power is increased until the desired temperature is achieved.

The volume that can be heated depends on the physical characteristics of the energy source and on the type of applicator [89]. During local hyperthermia, the tumor temperatures are increased to levels that are as high as possible, as long as the tolerance limits of the surrounding normal tissues are not exceeded [10].

Candidates for local hyperthermia include chest wall recurrences, superficial malignant melanoma lesions, and lymph node metastases of head and neck tumors. Advancement in the delivery of local hyperthermia requires development of additional techniques for heating, expansion the tumor locations that can be treated adequately, and improvement of the existing systems [90–92].

9.3.1.1 External Local Hyperthermia

Heating of small areas (usually up to 50 cm²) to treat tumors that are in or just below the skin (up to 4 cm) may be achieved quite easily today. External local hyperthermia therapy may be used alone or in combination with radiation therapy for the treatment of patients with primary or metastatic cutaneous or subcutaneous superficial tumors (e.g., superficial recurrent melanoma, chest wall recurrence of breast cancer, and

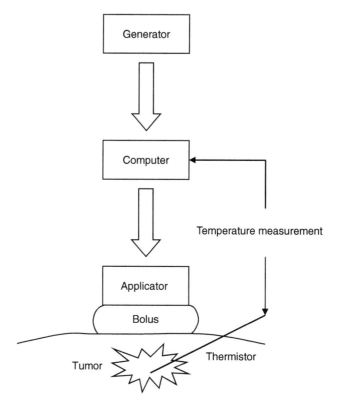

FIGURE 9.1   A diagram for local hyperthermia.

cervical lymph node metastases from head and neck cancer). Heat is usually applied using high-frequency energy waves generated from a source outside the body (such as a microwave or ultrasound source).

9.3.1.2   Intraluminal Local Hyperthermia

Intraluminal or endocavitary methods may be used to treat tumors within or near body cavities. Endocavitary antennas are inserted in natural openings of hollow organs. These include: (1) gastrointestinal (esophagus, rectum), (2) gynecological (vagina, cervix, and uterus), (3) genitourinary (prostate, bladder), and (4) pulmonary (trachea, bronchus) [51]. Very localized heating is possible with this technique by inserting an endotract electrode into lumens of the human body to deliver energy and heat the area directly. Various types of electrodes are available depending on the size of the lumen and the site of the lesion.

To improve the treatment results of locally advanced esophageal carcinoma, Sugimachi et al. [93–95], Kitamura et al. [96], and Saeki et al. [97] used intraluminal RF hyperthermia in addition to external irradiation and chemotherapy to treat inoperable cases and reported good therapeutic results. Fuwa et al. [98] developed an applicator enabling simultaneous intraluminal radiotherapy and intraluminal hyperthermia delivery to improve the treatment results for locally advanced esophageal carcinoma. Hyperthermia was delivered by a RF current thermotherapy instrument for 30 min at an output that raised the esophageal mucosal surface temperature to 42–43°C. Intraluminal radiotherapy was delivered to a submucosal depth of 5 mm after the first 15 min of hyperthermia. Four cases out of eight achieved complete response, with all demonstrating local control. Partial response was obtained in four cases and three of these patients died of local recurrence. There were no significant adverse side effects apart from a fistula in one case. The above work is a further improvement over previous work [99] involving a treatment by an applicator that simultaneously delivered an intraluminal high dose of iridium irradiation and intra-luminal RF hyperthermia.

Recently, Freudenberg et al. [100] measured the effect of hyperthermia applied through a heatable stent in the esophagus to investigate whether this procedure offers a therapeutic option for tumor treatment. The maximal heating temperature tolerated in the esophagi without transmural necrosis was 46.5°C, when applied twice for 60 min with a pause of 48 h. With this procedure, a tumor-damaging temperature of 42.5°C was achieved at a maximum distance of 12 mm surrounding the stent.

9.3.1.3   Interstitial Local Hyperthermia

Interstitial techniques are used to treat tumors deep within the body, such as brain tumors. Many types of interstitial hyperthermia equipment are used. These include local current field techniques utilizing RF energy (at frequency of 0.5 MHz); micro-wave techniques utilizing small microwave antennas inserted into hollow tubings with frequencies between 300 and 2450 MHz; ferromagnetic seed implants for delivering thermal energy to deep-seated tumors; hot water tubes; and laser fibers. Interstitial heating allows the tumor to be heated to higher temperatures than exter-nal techniques. Other advantages of this technique include better control of heat dis-tributions within the tumor as compared with external hyperthermia, and the sparing of normal tissues, especially the overlaying skin. However, the disadvantages are invasiveness, difficulty in repeated treatment, and limitation of applicable sites.

Under anesthesia, probes or small needles (thin antennas) are inserted into the body to produce localized deposition of EM energy in subcutaneous and deep-seated tumors. For treatment regions that are large compared to the field penetration depth of frequency used, the required SAR uniformity throughout a tumor volume cannot be achieved with a single antenna, and arrays of antennas are then employed [101,102]. Imaging techniques, such as ultrasound, may be used to ensure that the probe is prop-erly positioned within the tumor.

9.3.2   Regional Hyperthermia

Regional heating is indicated for patients with locally advanced deep-seated tumors such as those in the pelvis or abdomen. The application of regional hyperthermia is, however, more complex than local heating, particularly because of wide variation in physical and physiological properties. It requires more sophisticated planning, ther-mometry, and quality assurance. Since regional heating techniques apply energy to the adjacent deep-seated tumors in a focused manner, energy is also delivered to the adjacent normal tissues. Under such conditions, selective heating of tumors is only possible when heat dissipation by blood flow in normal tissue is greater than that in tumor tissue. Most clinical trials on regional hyperthermia have used the approach as an adjunct to radiotherapy [60]. Locally advanced or recurrent tumors of the pelvis are the major indications for regional hyperthermia, including rectal carcinoma, cervical carcinoma, bladder carcinoma, prostate carcinoma, or soft tissue sarcoma. Some of these indications were validated in prospective studies.

9.3.2.1 Deep Regional Hyperthermia

Heat delivery to deep-seated tumors is the most difficult problem and major efforts have been devoted to the development of external deep-heating equipment. The ideal heating device should be capable of raising the whole tumor volume to a therapeutic temperature without overheating adjacent normal tissues [41]. Treatments of deep-seated tumors are difficult because EM energy is rapidly absorbed by human tissue [103]. External applicators are positioned around the body cavity or organ to be treated, and EM energy is focused on the area to raise its temperature. Deep regional hyperthermia is usually performed using arrays of multiple applicators [104]. For example, annular phased-array systems delivering EM energy and RF capacitive heating apparatus are examples of regional heating devices. This system has the advantage that subcutaneous fat is not excessively heated and, thus, it is suitable for obese patients. However, this method causes systemic symptoms such as tachycardia and malaise, which result from the use of large-sized applicators [41]. Model calculations show significant improvements in control of power distribution by increasing the antenna number with the assumption of optimum adjustment of phases and amplitudes [105]. The Sigma-60 applicator is a widely spread applicator, which consists of four dipole antenna pairs arranged in a ring around the patient [60]. The Sigma-Eye applicator is one of the next generation of commercially available applicators, consisting of three shorter rings, each with four flat dipole-antenna pairs [106].

9.3.2.2 Regional Perfusion Hyperthermia

Regional perfusion techniques can be used to treat cancers in the arms and legs, such as melanoma, or cancer in some organs such as the liver or lung. In this procedure, some of the patient's blood is removed, heated, and then pumped (perfused) back into the limb or organ. Anticancer drugs are commonly given during this treatment. Regional hyperthermia is usually applied by perfusion of a limb, organ, or body cavity with heated fluids [107,108].

Much experience with hyperthermic chemoperfusion has been gained since 1970. In contrast to external heating methods, hyperthermic perfusion techniques carry the risk of severe and persisting adverse effects (e.g., neuropathy and amputation of limbs). However, both hyperthermic isolated limb perfusion and hyperthermic intraperitoneal perfusion at different temperatures achieve high response rates in comparison with historical control groups receiving systemic chemotherapy. This success is due to both the homogeneous and well-controlled heat application and the much higher (more than tenfold) drug concentration possible [60].

Hyperthermic isolated limb perfusion has been used mostly as a melphalan-based induction therapy in advanced stages of nonresectable melanomas and soft-tissue sarcomas (limited to one limb). Trials showed further improvement in response rates with the addition of high doses of TNF, whereas application of additional drugs (especially cisplatin) is not beneficial. Because of these high response rates, no prospective randomized trials on induction therapy with hyperthermic isolated limb perfusion have yet been done [109–111].

9.3.2.3 Other Regional Hyperthermic Techniques

Other hyperthermia approaches of clinical interest are under investigation for prostate cancer [112], preirradiated rectal cancer and, particularly, use of part-body hyperthermia for peritoneal carcinosis (for ovarian cancer) in conjunction with chemotherapy (liposomal doxorubicin) [60]. Continuous hyperthermic peritoneal perfusion is another technique used to treat cancers within the peritoneal cavity (the space within the abdomen that contains the intestines, stomach, and liver), including primary peritoneal mesothelioma and stomach cancer. During surgery, heated anticancer drugs flow from a warming device through the peritoneal cavity. The peritoneal cavity temperature reaches 41–42°C.

9.3.3 WHOLE-BODY HYPERTHERMIA

Early attempts at WBH go back to the 1890s [113]. WBH (to a limit of 42°C) is a distinctive and complex pathophysiological condition that has tremendous impact on tissue metabolism, blood flow, organ function, and tissue repair. For example, the basal metabolic rate of a patient weighing about 70 kg is 85 W at 37°C and double that at 42°C; this in itself is enough to raise the body temperature within 180 min from 37.5°C to 42°C, if thermal isolation is perfect [60]. WBH has been investigated since the 1970s as an adjuvant with conventional chemo- or radiotherapy for the treatment of various malignant diseases [114]. It is used to treat metastatic cancer that has spread throughout the body. To ensure that the desired temperature is reached, but not exceeded, the temperature of the tumor and surrounding tissue is monitored throughout hyperthermia treatment.

Three major methods are now available to achieve reproducible, controlled WBH—thermal conduction (surface heating), extracorporeal induction (blood is pumped out of the patient's body, heated to 42°C or more, then put back in the body while still hot), and radiant or EM induction [115–117]. The tolerance of liver and brain tissue limits the maximum temperature for using WBH from 41.8 to 42.0°C, but this temperature may be maintained for several hours. Heating can be accomplished with thermal conduction heat sources such as immersion in heated fluids [118], heated air [119], wrapping the patient in heated blankets [120], or using thermal chambers (similar to large incubators). WBH hyperthermia may also be used to treat AIDS. Extracorporeal hyperthermia treatment of bone followed by its reimplantation may be an optional treatment of bone tumors [121].

EM techniques are available that use radiant heat, microwave radiation, infrared radiation, or combinations of these to induce WBH with steady-state temperatures of 41–42°C. Although the power absorption patterns are nonuniform, redistribution of the thermal energy is rapid via the circulatory system. WBH can be combined with chemotherapy to increase tumor cell death without increasing bone marrow suppression [122]. A newer approach is to increase the temperature to ~40°C for a longer period, which, in combination with cytokines and cytotoxic drugs, is expected to lead to a greater therapeutic index than WBH at the maximum tolerated level [123].

WBH can be applied only to patients in a good general condition, and when combined with drugs the first step must evidently be to demonstrate its safety [10]. The toxicities associated with WBH may be significant; therefore, careful patient selection and supportive care are essential. Sedation or general anesthesia must be used and continuous monitoring of vital signs, core body temperature, cardiac functions (using ECG), and urine output is necessary.

9.3.4 EXTRACELLULAR HYPERTHERMIA

The classical hyperthermia effect is based on well-focused energy absorption targeting the malignant tissue. The treatment temperature has been considered as the main technical parameter. There are discussions about the mechanism and control of the process because of some doubts about the micromechanisms. The main idea of extracellular hyperthermia (electro-hyperthermia or oncothermia) is to heat up the targeted tissue by means of electric field, keeping the energy absorption in the extracellular liquid [124]. Extracellular hyperthermia is devoted to enhancing the efficiency of conventional hyperthermia by additional, nonequilibrium thermal effects with the aim of suppressing the existing disadvantages of classical thermal treatments. Although this new technique recognizes the benefits of increased tissue temperature and its biological consequences, it also argues that nonequilibrium thermal effects are partially responsible for the observed clinical deviations from the purely temperature-based treatment theory [49].

Extracellular hyperthermia is based on a capacitively coupled energy transfer applied at a frequency that is primarily absorbed in the extracellular matrix due to its inability to penetrate the cell membrane [125]. The energy absorption for these effects is more significant than the temperature, so it is important to characterize the hyperthermia by thermal dose and not by temperature. Thermal dose changes many energetic processes in the tissue and in their physiology. Most of the desired changes (structural and chemical) involve energy consumption [49].

9.4 HYPERTHERMIA HEATING DEVICES

Most clinical hyperthermia systems operate by causing a target volume of tissue to be exposed to EM fields or ultrasound radiation. A structure is needed that is capable of transferring energy into biological tissue and getting the best approximation of the area to be treated by 3D distribution of SAR. The majority of the hyperthermia treatments are applied using external devices (applicators) employing energy transfer to the tissue [87,88,126]. User needs require that the system be effective, safe, and robust. For a heating system to be effective, it must be able to produce final time and temperature histories that include a set of tumor temperatures that can be maintained for long enough times to result in clinically effective thermal doses without also producing unacceptable normal tissue temperatures [3].

9.4.1 Techniques

Facilitated by the enormous progression in computational power, the last decade has brought significant advances and innovations in the technology needed to develop RF, microwave, and ultrasound applicators. Applicators are positioned around or near the appropriate region, and energy is focused on the tumor to raise its temperature. Currently, hyperthermia systems can be interfaced with MRI systems, allowing noninvasive temperature monitoring of the treatment.

9.4.1.1 Ultrasound

Sound is vibration. Ultrasound waves involve the propagation of sound waves at a frequency of 2–20 MHz through soft tissues. Absorption of ultrasound waves results in heating of the medium. In terms of basic physics, ultrasound has the best combination of small wavelengths and corresponding attenuation coefficient that allow penetration to deep sites with the ability to focus power into regions of small size. The primary limitation of such systems is their inability to penetrate air and the difficulty in penetrating bone.

Early ultrasound systems used single-transducer applicators that showed increased tumor temperatures compared with microwave systems. Multiple elements and frequencies can be used to increase the energy focus while maintaining good penetration depth, thus making SAR shaping by either phasing or mechanical scanning clinically feasible for superficial sites [3]. Over the years, ultrasound devices capable of improved heating uniformity and controlled depth of penetration, mostly by using multiple applicators with phasing and power steering, have been designed [127–133].

9.4.1.2 Radiofrequency

The initial investigation of the use of RF waves in the body is credited to d'Arsonval in 1891, who showed that RF waves that pass through living tissue cause an elevation in tissue temperature without causing neuromuscular excitation. These observations eventually led to the development in the early to mid-1900s of electrocautery and medical diathermy [134–137]. To heat large tumors at depth, RF fields in the range of 10–120 MHz are generally used with wavelengths that are long compared to body dimensions and, thus, deposit energy over a sizeable region [64]. Schematically, a closed-loop circuit is created by placing a generator, a large dispersive electrode (ground pad), a patient, and a needle electrode in series. Both the dispersive electrode and needle electrode are active, while the patient acts as a resistor. Thus, an alternating electric field is created within the tissue of the patient. Given the relatively high electrical resistance of tissue in comparison with the metal electrodes, there is marked agitation of the ions present in the tumor tissue that immediately surrounds the electrode. This ionic agitation creates frictional heating within the body, which can be tightly controlled through modulation of the amount of RF energy deposited [138–140]. The tissue's resistance to current flow results in thermal lesions. The desiccated and coagulated tissue raises the resistance to current flow, impeding effective tissue heating and limiting the size of RF-induced lesions. Studies have shown that

RF-induced lesions increase rapidly in size during the initial period of power application, and then the rate of increase diminishes rapidly as the resistance rises at the electrode–tissue interface and the current flow falls [141,142].

9.4.1.3 Microwaves

One of the more promising hyperthermia techniques is the use of microwaves. Microwave hyperthermia has been used on thousands of patients suffering from prostate or breast cancer. Microwave-generated heat is used to shrink or destroy cancerous tumors. Microwave hyperthermia has generally utilized single-waveguide microwave antennas working at 434, 915, and 2450 MHz. A hyperthermia system includes the antenna and a noncontacting temperature sensor that scan a predetermined path over the surface of the tissue to be treated. The temperature sensor senses the temperature of the tissue and a controller closes a feedback loop, which adjusts the microwave power applied to the antenna in a manner which raises the temperature of the tissue uniformly. Microwave hyperthermia is frequently used in conjunction with other cancer therapies, such as radiation therapy. It can increase tumor blood flow, thereby helping to oxygenate poorly oxygenated malignant cells.

The early systems have had the heating disadvantage of having lateral SAR contours that are significantly smaller than the applicator dimensions, thus causing underheating problems in early trials, when investigators used applicators that covered the tumors visually but heated only their central region. Also, at the frequency of operation these systems have relatively long wavelengths, limiting their ability to focus on tumors. To overcome these limitations, improved antenna-based systems and multiple-applicator systems have been used clinically for large tumors and phasing in of such systems is a possibility [3].

9.4.2 EXTERNAL RF APPLICATORS

9.4.2.1 Capacitive Heating

An RF approach that has been used clinically is a capacitively coupled system. This name is due to the applicator shape, which is similar to a two-plate capacitor excited by an electric potential between the plates, as shown in Figure 9.2. Capacitor-plate applicators are typical electric field (E-type) applicators. These applicators are usually operated at either 13.56 or 27.12 MHz, two of the frequencies assigned to ISM use (ISM frequencies). Capacitive hyperthermia equipment generally consists of an RF generator, an RF power meter, an impedance matching network, a set of electrode applicators, a temperature control system for the applicators, a set of connecting cables, and a patient support assembly. The RF energy is transmitted from the generator via coaxial cables to electrodes placed on opposite sides of the body and the power is distributed locally or regionally through interaction of electric fields produced between the parallel-opposed electrodes. The adjustable positions of the electrodes permit heating at different angles and treatment sites.

RF-capacitive devices are convenient to apply to various anatomical sites. Tissues can be heated by displacement currents generated between the two capacitor plates. However, they are not robust in terms of positioning, because currents tend to concentrate around the closer electrode tips when they are nonparallel. Another

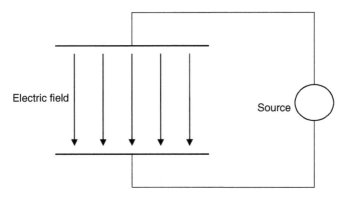

FIGURE 9.2   Capacitive heating system.

disadvantage is the excessive heating of subcutaneous fat. This is because the electric fields generated are normal to the skin surface and currents must pass through the high-resistance, low-blood-flow superficial fatty layers, causing substantial superficial heating. It has been shown that a patient with subcutaneous fat of more than 1.5–2 cm in thickness is difficult to heat with this heating modality, whose related pain levels are frequently treatment limiting, even when skin precooling is applied [3,143,144].

With multiple capacitor configurations [145], internal heating patterns can be adjusted by changing the relative voltages applied to various plates. Ring capacitors can produce deep internal heating without overheating the surface if a proper gap is maintained between the rings and the body surface. A number of researchers indicate the ability of RF-capacitive systems to achieve a good regional deep heating [144,146–159]. Results of a Japanese seven-institution trial employing the Thermotron RF-8 capacitive heating device (Yamamoto Vinyter, Osaka, Japan) are noteworthy. Treatment given to 177 patients with deep-seated tumors used hyperthermia in combination with radiation therapy alone (96 patients) or with radiochemotherapy (81 patients). Maximum intratumor or intracavitary temperatures greater than 42°C were obtained in 77 and 74% of the tumors, respectively. Response rates and symptomatic improvement were felt to be higher than expected for historical controls treated with radiation therapy or chemotherapy alone [149].

9.4.2.2   Inductive Heating

Inductive heating by coupled energy transfer from a coil carrying AC surrounding a biological object through air is used to achieve deeper hyperthermia (e.g., more than 5 cm). Magnetic fields in RF induction heating can penetrate tissues, such as subcutaneous fat, without excessive heating. Such magnetic fields induce eddy currents inside the tissues. Since the induced electric fields are parallel to the tissue interface, heating is maximized in muscle rather than in fat. However, the heating pattern is generally toroidal in shape with a null at the center of the coil.

The simplest inductive applicator is a single coaxial current loop [160]. Since the coaxial current loop produces eddy current type electric fields that circulate around the axis of the loop, heating in the center of the body is minimal. In general, inductive

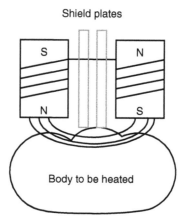

FIGURE 9.3   Inductive applicator for hyperthermia.

applicators seem not to couple as strongly to the body as capacitive applicators, and relatively high currents are usually needed to get adequate heating. Subsequent use of these devices shows that they still heat a large amount of normal tissue. These applicators are usually operated at ISM frequencies of 13.56, 27.12, and 40 MHz, with the depth of penetration being a few centimeters.

Induction hyperthermia equipment generally consists of an RF power generator, an RF power meter, an impedance matching network, one or more induction coil applicators, a set of connecting cables, and a patient support assembly. An inductive applicator for hyperthermia is shown in Figure 9.3. A pair of cylindrical ferrite cores is used for the applicator. The distance between the pair of ferrite cores is adjustable depending on the size of the region to be heated. The target is placed between or under the pair of ferrite cores. The time-varying magnetic field penetrating the body causes an eddy current. As a result, Joule's heat is produced. To effectively control the heating position vertically or horizontally, conductive plates to shield the magnetic field are introduced [161].

In response to demand for clinical use, various inductive heating applicator systems have been developed and used in the long history of hyperthermia [156,160–163].

9.4.2.3   Hybrid Heating Systems

A heating system combining a pair of capacitively coupled electrodes and induction-aperture-type applicators is also called a hybrid heating system. Figure 9.4 shows schematically the inductive heating system. In this case, the currents produced by the electrodes and applicators are substantially additive in the central region of the phantom, but are substantially opposed in the superficial regions beneath the apertures of the applicators [164].

9.4.3   EXTERNAL RADIATIVE EM DEVICES

One of the major problems of high-frequency EM devices is the limited depth of penetration due to the EM principle of skin-depth. Only tumors located 2–3 cm

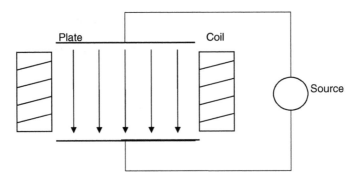

FIGURE 9.4   Capacitive and inductive heating system.

from the skin surface can, therefore, be heated with conventional surface applicators [165]. Different types of antennas can be used as applicators, including waveguides and horns [166–169], and microstrip patches [170–173]. To attain deeper localized heating, metal-plate lens applicators are used. These applicators can converge microwave energy in a lossy medium, such as human muscle of up to 6 cm [174].

9.4.3.1   Single Applicators

Early hyperthermia trials were conducted with single-aperture devices having no ability to steer or focus energy other than shifting patient position relative to the applicator. These trials included 27 MHz ridged waveguide [166], 82 MHz helix [175], 70 MHz coaxial TEM applicator [167–169], and 27–70 MHz evanescent-mode waveguide excited below cutoff frequency by entering resonant circuit (lumped capacity and inductance) with wave impedance build up band pass filter for the operating frequency [126,176]. Most of the microwave equipment includes a water bolus for surface cooling. Low-profile, lightweight microstrip applicators, which are easier to use clinically, are also used. The type of applicator selected depends on the production of sufficient thermal field distributions at different depths of the tumor in a variety of anatomical sites. Single-element applicators can safely deliver optimum thermal doses to relatively small superficial tumors. Over the years, several types of applicators for external local hyperthermia have been investigated by many researchers based on the principle of dielectric filled waveguide or horn antenna [177–185].

9.4.3.2   Multielement Array Applicators

To increase the value of SAR at a depth relative to the surface SAR in hyperthermia therapy, we must geometrically focus energy deposition from multiple electric fields generated by an array of applicators [186]. A basic array for external deep heating will likely consist of an annular ring of radiating apertures as shown in Figure 9.5. The parameters of interest are external electric fields within an array at the surface of the patient's body, the SAR pattern within the target volume, and the radiation leakage levels of the scattered fields around the applicator.

Several different RF electrode arrays have been investigated. Manning et al. [187] examined two arrays of needle electrodes arranged in two planes, with a bipolar RF

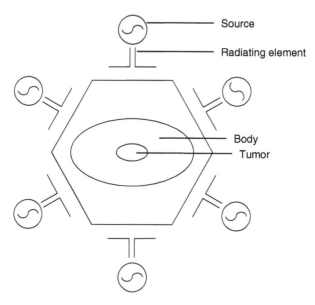

FIGURE 9.5   A ring of radiating elements.

current between the arrays. In the bipolar system, RF current is passed between two electrodes instead of between a single electrode and a ground path, so two electrodes heat the tissue instead of one, resulting in a larger ablation zone. Other groups investigated different array configurations [188,189] and segmented needle electrodes have been suggested to allow for better control of tissue heating [190].

An array of applicators with variations in phase, frequency, amplitude, and orientation of the applied fields can add more dimensions to controlling the heating patterns during hyperthermia cancer therapy [51]. Because of constructive interference of electric fields at the intended focus and destructive interference of electric fields away from the focus, multichannel coherent phased-array applicators can theoretically provide deeper tissue penetration and improved localization of the absorbed energy in deep-seated tumor regions without overheating the skin and superficial healthy tissues compared to single or incoherent array applicators.

Comparing array applicators with single applicators, array applicators provide deeper tissue penetration, reduce undesired heating of normal surrounding tissues between the applicator and tumor, and improve local control of the tumor temperature distribution. Heat generated by RF devices is delivered regionally across a much larger area. However, microwave array systems require target compression because of the shallow penetration of the higher microwave frequencies. RF array applicators surrounding the body are used in attempting to heat deep tumors. However, studies in external RF array thermotherapy have shown the difficulty of localizing RF energy in malignant tissue deep within the human body without damaging superficial healthy tissue due to hot spots. Improvements in RF energy deposition are achieved when the RF phased array is controlled by an adaptive algorithm to focus the RF energy in the tumor and tumor margins, while the superficial RF fields are nullified.

Clinically, the use of phased arrays as heating applicators has several advantages. Phased arrays can easily compensate for the effects of inhomogeneities of the treatment volume (which includes the tumor and the surrounding tissues). The heating pattern can be controlled electronically, thus eliminating the need for mechanical movement of the applicator head. This simplifies the machine–patient interface and allows for better use of the available power. Also, electronic switching can be performed rapidly, thus enabling swift response to changes in the tumor environment. However, clinicians cannot always accurately predetermine or manually adjust the optimum settings for output power and phase of each antenna to focus heat reliably into deep-seated tumors [186,191].

Two outstanding challenges in EM phased-array hyperthermia are (1) to selectively elevate the temperature in the cancerous tissue without excessively elevating the temperature of the surrounding healthy tissues in the presence of electrical and thermodynamic inhomogeneities, and (2) to react to unexpected changes in patient positioning and physiology (such as sudden change in blood flow in the tumor) that can significantly impact the quality of the delivered treatment [192,193].

Significant research progress has been obtained recently in heating devices appropriate for deep hyperthermia, including ultrasonic arrays [194–208], RF arrays [209–216], and microwave arrays [217–239].

Petrovich et al. [240] have reported the results of a 14-institution trial conducted in the United States that employed the annular phased-array system for regional hyperthermia production in 353 patients with advanced, recurrent, or persistent deep-seated tumors. Hyperthermia was used alone or in conjunction with radiation therapy or chemotherapy, chemotherapy, and radiation therapy in 4, 12, 13, and 69% of the patients, respectively. Complete responses (10%) and partial responses (17%) were obtained, with the highest complete response rates noted in patients receiving radiation therapy in conjunction with hyperthermia (12 versus 2%).

Better understanding of array applicators is always a requirement, not only in the design of single antenna in the near-field range (matching, symmetrization, efficiency) but also in combining these antennas in an array. The coupling between the antennas is the most essential and critical feature, which has to be as low as possible in a well-controllable array. Transforming networks are needed to link the amplifier system and antennas. A kind of feedback control must be established between the amplifier system (e.g., the single generators) and a patient-adapted power distribution [60].

9.4.4 Interstitial and Intracavitary Devices

As early as 1976, it was suggested that RF currents applied between groups of stainless-steel electrodes could be used to induce elevated temperatures in deep-seated (depth ≥ 3 cm) tumors [241]. The application of an alternating voltage of sufficient magnitude across planes comprising multiple pairs of such electrodes is capable of generating electrical currents through the tumor, leading to an increase of the tissue temperature. The simplicity of the basic concept accounts for increasing acceptance of interstitial probes by hyperthermia research groups, and its application to various anatomical tumor-bearing sites.

Interstitial hyperthermia is an invasive procedure in which a single or an array of interstitial antennas or electrodes is implanted in accessible tumors, which might be located in deep or superficial tissues. The invasiveness gives interstitial systems the clear advantage of being potentially effective, therefore potentially maximizing the tumor temperature while minimizing thermal damage to normal tissue. In addition to electrodes, the interstitial hyperthermia system includes a generator controlled with an automatic tuning system and temperature limitation system. Temperature measurements must be performed at the antennas and between them. In most systems, every single antenna is controlled by its own generator. Dedicated systems have in addition two or more segments per antenna or electrode controlled in phase or amplitude. One limitation of the interstitial heating approach is the inability of the system to vary the power deposition along the radial direction.

Although often compared to interstitial systems, intracavitary systems are really interior versions of superficial systems that, by using the appropriate body cavities, minimize both the amount of intervening normal tissue between the applicator and the tumor (compared with using a superficial system for the same tumor) and the amount of tissue trauma (compared with the more invasive interstitial system). Intracavitary systems are quite promising for a few important sites such as the prostate and the esophagus. More advances systems have been developed recently, including multiple applicators in a segmented, phased-array ultrasound system [3].

Accurate models of the power deposition patterns of specific applicators and the bioheat response of the tissue to these procedures are continually being developed and improved upon. These models have been important in developing treatment strategies and in the implementation of treatment planning [242]. Some examples of model development specific to interstitial applicator design and treatment planning include those for ultrasound [243–249], RF current sources [190,221,250–255], and microwave [256–261].

Clinically, interstitial hyperthermia has been applied for prostate carcinoma, recurrent breast cancer, and malignant brain tumors [101,102,190,261–266]. The development of partially insulated electrodes is helping significantly to reduce the temperatures in surrounding normal tissues, therefore improving the therapeutic gain. Multiple electrode multiplexing also provides added flexibility and the means for dynamic control of power deposition during treatments.

9.4.5 NANOTECHNOLOGY-BASED SOURCES

The major problem of actually applying hyperthermia treatments is to achieve a homogenous heat distribution in the treated tissue. The currently available modalities of hyperthermia are often limited by their inability to selectively target tumor tissue and, hence, they carry a high risk of collateral organ damage or they deposit heat in a much localized manner which can result in under-treatment of a tumor. Nanotechnology-based cancer therapy is a special form of interstitial thermotherapy with the advantage of selective heat deposition to the tumor cells. This new therapy is one of the first applications of nanotechnology in medicine and based on heating of ferric oxide nanoparticles in an AC magnetic field. The method is also known as magnetic fluid hyperthermia (MFH) or nanocancer therapy. This technique meets the requirement of maximal deposition of heat within the targeted region under maximal protection of the surrounding healthy tissue at the same time.

Deep local inductive heating can be achieved by using an implant material, which generates heat by its interaction with the magnetic field. However, since eddy currents are predominantly induced near the surface of the human body, the result is that both the implanted region and the superficial normal tissues are being heated. Eddy current absorbers consisting of silicon rubber that contains a fine carbon powder are used.

The concept of application of biocompatible magnetic nanoparticles (in the form of ferrofluids) with diagnosis and therapeutic purposes is being considered by a growing number of researchers in biomedical areas. Their applications in biology and medicine include: separation of biological materials using magnetically labeled beads [267]; drug delivery and medicine [45]; cell sorting, based on the fact that high magnetic flux density attracts magnetically labeled cells [268,269]; and hyperthermia [270–274]. Hyperthermia with magnetic nanoparticles enables the physician to select between different treatment temperatures for the first time, after only a single injection of the nanoparticles. The process involved in magnetic hyperthermia, which is based on the known hyper-sensibility of tumor cells to heating, is related to energy dissipation when a ferromagnetic material is placed in an external alternating magnetic field. The technique consists of the localization of magnetic particles or seeds within tumor tissue followed by exposure to an externally applied magnetic field to cause them to heat [44]. If particles are localized into the tumor tissues in the bone, it will be easy to heat the tumor because heat quenching by the blood flow is ignored and a high hyperthermic effect will be expected [274]. The success of such approach depends critically on the ability to specifically attach a given particle on certain types of cells, the ones that are to be killed. This is a very complex biochemical and biomedical subject. Other issues to be resolved (depending on the kind of organs to be treated) are: transportation to the target, neutralizing the body's immune system, minimizing the mass of magnetic material, and detection of possible accumulation of magnetic material in other organs.

Magnetically mediated hyperthermia using magnetic particles has been used against brain tumor, tongue cancer, kidney cancer, malignant melanoma, and a hamster osteosarcoma [274]. The physician may either choose hyperthermia conditions (up to 45°C) to intensify conventional therapies like radiation or chemotherapy, or thermoablation by using higher temperatures, up to 70°C. Clinically this technique may provide the potential to address many shortcomings of other delivery systems.

For clinical applications, magnetic materials should present low levels of toxicity, as well as a high saturation magnetic moment to minimize the doses required for temperature increase. Currently, magnetite (Fe_3O_4) is used in this process because it presents a high Curie temperature, high saturation magnetic moment (90–98 emu/g or ~450–500 emu/cm^3), and has shown the lowest toxicity index in pre-clinical tests. However, it should be carefully investigated whether long-term deposits of magnetite affects patient health, that is, whether they show acute or chronic toxicity by excess absorption of Fe ions, e.g., hemochromatosis [275].

9.5   HYPERTHERMIA WITH OTHER MODALITIES

Hyperthermia has been used for the treatment of resistant tumors of many kinds, but still with unsatisfactory results. Hyperthermia can be used by itself and results in shrinkage, sometimes even complete eradication, of tumors. However, these results may not last and the tumors regrow. Most tumor sites are unreachable with the present interstitial, superficial, and regional hyperthermia techniques, while for those limited sites which are heatable, all dosimetry studies indicate that the temperature distributions reached are highly inhomogeneous and that it is almost impossible to obtain the protocol temperature goals [242,276–280]. Accordingly, the most beneficial contribution of hyperthermia for oncological treatments will be based on enhancing the effectiveness of other treatment modalities (radiotherapy, chemotherapy, radiochemotherapy, gene therapy, immune therapy, etc.).

The biological rationale for hyperthermia applied in combination with radiotherapy or chemotherapy is well-established and extremely promising; in particular, the sensitivity of hypoxic cells to heating makes hyperthermia an ideal additive to standard radiotherapy [281]. Hyperthermia produces direct injury by damaging the entire cellular machinery, including nucleic acids, cytoskeleton, and cell membranes. Radiotherapy and many chemotherapeutic agents have similar mechanisms of action. There are reports of synergistic effects of regional or WBH for cancer treatments that include radiotherapy, bleomycin, mitomycin C, Adriamycin, 5-flurourical, cisplatin, and carboplatin [282,283].

Falk and Issels [59] conducted an extensive review on state-of-the-art hyperthermia in the year 2000, describing the effect of hyperthermia combined with radiotherapy, chemotherapy, or both. All the considered studies but two show a statistically significant higher (up to a doubling) tumor control or cure rate for the combined treatment modality. The positive results of most of the studies explain the renewed enthusiasm for hyperthermia, which is reflected in the growing number of institutes interested in the application of hyperthermia [57,69,283].

9.5.1   HYPERTHERMIA AND RADIATION

The synergistic effects of hyperthermia combined with radiation have been investigated and reported to yield higher complete and durable responses than radiation alone in superficial tumors. Several mechanisms are responsible for the supra-additive effect of the combination of radiotherapy and hyperthermia. The additive complementary effect comes from the sensitivity of cells in the hypoxic, low pH areas, and the cells in S-phase, which are both relatively radioresistant [4]. Hyperthermia may cause an increased blood flow, which may result in an improvement in tissue oxygenation, which then results in a temporally increased radiosensitivity [284]. Clinical data and experiments *in vivo* show hyperthermia at mild temperatures, easily achievable with the use of presently available clinical hyperthermia devices, increases perfusion in the tumor region, leading to a higher oxygen concentration. Higher perfusion can increase drug delivery and reoxygenation. Most human tumors have increased blood flow under hyperthermia, even hours later. Only a few cases of human tumors have shown vascular breakdown [285,286].

Biologically, hyperthermia has two different types of interactions with radiation. Firstly, heat has a radiosensitizing effect. This is most prominent with simultaneous application, but is of the same magnitude in both tumor and normal tissue and will not improve the therapeutic ratio unless the tumor is heated to a higher temperature than the normal tissue. Secondly, hyperthermia exhibits a direct cytotoxic effect, and a moderate heat treatment alone can almost selectively destroy tumor cells in a nutritionally deprived, chronically hypoxic and acidic environment. Because such cells are the most radioresistant, a smaller radiation dose is needed to control the remaining more radiosensitive cells. Clinically, heating of superficial tumors (e.g., breast, neck nodes, and malignant melanoma) has confirmed the biological rationale for using hyperthermia as an adjuvant to radiotherapy [287].

Combined hyperthermia and radiation offers potential clinical advantages for the treatment of tumors. Importantly, the synergy between radiation and heat is highly dependent on the application and highest when given simultaneously. It has been reported by many clinical trials that hyperthermia therapy has been shown to substantially improve local control of cancer, tumor clinical response, and survival rates when added to radiation treatments. It yields considerable therapeutic gain compared to radiation alone in treating various cancerous tumors [54,56,154,159,186,288–305]. However, not all studies have shown increased survival in patients receiving the combined treatments [2,59,60,306].

A disadvantage intrinsically associated with hyperthermia is that one heat treatment can cause a transient resistance against a subsequent treatment (thermotolerance). In radiotherapy, a standard treatment regimen consists of a 6-week course of radiation doses. If one would like to apply hyperthermia with each of these radiation treatments, this thermotolerance would certainly negatively interfere with the effectiveness of the treatment. Therefore, the mechanisms underlying thermotolerance are being extensively explored to find ways to minimize its development.

9.5.2   HYPERTHERMIA AND CHEMOTHERAPY

In clinical practice, it is difficult to deliver therapeutic amounts of infused chemotherapy to solid tumors deep in the body without incurring toxic effects in healthy body organs. Limited amounts of free chemotherapy infused into the bloodstream reach the tumor due to damaged vasculature in the vicinity of the tumor and due to tumor cell pressure that blocks the chemotherapy from passing through the cell membrane. A number of clinical studies have established that elevated cell tissue temperature, induced by EM energy absorption, significantly enhances the effectiveness of chemotherapy in the treatment of malignant tumors in the human body without increasing the infused amount of drug [59,95,307].

For the combination of hyperthermia and chemotherapy, spatial cooperation can again explain the additive effects. Drug concentration will be less in the insufficiently perfused tumor regions. When it comes to chemotherapy, there are indications that some chemotherapy can be potentiated by hyperthermia. This can, in some agents, increase toxicities and the incidence of damage associated with them at the usual doses, or it can be taken advantage of in the sense of getting the same results with lower doses of the drug. The important mechanisms for an interactive effect are an increased intracellular drug uptake, enhanced DNA damage, and higher intratumor drug concentrations, resulting from an increase in blood flow. An interactive effect was observed for virtually all cell lines treated at temperatures above 40°C for alkylating agents, nitrosureas, and platin analogues, with enhancement ratios depending on temperature and exposure time. The effect of these drugs can be enhanced by a factor of between 1.2 and 10, and an extremely high thermal enhancement ratio of 23 was even observed for *in vitro* application of melphalan to drug-resistant cells at 44°C [308]. In combination with chemotherapy, the type of drug, dose, temperature, and time of administration all play a role.

Improvement of local control by hyperthermia combined with systemic chemotherapy has been observed by many researchers [309–319]. There is insufficient information to make conclusions regarding the use of WBH as an adjunct to either radiation or chemotherapy, and inadequate data regarding the use of local hyperthermia in conjunction with chemotherapy alone. The policy is based, in part, on an initial body of evidence consisting of phase I and II clinical studies describing the technical feasibility of WBH [318,320–324]. Extensive reviews on the combination of hyperthermia with chemotherapy have been published [59,84].

9.5.3 HYPERTHERMIA AND RADIOCHEMOTHERAPY

Radiochemotherapy is a widely used means of treatment for patients suffering from primary, locally advanced, or recurrent rectal cancer. The efficacy of treatment can be enhanced by additional application of regional hyperthermia to this conventional therapy regime. Many researchers have conducted investigations on the effectiveness of hyperthermia combined with radiochemotherapy in the treatment of cancer [96,286,325–333]. An extensive review on the combination of hyperthermia with radiochemotherapy was published in 2001 [59].

9.5.4 HYPERTHERMIA AND GENE THERAPY

Gene therapy may be defined as the treatment in which genetic material is introduced in a cell to add or modify its function. This results in the manufacture of protein(s) which are either directly therapeutic or interact with other substances to exert a therapeutic effect. To treat cancer effectively, the genetic material must exert its effect only on tumor or tumor-associated cells, not on normal cells, and must not eliminate the body's immune response that is so critical in fighting cancer. To achieve these goals, an approach must be developed which combines fever-range WBH with a gene that only affects tumor cells spliced with additional genetic material designed to cause the suicide gene to be expressed predominantly in tumor cells. The hyperthermia is expected to help in opening up the pores of tumor blood vessels so that more liposomes reach the tumors and deliver their DNA content to tumor cells. It also increases the amount of protein created by the incorporated DNA and boosts the immune system so that it sends specialized cells into the tumors to help kill them.

Gene-infected cells were found to be more sensitive to hyperthermia [334–336]. In a murine system, intratumorally injected viral gene therapy encoding for interleukin-12, controlled with a heat shock promoter and followed by hyperthermia, was shown to be feasible and therapeutically effective, with no apparent systemic toxicity [337].

9.6 STATUS AND TRENDS

Hyperthermia is an emerging therapy method in oncology. It has been an effective modality of cancer treatment, showing significant improvements in clinical responses for many patients when used alone or in combination with other treatment methods, such as surgery, chemotherapy, radiation therapy, and gene therapy [49]. The clinical exploitation of hyperthermia was and is still hampered by various challenges including the high degree of interdependency between physiology and biology, technical and clinical limitations, and standardization.

9.6.1 BIOLOGICAL AND PHYSIOLOGICAL MECHANISMS

An important unresolved factor involves the biological and physiological mechanisms by which hyperthermia works [3]. Although hyperthermic cell killing has been demonstrated in many *in vitro* studies, the mechanisms underlying cell damage and death have not been fully elucidated. Further work is required toward this end and information from research studies on the effects of hyperthermia on tumors *in vivo* will be valuable. Until the underlying mechanisms by which positive clinical results have been obtained are understood, and the spatial and temporal distributions of the important biological and physiological variables are known, it will remain impossible to set precise engineering design goals [3,338].

9.6.2 TECHNICAL AND CLINICAL CHALLENGES

Realization of the potential of hyperthermia as a primary therapy depends on the advance that must be made in EM heating techniques and thermometry [34]. Many major technical advances have been applied in biological and clinical research; the resulting improvements in instrumentation have helped in conducting more accurate and elegant experiments to produce heat for hyperthermia treatment, including ultrasound, RF, and microwaves. Table 9.1 compares the major hyperthermia method [338].

Recent developments in hyperthermia have expanded the treatment options of patients with certain types of cancer. The effectiveness of hyperthermia treatment is related to the temperature achieved during the treatment, as well as the length of treatment and cell and tissue characteristics. Control of the heating process as a major part of hyperthermia should be improved to ensure that increased temperature levels can be properly maintained, delivered, and localized within the tumor region. To effectively control heating distribution will require (a) sophisticated controllers that can properly steer the power deposition to achieve close-to-optimal temperatures and (b) accurate measurements of the spatial and temporal distributions of temperature during the treatment. The theoretical evaluations and simulations of such controllers have been evolving from single-point controllers to more complex model-based controllers [192,193,339] that can control the complete temperature in the heated region.

The lack of necessary engineering tools can be viewed as a major stumbling block to hyperthermia's effective clinical implementation. Developing clinically effective systems will be difficult, however, because (a) it requires solving several complex

TABLE 9.1

Comparison of Major Hyperthermia Techniques

Heating Approach	Advantages	Disadvantages	Application
Ultrasound	Good focus performance in tissue. No hot spots in fatty tissues. Heating possible to 5–10 cm depth with single transducer and up to 20 cm depth with multiple transducers. Temperature is easy to measure and control.	Heating area is small. No penetration of tissue–air interfaces.	Treatment of superficial and deep regional tumors. Examples include surface lesions, head and neck, and lesions in extremities.
Radiofrequency	Simple instrumentation. No shield required. Large treatment area. Electrodes not limited in size and insulation can be accomplished.	Difficult to control electric fields. Only areas where fat is thin can be treated by capacitive systems. Heating regional, with external applicators.	Treatment for large and superficial tumors in neck, limb, chest, brain, abdomen, etc.
Microwaves	Technology very advanced. Heating large volumes is possible. Specialized antennas for heating from body cavities have been developed. Multiple applicators, coherent or incoherent, can be used. Can avoid hot spots in the fatty tissues.	Heating not localized at depth, limited penetration at high frequencies. Temperature measurement is difficult and thermometry requires noninteracting probes. Possible health effects on personnel. Shielding of treatment rooms required, except at medically reserved frequencies (e.g., 915 MHz).	For treatment of superficial tumors in breast, limb, prostate, brain, etc.

engineering problems, for which (b) setting appropriate design and evaluation goals is currently difficult owing to a lack of critical biological, physiological, and clinical knowledge, two tasks which must (c) be accomplished within a complicated social/political structure [3].

While hyperthermia requires investments in equipment and personnel training, the same is true for other types of cancer treatment modalities. Another obstacle for the acceptance of hyperthermia may be that it lacks public awareness. Most of the clinical studies are on its combination with radiotherapy. However, experimental and the few clinical results with combined chemotherapy and hyperthermia make clear that this combination is also worth further testing [10]. Carefully conducted phase III trials with rigorous quality assurance must employ prospective thermal dosimetry to validate the role of hyperthermia in multimodality therapy [68].

9.6.3 STANDARDIZATION

A number of challenges must be overcome before hyperthermia can be considered a standard treatment for cancer [2,10,60,68]. Hyperthermia suffers from a lack of dosing and treatment standardization and scientific consensus about its effects on malignant and healthy tissues. For hyperthermia to gain widespread approval and clinical use, the technique requires further research and standardization [49]. Standardization of equipment between centers must be achieved before large-scale trials can be realized [34]. Two major factors make hyperthermia difficult. First, there is no clear clinical thermal dose–effect relationship, which is coupled with the inability to produce consistently a uniform pattern of heat distribution throughout the tumor mass. Thermal dosimetry is the second major issue—the inability to predict or measure accurately the temperature throughout the tumor mass and the surrounding healthy tissues. Thermal dose formulations that have taken into account both the temperature distribution and time at various temperatures have shown good correlations with complete response rates [276] and duration of local tumor control [338,340]. These need to be confirmed in future clinical trials.

9.6.4 FUTURE RESEARCH

In conclusion, hyperthermia is not yet a fully developed modality; there are still problems with its routine clinical application and there is room for further technological improvements. Therefore, we believe that the development of hyperthermia is an example of a successful research program which is clearly important and from which physicians and patients will benefit.

REFERENCES

1. Ned B, Hornback MD. Is the community radiation oncologist ready for clinical hyperthermia? *Radiographics* 1987; 7: 139–149.
2. Kapp DS, Hahn GM, Carlson RW. Principles of hyperthermia. In: Bast RC Jr., Kufe DW, Pollock RE, Weichselbaum RR, Holland JF, Frei EF, Editors. *Cancer Medicine.* Hamilton: Decker, 2000.
3. Roemer RB. Engineering aspects of hyperthermia therapy. *Ann Rev Biomed Eng* 1999; 1: 347–376.
4. Raaphorst GP. Fundamental aspects of hyperthermic biology. In: Field SB, Hand JW, Editors. *An Introduction to the Practical Aspects of Clinical Hyperthermia.* London: Taylor & Francis, pp. 10–54, 1990.
5. Fajardo LF. Pathological effects of hyperthermia in normal tissues. *Cancer Res* 1984; 44: 4826s–4835s.
6. Dewey WC. Arrhenius relationships from the molecule and cell to the clinic. *Int J Hyperthermia* 1994; 10: 457–483.
7. Bush W. Über den Finfluss wetchen heftigere Eryspelen zuweilen auf organisierte Neubildungen dusuben. *Verh Natruch Preuss Rhein Westphal* 1886; 23: 28–30.
8. Westermark F. Über die Behandlung des ulcerirenden Cervix carcinoma mittels Knonstanter Warme. *Zentralbl Gynkol* 1898; 1335–1339.
9. Vander Vorst A, Rosen A, Kotsuka Y. *RF/Microwave Interaction with Biological Tissues.* Wiley–IEEE Press, 2006.

10. Van der Zee J. Heating the patient: a promising approach? *Ann Oncol* 2002; 13: 1173–1184.
11. Urano M, Double EB. *Hyperthermia and Oncology.* Vol. 1: Thermal effects on cells and tissues. VSP Utrecht: The Netherlands, 1988.
12. Urano M, Double EB. *Hyperthermia and Oncology.* Vol. 2: Biology of thermal potentiation of radiotherapy. VSP Utrecht: The Netherlands, 1989.
13. Urano M, Double EB. *Hyperthermia and Oncology.* Vol. 3: Interstitial hyperthermia: physics, biology and clinical aspects. VSP Utrecht: The Netherlands, 1992.
14. Urano M, Double EB. *Hyperthermia and Oncology.* Vol. 4: Chemopotentiation by hyperthermia: biology and clinical aspects. VSP Utrecht: The Netherlands, 1994.
15. Hahn GM. *Hyperthermia and Cancer.* New York: Plenum, 1982.
16. Handl-Zeller L, Editor. *Interstitial Hyperthermia.* Vienna: Springer-Verlag, 1992.
17. Gautherie M, Robins HI, Cohen, JD, Neville AJ, Editors. *Whole Body Hyperthermia: Biological and Clinical Aspects.* Berlin: Springer-Verlag, 1992.
18. Leibel SA, Phillips TL. *Textbook of Radiation Oncology.* Philadelphia, PA: Saunders, 1998.
19. Baronzio GF, Hager ED, Editors. *Locoregional Radiofrequency-Perfusional and Whole Body Hyperthermia in Cancer Treatment: New Clinical Aspects.* Eurekah.com and Springer Science Business Media, New York, 2005.
20. Baronzio GF, Hager ED, Editors. *Hyperthermia in Cancer Treatment: A Primer.* Berlin: Springer-Verlag, 2006.
21. Christensen DA. Thermometry and thermography. In: Storm FK, Editor. *Hyperthermia in Cancer Therapy.* Boston, MA: GK Hall Medical Publishers, pp. 223–232, 1983.
22. Dewhirst MW. Considerations for hyperthermia clinical trial designs. In: Seegenschmiedt MH, Fessenden P, Vernon CC, Editors. *Principles and Practice of Thermoradiotherapy and Thermochemotherapy.* Vol. 2. Berlin: Springer-Verlag, pp. 361–372, 1996.
23. Sneed PK, Stauffer PR, Li G, Steege G. Hyperthermia. In: Leibel SA, Phillips TL, Editors. *Textbook of Radiation Oncology.* 2nd ed. Philadelphia, PA: WB Saunders, pp. 1241–1262, 1998.
24. Stauffer PR. Thermal therapy techniques for skin and superficial tissue disease. In: Ryan TP, Editor. *Critical Reviews, Matching the Energy Source to the Clinical Need.* Bellingham: SPIE Optical Engineering Press, pp. 327–367, 2000.
25. Stauffer PR, Diederich CJ, Pouliot J. *Thermal Therapy for Cancer, Chapter in AAPM Monograph Series.* New York: American Institute of Physics, 2005.
26. Lele PP. Induction of deep, local hyperthermia by ultrasound and electromagnetic fields. Problems and choices. *Radiat Environ Biophys* 1980; 17: 205–217.
27. Schwan HP. Electromagnetic and ultrasonic induction of hyperthermia in tissue-like substances. *Radiat Environ Biophys* 1980; 17: 189–203.
28. Sterzer E. Localized hyperthermia treatment of cancer. *RCA Rev* 1981; 42: 727–751.
29. Christensen DA, Durney CH. Hyperthermia production for cancer therapy: a review of fundamentals and methods. *J Microw Power* 1981; 16: 89–105.
30. Oleson JR. A review of magnetic induction methods for hyperthermia treatment of cancer. *IEEE Trans Microw Theory Tech* 1982; 30: 1149–1157.
31. Strohbehn JW, Roemer RB. Survey of computer simulations of hyperthermia treatments. *IEEE Trans Biomed Eng* 1984; 31: 136–149.
32. Cheung AY, Neyzari A. Deep local hyperthermia for cancer therapy: external electromagnetic and ultrasound techniques. *Cancer Res* 1984; 44: 4736s–4744s.
33. Abe A, Hiraoka M. Localized hyperthermia and radiation in cancer therapy. *Int J Radat Biol* 1985; 47: 347–359.
34. Conway J, Anderson AP. Electromagnetic techniques in hyperthermia. *Clin Phys Physiol Meas* 1986; 7: 287–318.

35. Field SB. 1985 Douglas Lea Memorial Lecture. Hyperthermia in the treatment of cancer. *Phys Med Biol* 1987; 32: 789–811.
36. Stuchly MA, Stuchly SS. Measurements of electromagnetic fields in biomedical applications. *Crit Rev Biomed Eng* 1987; 14: 241–288.
37. Hand JW. Heat delivery and thermometry in clinical hyperthermia. *Recent Results Cancer Res* 1987; 104: 1–23.
38. Cheung AY. Microwave hyperthermia for cancer therapy. *IEE Proc* 1987; 134: 493–522.
39. Magin RL, Peterson AF. Noninvasive microwave phased arrays for local hyperthermia: a review. *Int J Hyperthermia* 1989; 5: 429–450.
40. Fessenden P, Hand JW. Hyperthermia therapy physics. In: Smith AR, Editor. *Medical Radiology: Radiation Therapy Physics.* Berlin: Springer-Verlag, pp. 315–363, 1995.
41. Hiraoka M, Mitsumori M, Hiroi N, Ohno S, Tanaka T, Kotsuka Y, Sugimachi K. Development of RF and microwave heating equipment and clinical applications to cancer treatment in Japan. *IEEE Trans Microw Theory Tech* 2000; 48: 1789–1799.
42. Vaezy S, Andrew M, Kaczkowski P, Crum L. Image-guided acoustic therapy. *Annu Rev Biomed Eng* 2001; 3: 375–90.
43. Gel'vich EA, Mazokhin VN. Technical aspects of electromagnetic hyperthermia in medicine. *Crit Rev Biomed Eng* 2001; 29: 77–97.
44. Moroz P, Jones SK, Gray BN. Magnetically mediated hyperthermia: current status and future directions. *Int J Hyperthermia* 2002; 18: 267–284.
45. Saiyed ZM, Telang SD, Ramchand CN. Application of magnetic techniques in the field of drug discovery and biomedicine. *BioMagn Res Technol* 2003; 1: 2.
46. Chou C-K. Evaluation of microwave hyperthermia applicators. *Bioelectromagnetics* 2005; 13: 581–597.
47. Haemmerich D, Lee FT. Multiple applicator approaches for radiofrequency and microwave ablation. *Int J Hyperthermia* 2005; 21: 93–106.
48. Szasz A, Szasz O, Szasz N. Physical background and technical realizations of hyperthermia. In: Baronzio GF, Hager ED, Editors. *Locoregional Radiofrequency-Perfusional and Whole-Body Hyperthermia in Cancer Treatment: New Clinical Aspects.* Eurokah.com and Springer Science Business Media, New York, 2005.
49. Giammaria F, Andras S. Hyperthermia today: electric energy, a new opportunity in cancer treatment. *J Cancer Res Ther* 2006; 2: 41–46.
50. Dutreix J, Le Bourgeois JP, Salama M. The treatment of the tumors by hyperthermia. *J Radiol Electrol Med Nucl* 1978; 59: 323–334.
51. Chou C-K. Application of electromagnetic energy in cancer treatment. *IEEE Trans Instrum Meas* 1988; 37: 547–551.
52. Valdagni R, Amichetti M. Report of long-term follow-up in a randomized trial comparing radiation therapy and radiation therapy plus hyperthermia to metastatic lymph nodes in stage IV head and neck patients. *Int J Radiat Oncol Biol Phys* 1994; 28: 163–169.
53. Pontiggia P, Rotella GB, Sabato A, Curto FC. Therapeutic hyperthermia in cancer and AIDS: an updated survey. *J Environ Pathol Toxicol Oncol* 1996; 15: 289–297.
54. Overgaard J, Gonzalez Gonzalez D, Hulshof MC, Arcangeli G, Dahl O, Mella O, Bentzen SM. Randomised trial of hyperthermia as adjuvant to radiotherapy for recurrent or metastatic malignant melanoma. *Lancet* 1995; 345: 540–543.
55. Seegenschmiedt MH, Fessenden P, Vernon CC. *Thermoradiotherapy and Thermochemotherapy.* Vol 2: Clinical Applications. Berlin: Springer-Verlag, 1996.
56. Vernon CC, Hand JW, Field SB, Machin D, Whaley JB, Van der Zee J, van Putten WL, van Rhoon GC, van Dijk JD, Gonzalez Gonzalez D, Liu FF, Goodman P, Sherar M. Radiotherapy with or without hyperthermia in the treatment of superficial localized breast cancer: results from five randomized controlled trials. International Collaborative Hyperthermia Group. *Int J Radiat Oncol Biol Phys* 1996; 35: 1117–1121.

57. Dewhirst MW, Prosnitz L, Thrall D, Prescott D, Clegg S, Charles C, MacFall J, Rosner G, Samulski T, Gillette E, LaRue S. Hyperthermic treatment of malignant diseases: current status and a view toward the future. *Semin Oncol* 1997; 24: 616–625.
58. Dewhirst MW, Kong MW. Review hyperthermia and liposomes. *Int J Hyperthermia* 1999; 15: 345–370.
59. Falk MH, Issels RD. Hyperthermia in oncology. *Int J Hyperthermia* 2000; 17: 1–18.
60. Wust P, Hildebrandt B, Sreenivasa G, Rau B, Gellermann J, Riess H, Felix R, Schlag PM. Hyperthermia in combined treatment of cancer. *Lancet Oncol* 2002; 3: 487–497.
61. Feldman AL, Libutti SK, Pingpank JF, Bartlett DL, Beresnev TH, Mavroukakis SM, Steinberg SM, Liewehr DJ, Kleiner DE, Alexander HR. Analysis of factors associated with outcome in patients with malignant peritoneal mesothelioma undergoing surgical debulking and intraperitoneal chemotherapy. *J Clin Oncol* 2003; 21: 4560–4567.
62. Dewhirst MW, Jones E, Samulski TV, Vujaskovic Z, Li C, Prosnitz L. Hyperthermia. In: Kufe D, Pollock R, Weischelbaum R, Gansler RBT, Holland J, Rei EF, Editors. *Cancer Medicine.* 6th ed. Hamilton: Decker, pp. 623–636, 2003.
63. Haveman J, Van der Zee J, Wondergem J, Hoogeveen JF, Hulshof MC. Effects of hyperthermia on the peripheral nervous system: a review. *Int J Hyperthermia* 2004; 20: 371–391.
64. Stauffer PR. Evolving technology for thermal therapy of cancer. *Int J Hyperthermia* 2005; 21: 731–744.
65. Diederich CJ. Thermal ablation and high-temperature thermal therapy: overview of technology and clinical implementation. *Int J Hyperthermia* 2005; 21: 745–753.
66. Kampinga HH. Cell biological effects of hyperthermia alone or combined with radiation or drugs: a short introduction to newcomers in the field. *Int J Hyperthermia* 2006; 22: 191–196.
67. Issels RD. High-risk soft tissue sarcoma: clinical trial and hyperthermia combined chemotherapy. *Int J Hyperthermia* 2006; 22: 235–239.
68. Jones E, Thrall D, Dewhirst MW, Vujaskovic Z. Prospective thermal dosimetry: the key to hyperthermia's future. *Int J Hyperthermia* 2006; 22: 247–253.
69. Van Rhoon GC, Wust P. Introduction: Non-invasive thermometry for thermotherapy. *Int J Hyperthermia* 2005; 21: 489–495.
70. Gerard C, Rhoon V, Wust P. Introduction: non-invasive thermometry for thermotherapy. *Int J Hyperthermia* 2005; 21: 489–495.
71. Dewhirst MW, Ozimek EJ, Gross J, Cetas TC. Will hyperthermia conquer the elusive hypoxic cell? Implications of heat effects on tumor and normal-tissue microcirculation. *Radiology* 1980; 137: 811–817.
72. Goldstein LS, Dewhirst MW, Repacholi M, Kheifets L. Summary, conclusions and recommendations: adverse temperature levels in the human body. *Int J Hyperthermia* 2003; 19: 373–384.
73. Lepock JR, Frey HE, Ritchie KP. Protein denaturation in intact hepatocytes and isolated cellular organelles during heat shock. *J Cell Biol* 1993; 122: 1267–1276.
74. Lepock JR. Role of nuclear protein denaturation and aggregation in thermal radiosensitization. *Int J Hyperthermia* 2004; 20: 115–130.
75. Lepock JR. How do cells respond to their thermal environment? *Int J Hyperthermia* 2005; 21: 681–687.
76. Spiro IJ, Denman DL, Dewey WC. Effect of hyperthermia on CHO DNA polymerases α and β. *Radiat Res* 1982; 89: 134–149.
77. Michels AA, Kanon B, Konings AWT, Ohtsuka K, Bensaude O, Kampinga HH. HSP70 and HSP40 chaperone activities in the cytoplasm and the nucleus of mammalian cells. *J Biol Chem* 1997; 272: 33283–33289.
78. Read RA, Bedford JS. Thermal tolerance. *Br J Radiol* 1980; 53: 920–921.

79. Armour EP, McEachern D, Wang Z, Corry P, Martinez A. Sensitivity of human cells to mild hyperthermia. *Cancer Res* 1993; 53: 2740–2744.

80. Morimoto RI, Tissieres A, Georgopoulos C. *Stress Proteins in Biology and Medicine.* New York: Cold Spring Harbor, 1990.

81. Hahn GM, Adwankar MK, Basrur VS, Anderson RL. Survival of cells exposed to anti-cancer drugs after stress. In: Pardue ML, Feramisco JR, Lindquist S, Editors. *Stress-Induced Proteins.* New York: Liss, pp. 223–233, 1989.

82. Kampinga HH, Dikomey E. Hyperthermic radiosensitization: mode of action and clinical relevance. *Int J Radiat Biol* 2001; 77: 399–408.

83. Kampinga HH, Turkel-Uygur N, Roti Roti JL, Konings AWT. The relationship of increased nuclear protein content induced by hyperthermia to killing of HeLa S3 cells. *Radiat Res* 1989; 117: 511–522.

84. Dahl O. Interaction of heat and drugs *in vitro* and *in vivo*. In: Seegenschmiedt MH, Fessenden P, Vernon CC, Editors. *Thermoradiotherapy and Thermochemotherapy.* Vol. 1. Berlin: Springer-Verlag, pp. 103–121, 1995.

85. Hettinga JVE, Konings ATW, Kampinga HH. Reduction of cisplatin resistance by hyperthermia: a review. *Int J Hyperthermia* 1997; 13: 439–457.

86. Hildebrandt B, Wust P, Ahlers O, Dieing A, Sreenivasa G, Kerner T, Felix R, Riess H. The cellular and molecular basis of hyperthermia. *Crit Rev Oncol Hemato* 2002; 43: 33–56.

87. Lee ER. Electromagnetic superficial heating technology. In: Seegenschmiedt MH, Fessenden P. Vernon CC, Editors. *Thermoradiotherapy and Thermochemotherapy.* Berlin: Springer-Verlag, pp. 193–217, 1995.

88. Wust P, Seebass M, Nadobny J, Felix R. Electromagnetic deep heating technology. In: Seegenschmiedt MH, Fessenden P, Vernon CC, Editors. *Thermoradiotherapy and Thermochemotherapy.* Berlin: Springer-Verlag, pp. 219–251, 1995.

89. Myerson RJ, Moros E, Roti Roti JL. Hyperthermia. In: Perez CA, Brady LW, Editors. *Principles and Practice of Radiation Oncology.* Philadelphia, PA: Lippincott-Raben Publishers, pp. 637–683, 1997.

90. Wust P, Gellermann J, Beier J, Wegner S, Tilly W, Troger J, Stalling D, Oswald H, Hege HC, Deuflhard P, Felix R. Evaluation of segmentation algorithms for generation of patient models in radiofrequency hyperthermia. *Phys Med Biol* 1998; 43: 3295–3307.

91. Van Rhoon GC, Rietveld PCM, Van der Zee J. A 433 MHz lucite cone waveguide applicator for superficial hyperthermia. *Int J Hyperthermia* 1998; 14: 13–27.

92. Rietveld PJM, Van Putten WLJ, Van der Zee J, Van Rhoon GC. Comparison of the clinical effectiveness of the 433 MHz Lucite cone applicator with that of a conventional waveguide applicator in applications of superficial hyperthermia. *Int J Radiat Oncol Biol Phys* 1999; 43: 681–687.

93. Sugimachi K, Inokuchi K. Hyperthermochemoradiotherapy and esophageal carcinoma. *Semin Surg Oncol* 1986; 2: 38–44.

94. Sugimachi K, Kitamura K, Baba K, Ikebe M, Ikebe M, Morita M, Matsuda H, Kuwano H. Hyperthermia combined with chemotherapy and irradiation for patients with carcinoma of the oesophagus—a prospective randomized trial. *Int J Hyperthermia* 1992; 8: 289–295.

95. Sugimachi K, Kuwano H, Ide H, Toge T, Saku M, Oshiumi Y. Chemotherapy combined with or without hyperthermia for patients with oesophageal carcinoma: a prospective randomized trial. *Int J Hyperthermia* 1994; 10: 485–493.

96. Kitamura K, Kuwano H, Watanabe M, Nozoe T, Yasuda M, Sumiyoshi K, Saku M, Sugimachi K. Prospective randomized study of hyperthermia combined with chemoradiotherapy for esophageal carcinoma. *J Surg Oncol* 1995; 60: 55–58.

97. Saeki H, Kawaguchi H, Kitamura K, Ohno S, Sugimachi K. Recent advances in pre-operative hyperthermochemoradiotherapy for patients with esophageal cancer. *J Surg Oncol* 1998; 69: 224–229.

98. Fuwa N, Nomoto Y, Shouji K, Kodaira T, Kamata M, Ito Y. Therapeutic effects of simultaneous intraluminal irradiation and intraluminal hyperthermia on oesophageal carcinoma. *Br J Radiol* 2001; 74: 709–714.

99. Fuwa N, Nomoto Y, Shouji K, Nakagawa T, Ito Y, Kikuchi Y. Simultaneous intraluminal irradiation and hyperthermia treatment for esophageal carcinoma. *Nippon Igaku Hoshasen Gakkai Zasshi* 1995; 55: 993–995.

100. Freudenberg S, Rewerk S, Bay F, Al Khouri C, Wagner A, Isaac M, Gebhard MM, Kähler G. Local application of hyperthermia in the esophagus with a heatable malleable thermoplastic stent. *Eur Surg Res* 2006; 38: 42–47.

101. Lin JC, Wang YJ. Interstitial microwave antennas for thermal therapy. *Int J Hyperthermia* 1987; 3: 37–47.

102. Lin JC, Wang YJ. An implantable microwave antenna for interstitial hyperthermia. *Proc IEEE* 1987; 75: 1132–1133.

103. Sullivan D. Mathematical methods for treatment planning in deep regional hyperthermia. *IEEE Trans Microw Theory Tech* 1991; 39: 864–872.

104. Turner PF. Regional hyperthermia with an annular phased array. *IEEE Trans Biomed Eng* 1984; 31: 106–114.

105. Seebass M, Beck R, Gellermann J, Nadobny J, Wust P. Electromagnetic phased arrays for regional hyperthermia—optimal frequency and antenna arrangement. *Int J Hyperthermia* 2001; 17: 321–336.

106. Wust P, Fahling H, Wlodarczyk W, Seebass M, Gellermann J, Deuflhard P, Nadobny J. Antenna arrays in the SIGMA-Eye applicator: interactions and transforming networks. *Med Phys* 2001; 28: 1793–1805.

107. Coit DG. Hyperthermic isolation limb perfusion for malignant melanoma: a review. *Cancer Invest* 1992; 10: 277–284.

108. Ceelen WP, Hesse U, De Hemptinne B, Pattyn P. Hyperthermic intraperitoneal chemoperfusion in the treatment of locally advanced intra-abdominal cancer. *Br J Surg* 2000; 87: 1006–1015.

109. Ghussen F, Nagel K, Groth W, Muller JM, Stutzer H. A prospective randomized study of regional extremity perfusion in patients with malignant melanoma. *Ann Surg* 1984; 200: 764–768.

110. Hafstrom L, Rudenstam CM, Blomquist E, Lindholm C, Ringborg U, Westman G, Ostmp. Regional hyperthermic perfusion with melphalan after surgery for recurrent malignant melanoma of the extremities. *J Clin Oncol* 1991; 9: 2091–2094.

111. Koops HS, Vaglini M, Suciu S, Kroon BB, Thompson JF, Gohl J, Eggermont AM, Di Filippo F, Krementz ET, Ruiter D, Lejeune FJ. Prophylactic isolated limb perfusion for localized, high-risk limb melanoma: results of a multicenter randomized phase III trial. *J Clin Oncol* 1998; 16: 2906–2912.

112. Anscher MS, Samulski TV, Dodge R, Prosnitz LR. Dewhirst MW. Combined external beam irradiation and external regional hyperthermia for locally advanced adenocarcinoma of the prostate. *Int J Radiat Oncol Biol Phys* 1997; 37: 1059–1065.

113. Coley WB. The treatment of malignant tumors by repeated inoculations of erysipelas: with a report of ten original cases. *Am J Med Sci* 1893; 33: 195–199.

114. Xi L, Tekin P, Phargava P, Kukreja RC. Whole body hyperthermia and preconditioning of the heart: basic concepts, complexity, and potential mechanisms. *Int J Hyperthermia* 2001; 17: 439–455.

115. Millian AJ. Whole-body hyperthermia induction techniques. *Cancer Res* 1984; 44(Suppl): 4869S.

116. Storm FK. Clinical hyperthermia and chemotherapy. *Radiol Clin North Am* 1989; 27: 621–627.

117. Robins HI, Hugander A, Cohen JD. Whole body hyperthermia in the treatment of neoplastic disease. *Radiol Clin North Am* 1989; 27: 603–610.

118. Pettigrew RT, Galt JM, Ludgate CM, Horn DN, Smith AN. Circulatory and biochemical effects of whole body hyperthermia. *Br J Med* 1974; 61: 727–730.
119. Pomp H. Clinical application of hyperthermia in gynecological malignant tunors. In: Strefer C, Editor. *Cancer Therapy by Hyperthermia and Radiation*. Baltimore: Urban and Schwarzenberg, pp. 326–327, 1978.
120. Bull JM, Lees D, Schuette W, Whang-Peng J, Smith R, Bynum G, Atkinson ER, Gottdiener JS, Gralnick HR, Shawker TH, DeVita VT, Jr. Whole body hyperthermia: a phase I trial of a potential adjuvant to chemotherapy. *Ann Intern Med* 1979; 90: 317–323.
121. Liebergall M, Simkin A, Mendelson S, Rosenthal A, Amir G, Segal D. Effect of moderate bone hyperthermia on cell viability and mechanical function. *Clin Orthop Relat Res* 1998; 349: 242–248.
122. Gerke P, Filejski W, Robins HI, Wiedemann GJ, Steinhoff J. Nephrotoxicity of ifosfamide, carboplatin and etoposide (ICE) alone or combined with extracorporeal or radiant-heat-induced whole-body hyperthermia. *J Cancer Res Clin Oncol* 2000; 126: 173–177.
123. Bull JCM. Clinical practice of whole-body hyperthermia: new directions. In: Seegenschmiedt MH, Fessenden P, Vernon CC, Editors. *Thermoradiotherapy and Thermochemotherapy*. Vol. 2. Berlin: Springer-Verlag, pp. 303–322, 1996.
124. Szasz A, Vincze GY, Szasz O, Szasz N. An energy analysis of extracellular hyperthermia. *Electromag Biol Med* 2003; 22: 103–115.
125. Kotnik T, Miklavcic D. Theoretical evaluation of the distributed power dissipation in biological cells exposed to electric field. *Bioelectromagnetics* 2000; 21: 385–94.
126. Vrba J. Medical applications of microwaves. *Electromag Biol Med* 2005; 24: 441–448.
127. Hynynen K, Shimm D, Anhalt D, Stea B, Sykes H, Cassady JR, Roemer RB. Temperature distributions during clinical scanned, focused ultrasound hyperthermia treatments. *Int J Hyperthermia* 1990; 6: 891–908.
128. Svensson GK, Hansen JL, Delli Carpini D, Bornstein B, Herman T. SAR and temperature diatributions from a spherical focused segmented ultrasound machine (FSUM). In: Gerner EW, Editor. *Hyperthermic Oncology* 1992. Vol. 1. Tucson, AZ: Arizona Board of Regents, p. 335, 1992.
129. Lindsley K, Stauffer PR, Sneed P, Chin R, Phillips TL, Seppi E, Shapiro E, Henderson S. Heating patterns of the Helios ultrasound hyperthermia system. *Int J Hyperthermia* 1993; 9: 675–684.
130. Lu XQ, Burdette EC, Bornstein BA, Hansen JL, Svensson GK. Design of an ultrasonic therapy system for breast cancer treatment. *Int J Hyperthermia* 1996; 12: 375–399.
131. Lee RJ, Buchanan M, Kleine LJ, Hynynen K. Arrays of multielement ultrasound applicators for interstitial hyperthermia. *IEEE Trans Biomed Eng* 1999; 46: 880–890.
132. Lee RJ, Suh H. Design and characterization of an intracavitary ultrasound hyperthermia applicator for recurrent or residual lesions in the vaginal cuff. *Int J Hyperthermia* 2003; 19: 563–574.
133. Sekins KM, Leeper DB, Hoffman JK, Keilman GW, Ziskin MC, Wolfson MR, Shaffer TH. Feasibility of lung cancer hyperthermia using breathable perfluorochemical (PFC) liquids. Part II: Ultrasound hyperthermia. *Int J Hyperthermia* 2004; 20: 278–299.
134. Beer E. Removal of neoplasms of the urinary bladder: a new method employing high frequency (oudin) currents through a cauterizing cystoscope. *JAMA* 1910; 54: 1768–1769.
135. Clark WL. Oscillatory desiccation in the treatment of accessible malignant growths and minor surgical conditions. *J Adv Therap* 1911; 29: 169–183.
136. Clark WL, Morgan JD, Asnia EJ. Electrothermic methods in treatment of neoplasms and other lesions with clinical and histological observations. *Radiology* 1924; 2: 233–246.

137. Fenn AJ, Diederich CJ, Stauffer PR. An adaptive-focusing algorithm for a microwave planar phased-array hyperthermia system. *Lincoln Lab J* 1993; 6: 269–288.

138. Organ LW. Electrophysiologic principles of radiofrequency lesion making. *Appl Neurophysiol* 1976–1977; 39: 69 –76.

139. Sackenheim MM. Radio frequency ablation: the key to cancer treatment. *J Diagn Med Sonogr* 2003; 19: 88–92.

140. Rhim, H, Goldberg SN, Dodd GD, Solbiati L, Lim HK, Tonolini M, Cho OK. Essential techniques for successful radio-frequency thermal ablation of malignant hepatic tumors. *Radiographics* 2001; 21: S17–S35.

141. Wittkampt FHM, Hauer RNW, Roblesde Medina EO. Control of RF lesions size by power regulation. *Circulation* 1989; 80: 962–968.

142. Blouin LT, Marcus FI. The effect of electrode design on the efficiency of delivery of RF energy to cardiac tissue in vitro. *PACE* 1989; 12: 136–143.

143. Reddy NM, Maithreyan V, Vasanthan A, Balakrishnan IS, Bhaskar BK, Jayaraman R, Shanta V, Krishnamurthi S. Local RF capacitive hyperthermia: thermal profiles and tumour response. *Int J Hyperthermia* 1987; 3: 379–387.

144. Hiraoka M. Radiofrequency capacitive hyperthermia for deep-seated tumors. I. Studies on thermometry. *Cancer* 1987; 60: 121–127.

145. Nussbaum GH, Sidi J, Rouhanizadeh N, Morel P, Jasmin C, Convert G, Mabire JB, Azam G. Manipulation of central axis heating patterns with a prototype, three-electrode capacitive device for deep-tumor hyperthermia. *IEEE Trans Microw Theory Tech* 1986; 34: 620–625.

146. Kato H, Ishida T. A new inductive applicator for hyperthermia. *J Microw Power* 1983; 18: 331–335.

147. Kato H, Hiraoka M, Nakajima T, Ishida T. Deep-heating characteristics of an RF capacitive heating device. *Int J Hyperthermia* 1985; 1: 15–28.

148. Song CW, Rhee JG, Lee CK, Levitt SH. Capacitive heating of phantom and human tumors with an 8 MHz radiofrequency applicator (Thermotron RF-8). *Int J Radiat Oncol Biol Phys* 1986; 12: 365–372.

149. Kakehi M, Ueda K, Mukojima T, Hiraoka M, Seto O, Akanuma A, Nakatsugawa S. Multi-institutional clinical studies on hyperthermia combined with radiotherapy or chemotherapy in advanced cancer of deep-seated organs. *Int J Hyperthermia* 1990; 6: 719–740.

150. Orcutt N, Gandhi OP. Use of the impedance method to calculate 3-D power deposition patterns for hyperthermia with capacitive plate electrodes. *IEEE Trans Biomed Eng* 1990; 37: 36–43.

151. Nishimura Y, Hiraoka M, Akuta K, Jo S, Nagata Y, Masunaga S, Takahashi M, Abe M. Hyperthermia combined with radiation therapy for primarily unresectable and recurrent colorectal cancer. *Int J Radiat Oncol Biol Phys* 1992; 23: 759–768.

152. Takeshita N, Tanaka Y, Matsuda T. Thermoradiotherapy for adenocarcinoma of the rectum and sigmoid—application to primarily inoperable and recurrent cases. *Nippon Igaku Hoshasen Gakkai Zasshi.* 1992; 52: 472–482.

153. Brown SL, Hill RP, Heinzl L, Hunt JW. Radiofrequency capacitive heaters: the effect of coupling medium resistivity on power absorption along a mouse leg. *Phys Med Biol* 1993; 38: 1–12.

154. Karasawa K, Muta N, Nakagawa K, Hasezawa K, Terahara A, Onogi Y, Sakata K, Aoki Y, Sasaki Y, Akanuma A. Thermoradiotherapy in the treatment of locally advanced nonsmall cell lung cancer. *Int J Radiat Oncol Biol Phys* 1994; 30: 1171–1177.

155. Imada H, Nomoto S, Tomimatsu A, Kosaka K, Kusano S, Ostapenko VV, Terashima H. Local control of non small cell lung cancer by radiotherapy combined with high power hyperthermia using an 8 MHz RF capacitive heating device. *Jpn J Hyperthermic Oncol* 1999; 15: 15–19.

156. Kuroda S, Uchida N, Sugimura K, Kato H. Thermal distribution of radio-frequency inductive hyperthermia using an inductive aperture-type applicator: evaluation of the effect of tumour size and depth. *Med Biol Eng Comput* 1999; 37: 285–290.
157. Kroeze H, Van de Kamer JB, De Leeuw AAC, Kikuchi M, Lagendijk JJW. Treatment planning for capacitive regional hyperthermia. *Int J Hyperthermia* 2003; 19: 58–73.
158. Ohguri T, Imada H, Yahara K, Kakeda S, Tomimatsu A, Kato F, Nomoto S, Terashima H, Korogi Y. Effect of 8-MHz radiofrequency-capacitive regional hyperthermia with strong superficial cooling for unresectable or recurrent colorectal cancer. *Int J Hyperthermia* 2004; 20: 465–475.
159. Ohguri T, Imada H, Kato F, Yahara T, Morioka T, Kakano K, Korogi Y. Radiotherapy with 8 MHz radiofrequency-capacitive regional hyperthermia for pain relief of unresectable and recurrent colorectal cancer. *Int J Hyperthermia* 2006; 22: 1–14.
160. Storm FK, Elliot RS, Harrison WH, Morton DL. Clinical RF hyperthermia by magnetic-loop induction: a new approach to human cancer therapy. *IEEE Trans Microw Theory Tech* 1982; 30: 1124–1158.
161. Kotsuka Y, Watanabe M, Hosoi M, Isono I, Izumi M. Development of inductive regional heating system for breast hyperthermia. *IEEE Trans Microw Theory Tech* 2000; 48: 1807–1814.
162. Minamimura T, Sato H, Kasaoka S, Saito T, Ishizawa S, Takemori S, Tazawa K, Tsukada K. Tumor regression by inductive hyperthermia combined with hepatic embolization using dextran magnetite-incorporated microspheres in rats. *Int J Oncol* 2000; 16: 1153–1158.
163. Trakic A, Liu F, Crozier S. Transient temperature rise in a mouse due to low-frequency regional hyperthermia. *Phys Med Biol* 2006; 51: 1673–1691.
164. Kato H, Hand JW, Prior MV, Furukawa M, Yamamoto O, Ishida T. Control of specific absorption rate distribution using capacitive electrodes and inductive aperture-type applicators: implications for radiofrequency hyperthermia. *IEEE Trans Biomed Eng* 1991; 38: 644–647.
165. Perez CA, Nussbaum G, Emami B, VonGerichten D. Clinical results of irradiation combined with hyperthermia. *Cancer* 1983; 52: 1597–1603.
166. Paglione R, Sterzer F, Mendecki J, Friedenthal E, Botstein C. 27 MHz ridged waveguide applicators for localized hyperthermia treatment of deep-seated malignant tumors. *Microwave J* 1981; 24: 71–80.
167. De Leeuw AA, Mooibroek J, Lagendijk JJ. Specific absorption rate by patient positioning in the "coaxial TEM" system: phantom investigation. *Int J Hyperthermia* 1991; 7: 605–611.
168. Van Es CA, Wijrdeman HK, De Leeuw AAC, Mooibroek J, Lagendijk JJW, Battermann JJ. Regional hyperthermia of pelvic tumours using the Utrecht coaxial TEM system: a feasibility study. *Int J Hyperthermia* 1995; 11: 173–186.
169. Van Vulpen M, De Leeuw AA, Van De Kamer JB, Kroeze H, Boon TA, Warlam-Rodenhuis CC, Lagendijk JJ, Battermann JJ. Comparison of intra-luminal versus intra-tumoural temperature measurements in patients with locally advanced prostate cancer treated with the coaxial TEM system: report of a feasibility study. *Int J Hyperthermia* 2003; 19: 481–497.
170. Gabriele P, Orecchia R, Tseroni V, Melano A, Fillini C, Ragona R, Bolla L, Ogno G. Three new applicators for hyperthermia. *Arch Geschwulstforsch* 1989; 59: 271–275.
171. Montecchia F. Microstrip-antenna design for hyperthermia treatment of superficial tumors. *IEEE Trans Biomed Eng* 1992; 39: 580–588.
172. Stauffer PR, Rossetto F, Leencini M, Gentilli GB. Radiation patterns of dual concentric conductor microstrip antennas for superficial hyperthermia. *IEEE Trans Biomed Eng* 1998; 45: 605–613.

173. Gelvich EA, Klimanov VA, Kramer-Ageev EA, Mazokhin VN. Computational evaluation of changes in ionizing radiation dose distribution in tissue caused by EM applicators when external radiation and hyperthermia act simultaneously. *Int J Hyperthermia* 2006; 22: 343–352.

174. Nikawa Y, Kikuchi M, Mori S. Development and testing of a 2450 MHz lens applicator for localized microwave hyperthermia. *IEEE Trans Microw Theory Tech* 1985; 33: 1212–1216.

175. Croghan MK, Shimm DS, Hynynen KH, Anhalt DP, Valencic SL, Fletcher AM, Kittleson JM, Cetas TC. A phase I study of the toxicity of regional hyperthermia with systemic warming. *Am J Clin Oncol* 1993; 16: 354–358.

176. Vrba J, Lapes M, Oppl L. Technical aspects of microwave thermotherapy. *Bioelectrochem Bioenerg* 1999; 48: 305–309.

177. Guy AW. Electromagnetic fields and relative heating patterns due to a rectangular aperture source in direct contact with bilayered biological tissue. *IEEE Trans Microw Theory Tech* 1971; 19: 214–223.

178. Antolini R, Cerri G, Cristoforetti L, De Leo R. Absorbed power distributions from single or multiple waveguide applicators during microwaved hyperthermia. *Phys Med Biol* 1986; 31: 1005–1019.

179. Nikita KS, Uzunoglu NK. Analysis of the power coupling from a waveguide hyperthermia applicator into a three-layered tissue model. *IEEE Trans Microw Theory Tech* 1989; 37: 1794–1800.

180. Andreuccetti D, Bini M, Ignesti A, Olmi R, Priori S, Vanni R. High permittivity patch radiator for single and multi-element hyperthermia applicators. *IEEE Trans Biomed Eng* 1993; 40: 711–715.

181. Surowiec A, Bicher HI. Heating characteristics of the TRIPAS hyperthermia system for deep seated malignancy. *J Microw Power Electromag Energy* 1995; 30: 135–140.

182. Samaras T, Rietveld PJM, Rhoon GCV. Effectiveness of FDTD in predicting SAR distributions from the Lucite cone applicator. *IEEE Trans Microw Theory Tech* 2000; 48: 2059–2063.

183. Siauve N, Nicolas L, Vollaire C, Marchal C. Optimization of the sources in local hyperthermia using a combined finite element-genetic algorithm method. *Int J Hyperthermia* 2004; 20: 815–833.

184. Gupta RC, Singh SP. Analysis of the SAR distributions in three-layered bio-media in direct contact with a water-loaded modified box-horn applicator. *IEEE Trans Microw Theory Tech* 2005; 53: 2665–2671.

185. Gupta RC, Singh SP. Development and analysis of a microwave direct contact water-loaded box-horn applicator for therapeutic heating of bio-medium. *Prog Electromag Res* 2006; 62: 217–235.

186. Fenn AJ, Sathiaseelan V, King G, Stauffer PR. Improved localization of energy deposition in adaptive phased-array hyperthermia treatment of cancer. *Lincoln Lab J* 1996; 9: 187–196.

187. Manning MR, Cetas TC, Miller RC, Oleson JR, Connor WG, Gerner EW. Clinical hyperthermia results of a phase I trial employing hyperthermia alone or in combination with external beam or interstitial radiotherapy. *Cancer* 1982; 49: 205–216.

188. Strohbehn JW. Temperature distribution from RF electrode hyperthermia system: theoretical predictions. *Int J Radiat Oncol Biol Phys* 1986; 12: 293.

189. Stauffer PR, Sneed PK, Suen SA, Satoh T, Matsumoto K, Fike JR, Phillips TL. Comparative thermal dosimetry of interstitial microwave and radiofrequency-LCF hyperthermia. *Int J Hyperthermia* 1989; 5: 307–318.

190. Leybovich LB, Dogan N, Sethi A. A modified technique for RF-LCF interstitial hyperthermia. *Int J Hyperthermia* 2000; 16: 405–413.

191. Fenn AJ, Wolf GL, Fogle RM. An adaptive microwave phased array for targeted heating of deep tumours in intact breast: animal study results. *Int J Hyperthermia* 1999; 15: 45–61.

192. Kowalski ME, Jin JM. Model-order reduction of nonlinear models of electromagnetic phased-array hyperthermia. *IEEE Trans Biomed Eng* 2003; 50: 1243–1254.

193. Kowalski ME, Jin JM. A temperature-based feedback control system for electromagnetic phased-array hyperthermia: theory and simulation. *Phys Med Biol* 2003; 48: 633–651.

194. Ocheltree KB, Benkeser PJ, Frizzell LA, Charles AC. An ultrasound phased array applicator for hyperthermia. *IEEE Trans Sonics Ultrasonics* 1984; SU-31: 526–531.

195. Cain CA, Umemura S. Concentric-ring and sector-vortex phased-array applicators for ultrasound hyperthermia. *IEEE Trans Microw Theory Tech* 1986; 34: 542–551.

196. Benkeser BJ, Frizzell LA, Ocheltree KB, Cain CA. A tapered phased array ultrasound transducer for hyperthermia treatment. *IEEE Trans Ultras Ferro Freq Contr* 1987; 34: 446–453.

197. Ebbini ES, Umemura SI, Ibbini M, Cain CA. A cylindrical-section ultrasound phased-array applicator for hyperthermia cancer therapy. *IEEE Trans on Ultrasonics* 1988; 35: 561–572.

198. Diederich CJ, Hynynen K. Induction of hyperthermia using an intracavitary multielement ultrasonic applicator. *IEEE Trans Biomed Eng* 1989; 36: 432–438.

199. Diederich, CJ, Hynynen K. The feasibility of using electrically focused ultrasound arrays to induce deep hyperthermia via body cavities. *IEEE Trans Ultras Ferro Freq Contr* 1991; 38: 207–219.

200. Quan KM, Shiran M, Watmough DJ. Applicators for generating ultrasound-induced hyperthermia in neoplastic tumours and for use in ultrasound physiotherapy. *Phys Med Biol* 1989; 34: 1719–1731.

201. Daum DR, Buchanan MT, Fjield T, Hynynen K. Design and evaluation of a feedback based phased array system for ultrasound surgery. *IEEE Trans Ultras Ferro Freq Contr* 1998; 45: 431–438.

202. Ibbini MS, Cain CA. The concentric-ring array for ultrasound hyperthermia: combined mechanical and electrical scanning. *Int J Hyperthermia* 1990; 6: 401–419.

203. McGough RJ, Kessler ML, Ebbini ES, Cain CA. Treatment planning for hyperthermia with ultrasound phased arrays. *IEEE Trans Ultras Ferro Freq Contr* 1996; 43: 1074–1084.

204. Daum DR, Hynynen K. A 256-element ultrasonic phased array system for the treatment of large volumes of deep seated tissue. *IEEE Trans Ultras Ferro Freq Contr* 1999; 46: 1254–1268.

205. Smith NB, Merilees NK, Hynynen K, Dahleh M. Control system for an MRI compatible intracavitary ultrasound array for thermal treatment of prostate disease. *Int J Hyperthermia* 2001; 17: 271–282.

206. Hynynen K, Pomeroy O, Smith DN, Huber PE, McDonnald NJ, Kettenbach J, Baum J, Singer S, Jolesz FA. MR imaging-guided focused ultrasound surgery of fibroadenomas in the breast: a feasibility study. *Radiology* 2001; 219: 176–185.

207. Ju K-C, Chen Y-Y, Lin W-L, Kuo T-S. One-dimensional phased array with mechanical motion for conformal ultrasound hyperthermia. *Phys Med Biol* 2003; 48: 167–182.

208. Connor CW, Hynynen K. Patterns of thermal deposition in the skull during transcranial focused ultrasound surgery. *IEEE Trans Biomed Eng* 2004; 51: 1693–1706.

209. Hand JW. Development of array applicators for superficial hyperthermia. *Int J Hyperthermia* 1991; 7: 209–210.

210. Francomi C, Raganella L, Tiberio CA, Begnozzi L. Low-frequency RF hyperthermia. IV. A 27 MHz hybrid applicator for localized deep tumor heating. *IEEE Trans Biomedical Eng* 1991; 38: 287–293.

211. Zhang Y, Joines WT, Jirtle RL, Samulski TV. Theoretical and measured electric field distribution within an annular phased array: consideration of source antennas. *IEEE Trans Biomed Eng* 1993; 40: 780–787.
212. Gopal MK, Cetas TC. Current sheet applicators for clinical microwave hyperthermia. *IEEE Trans Microw Theory Tech* 1993; 41: 431–437.
213. Wust P, Seebass M, Nadobny J, Deuflhard P, Monich G, Felix R. Simulation studies promote technological development of radiofrequency phased array hyperthermia. *Int J Hyperthermia* 1996; 12: 477–494.
214. Wiersma J, Van Dijk JD. RF hyperthermia array modelling; validation by means of measured EM-field distributions. *Int J Hyperthermia* 2001; 17: 63–81.
215. Nadobny J, Wlodarczyk W, Westhoff L, Gellermann J. Development and evaluation of a three-dimensional hyperthermia applicator with water-coated antennas (WACOA). *Med Phys* 2003; 30: 2052–2064.
216. Wu L, McGough RJ, Arabe OA, Samulski TV. An RF phased array applicator designed for hyperthermia breast cancer treatments. *Phys Med Bio* 2006; 51: 1–20.
217. Rappaport CM, Morgenthaler FR. Localized hyperthermia with electromagnetic arrays and the leaky-wave troughguide applicator. *IEEE Trans Microw Theory Tech* 1986; 34: 636–643.
218. Nikawa Y, Katsumata T, Kikuchi M, Mori S. An electric field converging applicator with heating pattern controller for microwave hyperthermia. *IEEE Trans Microw Theory Tech* 1986; 34: 631–635.
219. Jouvie F, Bolomey J-C, Gaboriaud G. Discussion of capabilities of microwave phased arrays for hyperthermia treatment of neck tumors. *IEEE Trans Microw Theory Tech* 1986; 34: 495–501.
220. Loane J, Ling H, Wang BF, Lee SW. Experimental investigation of a retro-focusing microwave hyperthermia applicator: conjugate-field matching scheme. *IEEE Trans Microw Theory Tech* 1986; 43: 490–494.
221. Zhang Y, Joines WT, Oleson JR. Heating patterns generated by phase modulation of a hexagonal array of interstitial antennas. *IEEE Trans on Biomed Eng* 1991; 38: 92–97.
222. Diederich CJ, Stauffer PR. Preclinical evaluation of a microwave array applicator for superficial hyperthermia. *Int J Hyperthermia* 1993; 9: 227–246.
223. Sherar MD, Clark H, Cooper B, Kumaradas J, Liu FF. A variable microwave array attenuator for use with single-element waveguide applicators. *Int J Hyperthermia* 1994; 10: 723–731.
224. Stauffer PR, Leoncini M, Manfrini V, Diederich CJ, Bozzo, D. Dual concentric conductor radiator for microwave hyperthermia with improved field uniformity to periphery of aperture. *IEICE Trans Comm* 1995; E78-B(6): 826–835.
225. Reuter CE, Taflove A, Sathiaseelan V, Piket-May M, Mittal BB. Unexpected physical phenomena indicated by FDTD modeling of the Sigma-60 deep hyperthermia applicator. *IEEE Trans Microw Theory Tech* 1998; 46: 313–319.
226. Fenn AJ, Sathiaseelan V, King GA, Stauffer PR. Improved localization of energy deposition in adaptive phased-array hyperthermia treatment of cancer. *J Oncol Manag* 1998; 7: 22–29.
227. Gavrilov LR, Hand JW, Hopewell JW, Fenn AJ. Pre-clinical evaluation of a two-channel microwave hyperthermia system with adaptive phase control in a large animal. *Int J Hyperthermia* 1999; 15: 495–507.
228. Jacobsen S, Stauffer PR, Neuman DG. Dual-mode antenna design for microwave heating and noninvasive thermometry of superficial tissue disease. *IEEE Trans Biomed Eng* 2000; 47: 1500–1509.
229. Rossetto F, Diederich CJ, Stauffer PR. Thermal and SAR characterization of dual concentric conductor array applicators for hyperthermia, a theoretical investigation. *Med Phys* 2000; 27: 745–753.

230. Rossetto F, Stauffer PR. Theoretical characterization of dual concentric conductor microwave applicators for hyperthermia at 433 MHz. *Int J Hyperthermia* 2001; 17: 258–270.

231. Jacobsen S, Stauffer PR. Non-invasive temperature profile estimation in a lossy medium based on multi-band radiometric signals sensed by a microwave dual-purpose body-contacting antenna. *Int J Hyperthermia* 2002; 18: 86–103.

232. Carlier J, Thomy V, Camart J-C, Dubois L, Pribetich J. Modeling of planar applicators for microwave thermotherapy. *IEEE Trans Microw Theory Tech* 2002; 50: 3036–3042.

233. Gardner RA, Vargas HI, Block JB, Vogel CL, Fenn AJ, Kuehl GV, Doval M. Focused microwave phased array thermotherapy for primary breast cancer. *Ann Surg Oncol* 2002; 9: 326–332.

234. Kumaradas JC, Sherar MD. Optimization of a beam shaping bolus for superficial microwave hyperthermia waveguide applicators using a finite element method. *Phys Med Biol* 2003; 48: 1–18.

235. Converse M, Bond EJ, Hagness SC, Van Veen BD. Ultrawide-band microwave space-time beamforming for hyperthermia treatment of breast cancer: a computational feasibility study. *IEEE Trans Microw Theory Tech* 2004; 52: 1876–1889.

236. Jaehoon K, Rahmat-Samii Y. Implanted antennas inside a human body: simulations, designs, and characterizations. *IEEE Trans Microw Theory Tech* 2004; 52: 1934–1943.

237. Vargas HI, Dooley WC, Gardner RA, Gonzalez KD, Venegas R, Heywang-Kobrunner SH, Fenn AJ. Focused microwave phased array thermotherapy for ablation of early-stage breast cancer: results of thermal dose escalatio. *Ann Surg Oncol* 2004; 11: 139–146.

238. Taschereau R, Stauffer PR, Hsu IC, Schlorff JL, Milligan AJ, Pouliot J. Radiation dosimetry of a conformal heat-brachytherapy applicator. *Technol Cancer Res Treat* 2004; 3: 347–358.

239. Sangster AJ, Sinclair KI. Multimode degenerate mode cavity for microwave hyperthermia treatment. *IEEE Proc Microw Antennas Propag* 2006; 153: 75–82.

240. Petrovich Z, Langholz B, Gibbs FA, Sapozink MD, Kapp DS, Stewart RJ, Emami B, Oleson J, Senzer N, Slater J, Astrahan M. Regional hyperthermia for advanced tumors: a clinical study of 353 patients. *Int J Radiat Oncol Biol Phys* 1989; 16: 601–607.

241. Doss JD, McCabe CW. A technique for localized heating in tissue: an adjunct to tumor therapy. *Ned Instrum* 1976; 10: 16–21.

242. Lagendijk JJW. Hyperthermia treatment planning. *Phys Med Biol* 2000; 45: R61–R76.

243. Van der Koijk JF, Crezee J, Van Leeuwen GMJ, Battermann JJ, Lagendijk JJW. Dose uniformity in MECS interstitial hyperthermia: the impact of longitudinal control in model anatomies. *Phys Med Biol* 1996; 41: 429–444.

244. Diederich CJ. Ultrasound applicators with integrated catheter-cooling for interstitial hyperthermia: theory and preliminary experiments. *Int J Hyperthermia* 1996; 12: 279–297.

245. Diederich CJ, Khalil IS, Stauffer PR, Sneed PK, Phillips TL. Direct-coupled interstitial ultrasound applicators for simultaneous thermobrachytherapy: a feasibility study. *Int J Hyperthermia* 1996; 12: 401–419.

246. Diederich CJ, Nau WH, Stauffer PR. Ultrasound applicators for interstitial thermal coagulation. *IEEE Trans Ultras Ferro Freq Contr* 1999; 46: 1218–1228.

247. Jarosz BJ, Kaytar D. Ultrasonic heating with waveguide interstitial applicator array. *IEEE Trans Instrumen Measur* 1998; 47: 703–707.

248. Nau WH, Diederich CJ, Burdette EC. Evaluation of multielement catheter-cooled interstitial ultrasound applicators for high-temperature thermal therapy. *Med Phys* 2001; 28: 1525–1534.

249. Jarosz BJ, St James S. Integrated temperature sensor for determination of ultrasound interstitial applicator heating effects. *IEEE Trans Instrumen Measur* 2005; 54: 1171–1174.
250. Deurloo IKK, Visser AG, Morawska M, Van Geel CAJF, Van Rhoon GC, Levendag PC. Application of a capacitive-coupling interstitial hyperthermia system at 27 MHz: study of different applicator configurations. *Phys Med Biol*; 36: 119–132.
251. Prior MV. A comparative study of RF-LCP and hot-source interstitial hyperthermia techniques. *Int J Hyperthermia* 1991; 7: 131–140.
252. Prionas SD, Kapp DS. Quality assurance for interstitial radiofrequency-induced hyperthermia. In: Handl-Zeller L, Editor. *Interstitial Hyperthermia*. Vienna: Springer-Verlag, pp. 77–94, 1992.
253. Kaatee RSJP, Crezee J, Kanis AP, Lagendijk JJW, Levendag PC, Visser AG. Design of applicators for a 27 MHz multielectrode current source interstitial hyperthermia system; impedance matching and effective power. *Phys Med Biol* 1997; 42: 1087–1108.
254. DeBree J, Lagendijk JJ, Raaymakers BW, Bakker CJ, Hulshof MC, Koot RW, Hanlo PW, Struikmans H, Ramos LM, Battermann JJ. Treatment planning of brain implants using vascular information and a new template technique. *IEEE Trans Med Imaging* 1998; 17: 729–736.
255. Crezee J, Kaatee RS, Van der Koijk JF, Lagendijk JJ. Spatial steering with quadruple electrodes in 27 MHz capacitively coupled interstitial hyperthermia. *Int J Hyperthermia* 1999; 15: 145–156.
256. Sathiaseelan V, Leybovich L, Emami B, Stauffer P, Straube W. Characteristics of improved microwave interstitial antennas for local hyperthermia. *Int J Radiat Oncol Biol Phys* 1991; 20: 531–539.
257. Hurter W, Reinbold F, Lorenz WJ. A dipole antenna for interstitial microwave hyperthermia. *IEEE Trans Microw Theory Tech* 1991; 39: 1048–1054.
258. Schaller G, Erb J, Engelbrecht R. Field simulation of dipole antennas for interstitial microwave hyperthermia. *IEEE Trans Microw Theory Tech* 1996; 44: 887–895.
259. Hamada L, Saito K, Yoshimura H, Ito K. Dielectric-loaded coaxial-slot antenna for interstitial microwave hyperthermia: longitudinal control of heating patterns. *Int J Hyperthermia* 2000; 16: 219–229.
260. Camart JC, Despretz D, Prevost B, Sozanski JP, Chive M, Pribetich J. New 434 MHz interstitial hyperthermia system monitored by microwave radiometry: theoretical and experimental results. *Int J Hyperthermia* 2000; 16: 95–111.
261. Saito K, Yoshimura H, Ito K, Aoyagi Y, Horita H. Clinical trials of interstitial microwave hyperthermia by use of coaxial-slot antenna with two slots. *IEEE Trans Microw Theory Tech* 2004; 52: 1987–1991.
262. Satoh T, Stauffer PR. Implantable helical coil microwave antenna for interstitial hyperthermia. *Int J Hyperthermia* 1988; 4: 497–512.
263. Iskander MF, Tumeh AM. Design optimization of interstitial antennas. *IEEE Trans Biomed Eng* 1989; 36: 238–246.
264. Schreier K, Budihna M, Lesnicar H, Handl-Zeller L, Hand JW, Prior MV, Clegg ST, Brezovich IA. Preliminary studies of interstitial hyperthermia using hot water. *Int J Hyperthermia* 1990; 6: 431–444.
265. Van Hillegersberg HR, Jzermans JNM. Interstitial laser coagulation for hepatic tumours. *Br J Surg* 1999; 86: 1365–2168.
266. Ikeda H, Tanaka M, Marsuo R, Fukuda H, Yamada R, Yamamoto I. Development of a new heating needle for interstitial hyperthermia compatible with interstitial radiotherapy. *Radiat Med* 2001; 19: 285–289.
267. Safarikova M, Safarik I. The application of magnetic techniques in biosciences. *Magn Electr* 2001; 10: 223–252.

268. Miltenyi S, Muller W, Weichel W, Radbruch A. High gradient magnetic cell separation with MACS. *Cytometry.* 1990; 11: 231–238.

269. Radbruch A, Mechtold B, Thiel A, Miltenyi S, Pfluger E. High-gradient magnetic cell sorting. *Methods Cell Biol* 1994; 42: 387–403.

270. Shinkai M, Yanase M, Honda H, Wakabayashi T, Yoshida J, Kobayashi T. Intracellular hyperthermia for cancer using magnetite cationic liposomes: *in vitro* study. *Jpn J Cancer Res* 1996; 87: 1179–1183.

271. Takegami K, Sano T, Wakabayashi H, Sonoda J, Yamazaki T, Morita S, Shibuya T, Uchida A. New ferromagnetic bone cement for local hyperthermia. *J Biomed Mater Res* 1998; 43: 210–214.

272. Sato F, Jojo M, Matsuki H, Sato T, Sendoh M, Ishiyyama K, Arai I. The operation of a magnetic micromachine for hyperthermia and its exothermic characteristic. *IEEE Trans Magnet* 2002; 38: 3362–3364.

273. Ito A, Tanaka K, Kondo K, Shinkai M, Honda H, Matsumoto K, Saida T, Kobayashi T. Tumor regression by combined immunotherapy and hyperthermia using magnetic nanoparticles in an experimental subcutaneous murine melanoma. *Cancer Sci* 2003; 94: 308.

274. Matsuoka F, Shinkai M, Honda H, Kubo T, Sugita T, Kobayashi T. Hyperthermia using magnetite cationic liposomes for hamster osteosarcoma. *Biomagn Res Technol* 2004; 2: 3.

275. Ohura K, Ikenaga M, Nakamura T, Yamamuro T, Ebisawa Y, Kokudo T, Kotoura Y, Oka M. A heat-generating bioactive glass-ceramic for hyperthermia. *J Appl Biomater* 1991; 2: 153–159.

276. Oleson JR, Samulski TV, Leopold KA, Clegg ST, Dewhirst MW, Dodge RK, George SL. Sensitivity of hyperthermia trial outcomes to temperature and time: implications for thermal goals of treatment. *Int J Radiat Oncol Biol Phys* 1993; 25: 289–297.

277. Prionas SD, Kapp DS, Goffinet DR, Ben-Yosef R, Fessenden P, Bagshaw MA. Thermometry of interstitial hyperthermia given as an adjuvant to brachytherapy for the treatment of carcinoma of the prostate. *Int J Radiat Oncol Biol Phys* 1994; 28: 151–162.

278. Emami B, Scott C, Perez CA et al. Phase III study of interstitial thermoradiotherapy compared with interstitial radiotherapy alone in the treatment of recurrent or persistent human tumors. A prospectively controlled randomized study by the Radiation Therapy Group. *Int J Radiat Oncol Biol Phys* 1996; 34: 1097–1104.

279. Hand JW, Machin D, Vernon CC, Whaley JB. Analysis of thermal parameters obtained during phase III trials of hyperthermia as an adjunct to radiotherapy in the treatment of breast carcinoma. *Int J Hyperthermia* 1997; 13: 343–364.

280. Wust P, Rau B, Gellerman J, Pegios W, Loffel J, Riess H, Felix R, Schlag PM. Radiochemotherapy and hyperthermia in the treatment of rectal cancer. *Recent Results Cancer Res* 1998; 146: 175–191.

281. Konings AW. Interaction of heat and radiation in vitro and in vivo. In: Seegendchmiedt MH, Fessenden P, Vernon CC, Editors. *Radiothermotherapy and Thermochemotherapy.* Vol 1. New York: Springer-Verlag, pp. 89–102, 1995.

282. Takahashi I, Emi Y, Hasuda S, Kakeji Y, Maehara Y, Sugimachi K. Clinical application of hyperthermia combined with anticancer drugs for the treatment of solid tumors. *Surgery* 2002; 131: S78–S84.

283. Dahl O, Dalene R, Schem BC, Mella O. Status of clinical hyperthermia. *Acta Oncol* 1999; 38: 863–873.

284. Song CWM, Shakil A, Griffin RJ, Okajima K. Improvement of tumor oxygenation status by mild temperature hyperthermia alone or in combination with carbogen. *Semin Oncol* 1997; 24: 626–632.

285. Song CW, Shakil A, Osborn JL, Iwata K. Tumour oxygenation is increased by hyper-thermia at mild temperatures. *Int J Hyperthermia* 1996; 12: 367–373.
286. Rau B, Wust P, Tilly W, Gellermann J, Harder C, Riess H, Budach V, Felix R, Schlag PM. Preoperative radiochemotherapy in locally advanced or recurrent rectal cancer: regional radiofrequency hyperthermia correlates with clinical parameters. *Int J Radiat Oncol Biol Phys* 2000; 48: 381–391.
287. Overgaard J. The current and potential role of hyperthermia in radiotherapy. *Int J Radiat Oncol Biol Phys* 1989; 16: 535–549.
288. Kim JH, Hahn EW, Tokita N, Nisce LZ. Local tumor hyperthermia in combination with radiation therapy. 1. Malignant cutaneous lesions. *Cancer* 1977; 40: 161–169.
289. Kim JH, Hahn EW, Benjamin FJ. Treatment of superficial cancers by combination hyperthermia and radiation therapy. *Clin Bull* 1979; 9: 13–16.
290. Bicher HI, Sandhu TS, Hetzel FW. Hyperthermia as an adjuvant to radiation: proposal for an effective fractionation regime. *Int J Radiat Oncol Biol Phys* 1980; 6: 867–870.
291. González González D, Van Dijk JDP, Blank LECM, Rümke PH. Combined treatment with radiation and hyperthermia in metastatic malignant melanoma. *Radiother Oncol* 1986; 6: 105–113.
292. Van der Zee J, Treurniet-Donker AD, The SK, et al. Low dose reirradiation in combina-tion with hyperthermia: a palliative treatment for patients with breast cancer recurring in previously irradiated areas. *Int J Radiat Oncol Biol Phys* 1988; 15: 1407–1413.
293. Van der Zee J, Peer-Valstar JN, Rietveld PJ, de Graaf-Strukowska L, Van Rhoon GC. Practical limitations of interstitial thermometry during deep hyperthermia. *Int J Radiat Oncol Biol Phys* 1998; 40: 1205–1212.
294. Van der Zee J, Van der Holt B, Rietveld PJM, Hele PA, Wijnmaalen AJ, Van Putten WL, Van Rhoon GC. Reirradiation combined with hyperthermia in recurrent breast cancer results in a worthwhile local palliation. *Br J Cancer* 1999; 79: 483–490.
295. Van der Zee J, González, González D, Van Rhoon GC, Van Dijk JDP, Van Putten WLJ, Hart AAM. Comparison of radiotherapy alone with radiotherapy plus hyperthermia in locally advanced pelvic tumours: a prospective, randomised, multicentre trial. *Lancet* 2000; 355: 1119–1125.
296. Hiraoka M, Masunaga S, Nishimura Y, Nagata Y, Jo S, Akuta K, Li YP, Takahashi M, Abe M. Regional hyperthermia combined with radiotherapy in the treatment of lung cancers. *Int J Radiat Oncol Biol Phys* 1992; 22: 1009–1014.
297. Masunaga S, Hiraoka M, Akuta K. The phase I/II trial of preoperative thermotherapy in the treatment of urinary bladder cancer. *Int J Hyperthermia* 1994; 10: 31–40.
298. Overgaard J, González González D, Hulshof MC, Arcangeli G, Dahl O, Mella O, Bentzen SM. Hyperthermia as an adjuvant to radiation therapy of recurrent or meta-static malignant melanoma. A multicentre randomized trial by the European Society for Hyperthermic Oncology. *Int J Hyperthermia* 1996; 12: 3–20.
299. Van der Zee J, González González D. Radiotherapy and hyperthermia in inoper-able pelvic tumours: Results of Dutch randomized studies. *Eur J Cancer* 1997; 33: S205–S206.
300. Myerson RJ, Strauble WL, Moros EG, Emami BN, Lee HK, Perez CA, Taylor ME. Simultaneous superficial hyperthermia and external radiotherapy: report of thermal dosimetry and tolerance to treatment. *Int J Hyperthermia* 1999; 15: 251–266.
301. Amichetti M, Romano M, Cristoforetti L, Valdagni R. Hyperthermia and radiotherapy for inoperable squamous cell carcinoma metastatic to cervical lymph nodes from an unknown primary site. *Int J Hyperthermia* 2000; 16: 85–93.
302. Van der Zee J, González González D. The Dutch deep hyperthermia trial: results in cervical cancer. *Int J Hyperthermia* 2002; 18: 1–12.
303. Van der Zee J. Lessons learned from hyperthermia. *Int J Radiat Oncol Biol Phys* 2003; 57: 596–597.

304. Van Vulpen M, De Leeuw AAC, Raaymakers BW, Van Moorselaar RJA, Hofman P, Lagendijk JJW, Battermann JJ. Radiotherapy and hyperthermia in the treatment of patients with locally advanced prostate cancer: preliminary results. *BJU Int* 2004; 93: 36–41.

305. Van der Zee J, Van Rhoon GC. Cervical cancer: radiotherapy and hyperthermia. *Int J Hyperthermia* 2006; 22: 229–234.

306. Vasanthan, A, Mitsumori, M, Park, JH, Zhi-Fan Z, Yu-Bin, Z, Oliynychenko, P, Tatsuzaki H, Tanaka Y, Hiraoka M. Regional hyperthermia combined with radiotherapy for uterine cervical cancers: a multi-institutional prospective randomized trial of the international atomic energy agency. *Int J Oncol Biol Phys* 2005; 61: 145–153.

307. Takahashi M, Fujimoto S, Kobayashi K, Mutou T, Kure M, Masaoka H, Shimanskaya RB, Takai M, Endoh F, Ohkubo H. Clinical outcome of intraoperative pelvic hyperthermochemotherapy for patients with Dukes' C rectal cancer. *Int J Hyperthermia* 1994; 10: 749–754.

308. Skibba JL, Jones FE, Condon RE. Altered hepatic disposition of doxorubicin in the perfused rat liver at hyperthermic temperatures. *Cancer Treat Rep* 1982; 66: 1357–1363.

309. Zimmer RP, Ecker HA, Popovic VP. Selective electromagnetic heating of tumors in animals in deep hypothermia. *IEEE Trans Microw Theory Tech* 1971; 19: 232–238.

310. Ghussen F, Krüger I, Smalley RV, Groth W. Hyperthermic perfusion with chemotherapy for melanoma of the extremities. *World J Surg* 1989; 13: 598–602.

311. Issels RD, Mittermüller J, Gerl A, Simon W, Ortmaier A, Denzlinger C, Sauer H, Wilmanns W. Improvement of local control by regional hyperthermia combined with systemic chemotherapy (ifosfamide plus etoposide) in advanced sarcomas: updated report on 65 patients. *J Cancer Res Clin Oncol* 1991; 117: S141–S147.

312. Kondo M. Therapeutic effects of chemoembolization using degradable starch microspheres and regional hyperthermia on unresectable hepatocellular carcinoma. In: Matsuda T, Editor. *Cancer Treatment by Hyperthermia, Radiation and Drugs.* New York: Taylor & Francis, pp. 317–327, 1993.

313. Zaffaroni N, Fiorentini G, De Giorgi U. Hyperthermia and hypoxia: new developments in anticancer chemotherapy. *Eur J Surg Oncol* 2001; 27: 340–342.

314. Prosnitz L, Jones E. Counterpoint: test the value of hyperthermia in patients with carcinoma of the cervix being treated with concurrent chemotherapy and radiation. *Int J Hyperthermia* 2002; 18: 13–18.

315. Sagowski C, Jaehne M, Kehrl W, Hegewisch-Becker S, Wenzel S, Panse J, Nierhaus A. Tumor oxygenation under combined whole-body-hyperthermia and polychemotherapy in a case of recurrent carcinoma of the oral cavity. *Eur Arch Otorhinolaryngol* 2002; 259: 27–31.

316. Morita K, Tanaka R, Kakinuma K, Takahashi H, Motoyama H. Combination therapy of rat brain tumours using localized interstitial hyperthermia and intra-arterial chemotherapy. *Int J Hyperthermia* 2003; 19: 204–212.

317. Mauz-Körholz C, Dietzsch S, Banning U, Tröbs RB, Körholz D. Heat- and 4-hydroperoxy-ifosfamide-induced apoptosis in B cell precursor leukaemias. *Int J Hyperthermia* 2003; 19: 444–460.

318. Hildebrandt B, Drager J, Kerner T, Deja M, Löffel J, Stroszczynski C, Ahlers O, Felix R, Riess H, Wust P. Whole-body hyperthermia in the scope of von Ardenne's systemic cancer multistep therapy (sCMT) combined with chemotherapy in patients with metastatic colorectal cancer: phase I/II study. *Int J Hyperthermia* 2004; 20: 317–333.

319. Ismail-Zade RS, Zhavrid EA, Potapnev MP. Whole body hyperthermia in adjuvant therapy of children with renal cell carcinoma. *Ped Blood Cancer* 2005; 44: 679–681.

320. Kraybill WG, Olenki T, Evans SS, Ostberg JR, O'Leary KA, Gibbs JF, Repasky EA. A phase I study of fever-range whole body hyperthermia (FR-WBH) in patients with advanced solid tumors: correlation with mouse models. *Int J Hyperthermia* 2002; 19: 253–266.

321. Hegewisch-Becker S, Gruber Y, Corovic A, Pichlmeier U, Atanackovic D, Nierhaus A, Hossfeld DK. Whole-body hyperthermia (41.8°C) combined with bimonthly oxaliplatin, high-dose leucovorin and 5-fluorouracil 48-hour continuous infusion in pretreated metastatic colorectal cancer: a phase II study. *Ann Oncol* 2002; 13: 1197–1204.
322. Bakhshandeh A, Bruns I, Traynor A, Robins HI, Eberhardt K, Demedts A, Kaukel E, Koschel G, Gatzemeier U, Kohlmann Th, Dalhoff K, Ehlers EM, Gruber Y, Zumschlinge R, Hegewisch-Becker S, Peters SO, Wiedemann GJ. Ifosfomide, carboplatin, and etoposide combined with 41.8 degrees centigrade whole body hyperthermia for malignant pleural mesothelioma. *Lung Cancer* 2003; 39: 339–345.
323. Hegewisch-Becker S, Braun K, Otte M, Corovic A, Atanackovic D, Nierhaus A, Hossfeld DK, Pantel K. Effects of whole body hyperthermia (41.8 degrees centigrade) on the frequency of tumor cells in the peripheral blood of patients with advanced malignancies. *Clin Cancer Res* 2003; 9: 2079–2084.
324. Richel O, Zum Vorde Sive Vording PJ, Rietbroek R, Van der Velden J, Van Dijk JD, Schilthuis MS, Westermann AM. Phase II study of carboplatin and whole body hyperthermia (WBH) in recurrent and metastatic cervical cancer. *Gynecol Oncol* 2004; 95: 680–685.
325. Kai H, Matsufuji H, Okudaira Y, Sugimachi K. Heat, drugs and radiation given in combination is palliative for unresectable esophageal cancer. *Int J Radiat Oncol Biol Phys* 1988; 14: 1147–1152.
326. Kuwano H, Matsuura H, Mori M. Hyperthermia combined with chemotherapy and irradiation for the treatment of patients with carcinoma of the oesophagus and the rectum. In: Matsuda T, Editor. *Cancer Treatment by Hyperthermia, Radiation and Drugs.* New York: Taylor & Francis, pp. 353–364, 1993.
327. Sakamoto T, Katoh H, Shimizu T, Yamashita I, Takemori S, Tazawa K, Fujimaki M. Clinical results of treatment of advanced esophageal carcinoma with hyperthermia in combination with chemoradiotherapy. *Chest* 1997; 112: 1487–1493.
328. Ohno S, Tomoda M, Tomisaki S, Kitamura K, Mori M, Maehara Y, Sugimachi K. Improved surgical results after combining preoperative hyperthermia with chemotherapy and radiotherapy for patients with carcinoma of the rectum. *Dis Colon Rectum* 1997; 40: 401–406.
329. Rau B, Wust P, Hohenberger P, Loffel J, Hunerbein M, Below C, Gellermann J, Speidel A, Vogl T, Riess H, Felix R, Schlag PM. Preoperative hyperthermia combined with radiochemotherapy in locally advanced rectal cancer. A phase II clinical study. *Ann Surg* 1998; 227: 380–389.
330. Sakurai H, Mitsuhashi N, Tamaki Y, Akimoto T, Murata O, Kitamoto Y, Maebayashi K, Ishikawa H, Hayakawa K, Niibe H. Interaction between low dose-rate irradiation, mild hyperthermia and low-dose caffeine in a human lung cancer cell line. *Int J Rad Biol* 1999; 75: 739–745.
331. Feyerabend T, Wiedemann GJ, Jäger B, Vesely H, Mahlmann B, Richter E. Local hyperthermia, radiation, and chemotherapy in recurrent breast cancer is feasible and effective except for inflammatory disease. *Int J Radiat Oncol Biol Phys* 2001; 49: 1317–1325.
332. Kouloulias V, Plataniotis G, Kouvaris J, Dardoufas C, Gennatas C, Uzunoglu N, Papavasiliou C, Vlahos L. Chemoradiotherapy combined with intracavitary hyperthermia for anal cancer: feasibility and long-term results from a phase II randomized trial. *Am J Clin Oncol* 2005; 28: 91–99.
333. Song CW, Park HJ, Lee CK, Griffin R. Implications of increased tumor blood flow and oxygenation caused by mild temperature hyperthermia in tumor treatment. *Int J Hyperthermia* 2005; 21: 761–767.
334. Gerner EW, Hersh EM, Pennington M, Tsang TC, Harris D, Vasanwala F, Brailey J. Heat-inducible vectors for use in gene therapy. *Int J Hyperthermia* 2000; 16: 171–181.

335. Huang Q, Hu JK, Lohr F, Zhang L, Braun R, Lanzen J, Little JB, Dewhirst MY, Li CY. Heat-induced gene expression as a novel targeted cancer gene therapy strategy. *Cancer Res* 2000; 60: 3435–3439.

336. Okamota K, Shinoura N, Egawa N, Asai A, Kirino T, Shibasaki F, Shitara N. Adenovirus-mediated transfer of p53 augments hyperthermia-induced apoptosis in U251 glioma cells. *Int J Radiat Oncol Biol Phys* 2001; 50: 525–531.

337. Lohr F, Hu K, Huang Q, Zhang L, Samulski TV, Dewhirst MW, Li CY. Enhancement of radiotherapy by hyperthermia-regulated gene therapy. *Int J Radiat Oncol Biol Phys* 2000; 48: 1513–1518.

338. Habash RWY, Bansal R, Krewski D, Alhafid HT. Thermal therapy, Part 2: Hyperthermia techniques. *Crit Rev Biomed Eng* 2006; 34: 491–542.

339. Mattingly M, Bailey EA, Dutton AW, Roemer RB, Devasia S. Reduced-order modeling for hyperthermia: an extended balanced-realization-based approach. *IEEE Trans Biomed Eng* 1997; 45: 1154–1161.

340. Kapp DS, Cox R. Thermal treatment parameters are most predictive of outcome in patients with single tumor nodules per treatment field in recurrent adenocarcinoma of the breast. *Int J Radiat Oncol Biol Phys* 1995; 33: 887–899.

10 Radio Frequency and Microwave Ablation

10.1 INTRODUCTION

The term "ablation" is defined as the direct application of chemical or thermal therapies to a specific tumor (or tumors) in an attempt to achieve eradication or substantial tumor destruction. The methods of ablation most commonly used in current practice are divided into two main categories: chemical ablation and thermal ablation. Chemical ablation includes therapies, which are classified on the basis of universally accepted chemical nomenclature of the agent(s), such as ethanol and acetic acid that induce coagulation necrosis and cause tumor ablation [1,2]. Thermal ablation is performed by interventional radiologists and is much less invasive than open surgery. Recent developments in thermal ablation have expanded the treatment options for certain oncology patients. Minimally invasive, image-guided therapy may now provide effective local treatment of isolated or localized neoplastic disease, and may also be used as an adjunct to conventional surgery, systemic chemotherapy, or radiation. Thermal ablation can be an alternative to risky surgery, and sometimes it can change a patient from having an inoperable tumor to being a candidate for surgery.

Ablation using RF or microwave techniques is gaining rapid clinical acceptance as a treatment modality enabling tissue heating and ablation for numerous applications. Such treatments are usually carried out with the patient either fully conscious, lightly sedated or under light general anaesthesia. Given the wide-ranging applicability of RF and microwave energy, numerous devices have been designed to optimize application-specific treatment delivery. Their principle of operation is described in this chapter, alongside an overview of the physical mechanisms governing energy propagation and induced heating.

This chapter discusses the engineering principles and biological responses by which RF and microwave ablation techniques can provide the desired changes in temperature in organs within the human body. Aspect of each ablation technique including mechanisms of action, equipment, patient selections, treatment approaches and outcomes, limitations and complications are presented, along with a discussion of future research directions.

10.2 THERMAL ABLATION THERAPY

The main aim of thermal tumor ablation is to destroy an entire tumor by using heat to kill the malignant cells in a minimally invasive fashion without damaging adjacent vital structures. Heat from various sources can be used with equal effectiveness to destroy tumor cells. As long as adequate heat can be generated throughout the tumor volume, it is possible to eradicate the tumor [3]. Multiple energy sources can be used to provide the heat necessary to induce coagulation of malignant tissue by causing direct cell destruction. The bioheat equation describing induced heat transfer through tissue, previously expressed by Pennes et al. [4], and described in Chapter 11, has been further simplified by Goldberg et al. [5] to

coagulation necrosis = energy deposited × local tissue interactions − heat loss (10.1)

Based on this, much attention has centered on increasing coagulation volume with use of multiple probes simultaneously to increase overall energy deposition [6–8], but this approach by itself may not produce the desired outcome of increased tumor destruction, given biologic limitations to energy deposition and tissue physiology (such as blood flow and poor thermal conductivity) that limit the effectiveness of increased energy deposition for *in vivo* coagulation [9,10].

10.2.1 Minimally Invasive Procedures

Some authors have referred to the procedures of thermal ablation as "minimally invasive" or "percutaneous" therapies; however, these terms should be used only where appropriate. Minimally invasive therapies refer to all therapeutic procedures that are less invasive than conventional open surgery. All percutaneous procedures are therefore minimally invasive; however, not all minimally invasive therapies are performed or applied percutaneously. Indeed, the term "minimally invasive" is often used by surgeons to refer to procedures performed with minilaparotomy or laparoscopy [11]. Although less invasive than open surgery, these procedures are clearly more invasive than are percutaneous image-guided tumor ablation procedures. Inclusion of the term "percutaneous" as a prefix to "image-guided tumor ablation" is often too limiting because it does not reflect the fact that tumor ablation procedures can also be performed by laparoscopy, endoscopy, or surgery [12,13]. The choice of the approach for ablation is usually dictated by the training of the physician who is going to perform the ablation and suitability of the approach for patients.

Whenever possible, ablation is performed percutaneously. Percutaneous treatment has several advantages over other approaches. The percutaneous approach is the least invasive, produces minimal morbidity, can be performed on an outpatient basis, requires only conscious sedation, is relatively inexpensive, and can be repeated as necessary to treat recurrent tumor. However, advocates of laparoscopic thermal ablation claim that the laparoscopic approach provides some distinct advantages over the percutaneous approach [14]. General anesthesia is required for laparoscopy or open surgical treatment. However, conscious sedation is usually sufficient for a percutaneous approach.

Traditionally, local tumor removal has required major surgery. Recently, improvements in imaging technologies have enabled the development of minimally invasive tumor therapies, which rely on imaging guidance for the accurate percutaneous placement of needle-like applicators [5,15]. The potential benefits of minimally invasive, image-guided ablation of focal neoplasms, as compared with conventional surgical options, include (a) the ability to ablate or palliate tumors in nonsurgical candidates; (b) reduced morbidity and costs and improved quality of life; and (c) the ability to perform these procedures on an outpatient basis [16].

10.2.2 ABLATION TECHNIQUES

Ablation strategies, including cryoablation and the use of RF, microwaves, lasers, and high-intensity focused ultrasound (HIFU), are gaining increasing attention as an alternative to standard surgical therapies. Williams et al. [17] reviewed the above techniques to facilitate the creation of electrically isolated lesions within the atria. Although each of these techniques works slightly differently, the goal of all thermal sources is to heat tissue to a temperature (50°C) above which irreversible electrical isolation occurs.

Although ablation devices are often referred to as "needles" or other nonspecific terms, they do not always conform to these precise classifications. Hence, the term "applicator" should be used generally to describe all devices. For specificity, RF applicators are electrodes, microwave applicators are antennas, and laser applicators are fibers. On the basis of convention and consensus, cryoprobes are used to freeze tissue during cryoablation. For reporting completeness, a reference describing the appropriate applicator(s) should be cited unless the report describes a new prototype device, in which case an appropriate figure or schematic should be provided [1].

A thermal ablation device generally consists of an applicator that is introduced into the tumor under imaging guidance. Energy deposited by this applicator results in heating of the surrounding tissue. The SAR is only significantly very close (within a few millimeter) to the applicator and, contrary to many hyperthermia devices, most of the tissue is heated mainly by thermal conduction from the hot region near the applicator [18]. Catheters are commonly used to insert devices such as angioplasty balloons, through blood vessels into various sites within the body [19]. In some cases, a catheter with multiple needle electrodes is designed [20].

Typically, thermal ablation is applied by surgeons, gastro-oncologists or radiologists using minimally invasive procedures (laparoscopy or percutaneously) under accurate monitoring systems (magnetic resonance [MR], CT, thermal mapping, etc.) used to guide the percutaneous placement of applicators into the selected target [21,22]. Because in most cases adequate lesion conspicuity and visualization of the applicator can be achieved with any of these methods, the choice of imaging technique is often dictated by personal preference or research interests [5].

Efforts to generate specific interactions with tissue in a safe and reproducible manner have been restricted by the availability of controllable energy sources, accurate monitoring systems, and complications unique to treating each specific organ [23].

10.2.3 CLINICAL APPLICATIONS

Thermal ablation has been most commonly employed for the treatment of liver tumors; however, interest is growing for treatment of tumors in the kidney, lung, rectum, breast, prostate and muscculosketal system. Thermal ablation is also being investigated for several other malignancies including carcinoma of the thyroid, primary breast tumors and adrenal neoplasms [18]. A major advantage of thermal ablation is the ability to treat a tumor with a defined volume in sites where surgery itself is difficult (e.g., liver) or where organ function preservation is needed or desired (e.g., prostate, uterus). However, this form of therapy may find little use for large bulky tumors such as bone [24,25], colorectal cancer primaries, soft tissue sarcomas, head and neck nodules, and superficial disease involving the skin.

The clinical application of thermal ablation usually includes the following steps: preoperative evaluation; choice of approach—percutaneous, laparoscopy, or laparotomy; anesthesia and medications; applicator placement and treatment strategy; and follow-up. The preoperative evaluation begins with a review of the pertinent imaging studies. Good-quality imaging is the fundamental imaging examination on which the candidacy of a patient for thermal ablation is based. These preoperative imaging studies are used to determine the number and size of tumors and their relationship to surrounding structures such as blood vessels, bile ducts, gallbladder, diaphragm, and bowel. Patients are considered potential candidates if they have fewer than five tumors, each less than 5 cm in diameter, and no evidence of extrahepatic tumor [26].

Given the large number of potential energy sources to achieve thermal therapy and different strategies for applying them, important questions have emerged as to which modalities and modifications are most appropriate for given clinical scenarios. In this section, we provide a brief overview of the use of thermal ablation and other clinical modalities in the treatment of organ systems to date.

10.2.3.1 Liver

Cancerous (malignant) tumors in the liver have either originated in the liver (primary liver cancer) or spread from cancer sites elsewhere in the body (metastatic liver cancer). Most cancerous tumors in the liver are metastatic. While there are other types of liver cancer, the most common form in adults is called hepatocellular carcinoma (HCC). It begins in the hepatocytes, the main type of liver cell. About 3 out of 4 primary liver cancers are of this type. HCC is the fourth most common cause of cancer-related deaths worldwide and approximately one million new cases are reported annually [27]. Mortality is essentially 100% when these tumors are not treated. Surgical resection is currently the standard treatment of choice because it has been shown to provide survival benefits, while systemic chemotherapy and radiotherapy are largely ineffective. However, only 5–15% of patients with HCC or hepatic metastasis are candidates for curative surgery due to a variety of criteria such as multifocal disease, tumor size, too many tumors, location of tumor in relation to key vessels, and underlying medical problems that increase the surgical risk. Other treatment options include intraarterial chemotherapy, transcatheter arterial chemoembolization, percutaneous ethanol injection, cryotherapy, thermotherapy, proton therapy, or a wide range of their possible combinations [28–32]. There is also significant perioperative morbidity and mortality. The average 5-year survival rate after successful resection for both HCC and metastasis is only 20–40% [30]. A considerable number of patients will develop recurrence of tumor, which is usually fatal [33].

Today, there is a demand for minimally invasive techniques for treating hepatic malignancies with an increasing number of relevant scientific articles in high-ranked journals that provide a good review on treatment of primary and secondary malignant hepatic tumors by thermal ablation [3,15,34–43].

10.2.3.2 Lung

The lung is the most common site for primary cancer worldwide as well as being a common site of metastases for various malignancies [44]. The majority of patients with primary and secondary lung malignancies are not candidates for surgery owing to poor cardiorespiratory reserve. Conventional treatments for such patients typically include external-beam radiation therapy, with or without systemic chemotherapy [45]. One of the most promising alternatives to surgical removal of lung tumors is eliminating the tumor cells using heat, especially through EM energy. Thermal ablation is a useful alternative treatment for patients with small, early-stage lung cancer who wish to avoid conventional surgery or are considered not fit to undergo surgery. The same applies to patients who have a small number of metastases in their lungs, which are tumors that have spread from a cancer somewhere else in the body, such as the kidney, intestine, or breast. Thermal ablation may be used to debulk a lung tumor that is too large to remove surgically. Thus, the tumor is reduced in size so that the remaining tumor cells are more easily eliminated by chemotherapy or radiation therapy.

10.2.3.3 Prostate

The prostate is a walnut-sized gland that forms part of the male reproductive system. The gland is made of two regions, enclosed by an outer layer of tissue. It is located in front of the rectum and just below the bladder. It is common for the prostate gland to become enlarged as a man ages, a condition referred to as benign prostatic hyperplasia (BPH). The pathological evidence of BPH is seen in more than 80% of the population aged 75 or older [46]. The conventional treatment of prostate diseases can be associated with significant side effects and complications, and less invasive treatment alternative has always been searched for. Because of the anatomical location and easy accessibility of the prostate, many newer treatment modalities using thermal ablation have been applied to the organ. These include not only heating of the pathological tissue but also freezing. Some of such treatment techniques have been shown to be effective and safe and been widely used clinically [47]. The current concept of thermal therapy for BPH is to destroy the hypertrophic tissue in the preurethral area (transition zone) by increasing tissue temperature to more than 45°C.

10.2.3.4 Kidney

The kidneys are each filled with tiny tubules that clean and filter the blood to remove waste and make urine. Renal cell cancer is a malignancy involving these tubules of the kidney. Renal tumor ablation is considered to be an effective, safe procedure for treating renal cell cancer. Indications include a prior partial or total nephrectomy, preexisting renal insufficiency, various comorbidities making the patient a high surgical risk, or syndromes with multiple tumors. The retroperitoneal location minimizes the risk of major bleeding, while the exophytic (peripheral) location of many renal tumors decreases the chance of injury to the central collecting system [18]. Solid renal masses have been traditionally removed surgically with either total or, if possible, partial nephrectomy. Many patients who present with small incidental solid renal masses are in their later stages of life. These masses are often exophytic, slowly growing renal cell carcinomas that will not often affect patient longevity [48]. Although resection currently remains the standard of care for renal carcinoma, the search for less invasive treatments has led to alternative surgical approaches. Even less invasive, and appropriate for many groups of patients, is percutaneous thermal ablation, which induces tumor necrosis via lethal hyperthermia [49].

There are a number of relevant scientific articles that provide a good review of various ablation techniques as they apply to the management of renal tumors [50,51].

10.2.3.5 Breast

At least 10% of the women in the Western world face the prospect of developing breast cancer. The tendency in modern treatment of these tumors is toward less invasive local treatment. Today breast-conserving surgery (BCS) has become more common than mastectomy in many countries. BCS and mastectomy combined with radiation are associated with satisfactory long-term outcome. The survival rates after BCS of ductal carcinoma *in situ* is approximately 98%, whereas approximately 100% of these patients are cancer free after mastectomy [52,53]. However, multiple treatments and additional adjuvant care are needed in up to 50% of the BCS cases, resulting in higher associated costs compared with mastectomy alone. Recently, approaches other than traditional surgery have been explored to satisfy these demands [54–56]. These techniques include cryosurgery, laser ablation, focused ultrasound, and RF ablation. Potential benefits with these techniques are reduced morbidity rates, reduced treatment duration, and the ability to perform therapy for patients in poor medical condition on an outpatient basis [57].

10.2.3.6 Bone

Surgical treatment of bone tumors often requires a generous resection of bone, leaving defects that are difficult to span. Within the musculoskeletal system, tumor ablation has become a common treatment for osteomas (small benign tumors that are often painful and usually occur in the extremities of children and young adults) and to relieve symptoms from painful bone metastases [58,59]. With thermal ablation, painful bone tumors like osteoid osteoma and metastases in vertebrae can be treated effectively. The procedure is performed under local anesthesia/conscious sedation as there may be some bone drilling required.

10.2.3.7 Cardiac Diseases

There are a variety of clinical conditions that can cause cardiac arrhythmia (abnormal heart rate or rhythm) [60]; however, all arrhythmias have at their root an abnormal focus of electrical activity or an abnormal conducting pathway within the heart. They all prevent the heart from pumping blood into the circulatory system at a rate sufficient to meet the body's needs [61–62]. The most common sources for this abnormality lie above the atrioventricular (AV) node and are, therefore, referred to as supraventricular tachyarrhythmias (SVTs) [63]. Atrial fibrillation (AF) is the most commonly encountered sustained arrhythmia in men. It is associated with a twofold mortality risk and an increased cost for health care providers. The relative inefficacy and the risks of pharmacologic approaches to AF therapy have contributed to increasing efforts to address AF with curative ablative strategies.

Until recently, the treatment of patients with cardiac arrhythmias was mostly palliative, involving lifelong dependence on medication. However, in a significant portion (10–15%) of these patients, available drug therapy has been found unsatisfactory because of a lack of meaningful response or unacceptable side effects. Surgical intervention has been the principal method of treatment in these cases [61]. In the last decade, minimally invasive thermal ablation has revolutionized the treatment of patients with cardiac diseases. The success of this therapy depends upon two factors: cardiac mapping and lesion formation. In cardiac ablation, energy is delivered to the myocardium via a catheter to create thermal lesions, in order to disrupt or eliminate conduction pathways supporting the arrhythmia, instead of using a surgical blade [64,65]. Ablation approaches for AF focus on two alternate strategies: ablation of the substrate for initiation and ablation of the substrate for maintenance of AF [66].

There is an increasing number of published articles that provide a good review on thermal ablation for cardiac treatments [17,64,66–75].

10.3   RF ABLATION

The use of RF energy to produce thermal tissue destruction has been the focus of increasing research and practice for the past several years [14,76]. The term "RF ablation" applies to coagulation induction from all EM energy sources with frequencies less than 30 MHz, although most currently available devices function in the 375–500 kHz range [48].

RF is the most commonly used technique for ablation in the United States [77], with an increasing number of worldwide relevant scientific articles reviewing physical background, technical realization, and clinical trials of this technique [33,78–89].

10.3.1   TECHNICAL CONSIDERATIONS

RF ablation is an electrosurgical technique that uses a high-frequency alternating current to heat tissues to the point of desiccation (thermal coagulation) [10].

10.3.1.1   Mechanisms

The RF generators approved for clinical catheter ablation are limited to around 200 W output (although there are investigational 150 W units). While in hyperthermia literature different frequencies in the kilohertz–megahertz range have been used, all recent studies on RF ablation use RF in the range of 460–480 kHz [90]. The ability of RF applicators to cause ablation depends on the conduction of localized RF energy and heat convection by blood [91]. RF energy is capable of creating therapeutic tissue ablation by achieving higher temperatures ($>60°C$) over a shorter duration (3–5 min) when compared with other thermal modalities. This offers an advantage over other systems, especially when compared with the conventional 30–60 min of treatment needed for tissue effect in hyperthermia (40–44°C) and for low-range microwave thermal therapy (in the range of 45–55°C) [92].

With RF ablation, relatively small probes are placed into the tumor and RF energy deposited. The RF energy causes the tissue around the tip of the probe to heat up to a high temperature above which cells break apart and die. Since RF energy kills both tumor and nontumor cells, the goal is to place the probes so that they destroy the entire tumor plus an adequate "rim" of nontumorous tissue around it. This procedure is usually performed by placing one or more probes through small (less than 1 cm) incisions in the skin and using either ultrasound or a CT scanner to guide the tip into the tumor. For those tumors difficult to visualize, this procedure can also be performed in the operating room using a standard and much larger upper abdominal incision.

An effective approach to increase the efficacy of RF ablation is to modulate the biologic environment of treated tissues [5]. Along these lines, several investigators have demonstrated the possibility of increasing RF tissue heating and coagulation during RF ablation by altering electrical or thermal conduction by injecting concentrated NaCl solution into the tissues during RF application [93,94].

In two animal studies alone [95,96], vascular occlusion combined with RF ablation increased the volume of necrosis in a short period of time, created a more spherical lesion, and increased the time tissue is exposed to lethal temperatures when compared with RF. This technique could therefore be applied to humans to destroy large tumor nodules.

10.3.1.2   Electrodes and Approaches

The first generation of monopolar electrodes was introduced in 1990 by McGahan et al. [97]. They showed that RF electrocautery could ablate hepatic lesions up to 10 mm in diameter. However, larger lesions could not be coagulated with a single probe because of charring, which limits the effectiveness of the probe by preventing a thermal destruction of liver parenchyma beyond the region of ablation. Technical developments of probes aim to maintain high probe-tip temperatures (around 90°C), without loss of contact caused by tissue desiccation or increased impedance resulting from passage of current through charred tissue.

Today, RF ablation can be performed through percutaneous, laparoscopic, thoracoscopic, and open approaches. The percutaneous approach is the least invasive route for RF ablation [40]. The probe placement can be guided by use of CT, MRI, or ultrasonography. Commercially available RF probes have an insulated shaft with the high-temperature component confined to the tip. The insulated shaft of the RF probe broadens the applicability of the technique for use in percutaneous and laparoscopic procedures. Early expandable electrodes had few prongs, no saline infusion, and low power (i.e., 50 W) generators [83]. The increase in RF power is in response to the small irregular lesions created with less powerful devices that led to a high local recurrence rate and the need for multiple, overlapping ablations, even when treating small tumors. This problem is exacerbated when attempting to ablate lesions near major blood vessels.

Several innovations, such as pulsed energy deposition [98], umbrella-shaped or multiprong electrodes [5], saline infusion [99], bipolar electrodes [100–104], multipolar systems [105–107], internally cooled electrodes and an expandable electrode [108], and multiple probes [109], have been introduced. The aim of the above innovations is to improve the effectiveness of RF ablation devices and enable the creation of larger lesions and therefore expand the potential clinical applications of RF ablation.

10.3.1.3 Multiple Applicators

Both RF ablation and microwave ablation necessitate multiple applications or multiple applicators to treat tumors greater than 2 cm, including a 1 cm ablation margin. For example, adequate treatment of a 3 cm tumor would require creation of a 5 cm zone of ablation, assuming perfect placement of the probes. Since current clinically used RF devices can drive only a single applicator (electrode) at a time, large tumors have to be treated by multiple sequential applications [110]. Larger tumors can, thus, be treated by either sequential application or simultaneous application. Three distinct methods have been investigated by different groups that allow the simultaneous employment of multiple electrodes during RF ablation: bipolar RF, simultaneous RF, and rapidly switched RF, as shown in Figure 10.1 [90]. Laeseke et al. [111] developed a multiple-electrode RF system based on rapid switching between electrodes that allows for the simultaneous use of as many as three electrically independent electrodes. This system would allow physicians to simultaneously treat multiple tumors, substantially reducing procedure time and anesthesia risk.

Effective local ablation of different sizes of tumors with RF energy has been made possible by recent advancements in biomedical engineering. An RF interstitial tumor ablation (RITA) system has been applied to various tumors such as hepatoma or renal cell carcinoma [12,112,113]. This system consists of a small needle with multiple antennas extending from the tip of the needle, once the needle is inserted in the tissue. The energy heats the tissues surrounding the multihook antenna to 100°C, resulting in thermal damage and subsequent necrosis of spherical shape tissue 2 cm in diameter. Multiple needles can be inserted in the tissue to achieve a larger area of necrosis [47]. If multiple needle units become clinically available, large or irregularly shaped lesions could be treated more effectively than with conventional single

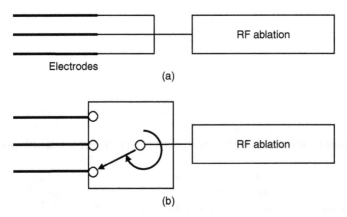

FIGURE 10.1 (a) Setup for simultaneous power application method. (b) Setup for rapidly switched power application method.

probe units, and multiple tumors could be ablated simultaneously, thus potentially decreasing procedure time and anesthetic complications [108].

10.3.1.4 Localization

The most difficult aspect of RF catheter ablation is localization of the correct ablation site. A method known as "entrainment mapping" can be employed for localization of reentrant pathways for hemodynamically stable reentrant arrhythmias. In this technique, the target tachyarrhythmia is first induced using stimulation approaches. Next, the ablation catheter is repeatedly repositioned within the suspected region of the heart. Trains of low-energy stimuli are then delivered at various sites while the arrhythmia continues, at a rate slightly faster (10–50 ms) than the intrinsic rate of the tachyarrhythmia. Certain criteria must be met before the catheter location is achieved. Pace mapping is another localization method that may be used for either focal or reentrant arrhythmias. In this technique, trains of low-energy stimuli are also delivered from multiple catheter positions within the suspected target region. The location in which the observed surface electrocardiogram is morphologically identical to that of the targeted tachyarrhythmia is considered to be at, or in very close proximity to, the site of initiation of the arrhythmia. Electroanatomical mapping, analogous to the use of a GPS, represents another localization method. This technique combines electrophysiological and spatial information and allows visualization of atrial activation in a 3D anatomical reconstruction of the atria. A catheter with a localization sensor on its top is repeatedly repositioned within the heart. Electrophysiological recordings from each site are recorded and associated with a specific spatial location relative to a system of localization sensors located under the patient [62,114].

10.3.1.5 Thermal–Electrical Modeling

To investigate and develop new techniques, and also to improve those currently employed, theoretical models and computer simulations are a powerful tool since they provide vital information on the electrical and thermal behavior of ablation rapidly and at low cost. In the future they could even help to plan individual treatment for each patient [115]. Temperature is a frequently used parameter to describe the predicted size of lesions computed by computational models. In many cases, however, temperature correlates poorly with lesion size [116]. Many computational studies have been reported in the literature to predict the growth of lesion size during ablation [117–119]. However, the majority of these models do not directly calculate lesion size. Surrogate endpoints such as temperature [94,98] are calculated and are interpreted as being equivalent to lesion size. In many cases, these surrogate endpoints do not correlate well with clinical outcome and vary considerably. Many computational studies justify these surrogate endpoints by showing a high correlation between temperature isotherms and lesion size. However, temperature isotherms and lesion size have never actually been shown to be equivalent. On the other hand, there have been many FEM studies of cardiac RF ablation [120–122]. Fewer FEM modeling studies were conducted on hepatic ablation [123], blood, myocardium, and torso tissues [124].

Gopalakrishnan [125] proposed a theoretical model for epicardial RF ablation. However, this model does not consider a dry ablation, but an irrigated electrode similar to the "pen electrode" introduced by Medtronics, Inc. (Minneapolis, MN) for endocardial ablation [126]. Results from a computer implementation of the model using a FEM suggest that transmural ablation lesions can be made in 4-mm-thick tissue. Effects of parameters such as tissue and saline layer thickness, irrigation rate, blood flow rate, and applied power are investigated. Saline is found to irrigate as well as ablate. Rise in saline temperature and consequent ablation by saline is more pronounced as saline layer becomes thicker. Electrode-tip temperatures as much as 40°C lower than maximum tissue temperature were found in simulations.

10.3.2 Clinical Advantages and Applications

RF ablation remains the most widely accepted thermoablative technique worldwide, presumably because of its ability to create a well-controlled focal thermal injury and its superior relation between probe diameter and size of ablated tissue. It is currently receiving the greatest clinical attention in Italy and the Far East, where HCC is more prevalent [3,48,127]. RF ablation is especially useful for patients who are not ideal surgical candidates, cannot undergo surgery, have recurrent tumors, or do not respond to conventional therapies. RF ablation may be reserved for patients at high risk for anesthesia, those with recurrent or progressive lesions, and those with smaller lesions sufficiently isolated from adjacent organs [20].

Potential advantages of RF ablation include low complication rates (0–12%), reduced morbidity and mortality rates compared with standard surgical resection, and the ability to treat nonsurgical patients [37,82]. RF ablation may be performed as an open [128], laparoscopic [129], or percutaneous [130] procedure.

10.3.2.1 Cancer Treatment

RF ablation is an effective technique for treating tumors localized to certain organs such as the liver, lung, kidney, prostate, and other cancer tumors.

Liver
RF ablation has gained enthusiasm in modern management of unresectable malignant liver tumors [40]. It was first proposed in 1990 for liver tumors [41]. Although surgery and liver transplant are considered the only curative treatment for HCC, few patients are eligible for RF ablation [131]. Eligibility criteria tend to vary by institution and physician. Contraindications include multiple tumors, decreased liver function, or multiple medical problems.

Percutaneous RF ablation of liver tumors is used in patients who have fewer than five hepatic tumors, each measuring <5 cm, all of which are visible by sonography (or CT scan) with a safe and acceptable route of access. RF ablation by laparoscopy or laparotomy is reserved for patients with tumors that are not accessible by percutaneous RF ablation, tumors >5 cm, and tumors in direct contact with the bowel. The laparoscopy approach offers the advantages of a quick recovery combined with the advantages of a surgical approach. The procedure requires experience in laparoscopic ultrasound as well as laparoscopic, ultrasound-guided needle placement [13,132].

There are several groups of patients who may derive benefit from RF ablation of liver tumors, such as cirrhotic patients with early-stage HCC. Patients with bilobar, otherwise unresectable colorectal carcinoma liver metastases, unresectable colorectal carcinoma liver metastases who are treated on protocol with adjuvant hepatic artery infusion chemotherapy, patients with symptomatic neuroendocrine tumor liver metastases may also benefit from this technique, along with selected patients with otherwise unresectable, nonneuroendocrine liver metastases with disease confined to the liver [132].

Although many clinical investigations and trials have suggested that RF ablation could represent a viable and safe treatment option for nonsurgical patients with HCC or colorectal hepatic metastases [13,76,77,133–150], the technique did not achieve general consensus until recently, given the paucity of studies reporting long-term outcomes of treated patients. Shiina et al. [138], who reported the largest single series study in Japan, recommended RF ablation to be used as the first line nonsurgical treatment of choice because it requires fewer treatment sessions and a shorter hospital stay to achieve complete necrosis of tumor.

Allgaier et al. [151], Mulier et al. [152,153], and Lencioni [42] reviewed the status of RF thermal ablation as a new minimally invasive and discussed techniques for the nonsurgical treatment of HCCs. They indicated that preliminary short-term results are promising; however, studies are underway to evaluate the long-term efficacy of RF ablation for liver tumors. Ng and Poon [40] reviewed the subject and focused on the role of RF ablation for liver malignancies, with special attention to the indication, approaches, complications, survival benefits, combination therapies, and comparison with other treatment modalities.

In the Netherlands, single-center reports suggest that RF ablation may be used successfully to control HCC in those patients awaiting liver transplantation. RF ablation is being increasingly used for colorectal liver metastases (CLM) as an adjunct to surgical resection in case of unresectable lesions. However, to date, there are still no data showing that such an approach is beneficial. For this reason, in the Netherlands, RF ablation for unresectable CLM is mainly used within a clinical trial. Within the multimodality treatment of neuroendocrine metastases, RF ablation may deserve a place for either intention to cure (rare) or debulking with the aim of reduction of symptoms or prolongation of life [146].

In addition to the low complication rate, most, if not all, percutaneous ablation procedures can be performed in the outpatient setting under conscious sedation. However, optimal sedation regimens are required to minimize patient discomfort. The early clinical studies are very promising and it is clear that RF ablation is and will be a major therapeutic intervention in the treatment of liver neoplasms for local cure [48].

Rhim [39] reviewed the Asian experience in the field of tumor ablation. Based on the survey data from Asian physicians who are currently performing image-guided tumor ablation, thermal ablation has been mainly performed for patients with unresectable liver tumors. RF ablation has replaced many other local ablation techniques such as microwave or ethanol ablation in treating small focal hepatic tumors for the last few years.

Lung

Success in treating liver malignancies with a percutaneous approach has created interest in active ongoing research on the ablation of tumors outside of the liver. Lung tumors are well suited to RF ablation because the surrounding air in adjacent normal lung parenchyma provides an insulating effect and concentrates the RF energy within the tumor tissue [5]. Hence, less RF energy deposition is required to achieve adequate tumor heating than with intrahepatic pathology.

In patients with nonsmall cell lung malignancy that are not candidates for surgery owing to poor cardiorespiratory reserve, RF ablation alone or followed by conventional radiation therapy with or without chemotherapy may prove to be a treatment option. In patients with metastatic disease, RF ablation may be suitable for treatment of a small tumor burden or for palliation of larger tumors that cause symptoms such as cough, hemoptysis, or pain. Patients with chest wall or osseous metastatic tumors in whom other therapies have failed may benefit from RF ablation as an alternative to radiation therapy [80].

Several hundred treatments of lung tumors have been performed worldwide, a sufficient number to develop reasonable safety profile with negligible mortality, little morbidity, short hospital stay, and enhanced quality of life [44,88,154–165].

Kidney

RF ablation is also being studied as a minimally invasive treatment for patients with kidney cancer. An effective, minimally invasive therapy could postpone kidney failure and prolong kidney function in patients with multiple or hereditary kidney cancer such as von Hippel–Lindau disease, which causes multiple, recurrent, and diffuse tumors. RF ablation may also provide a useful option for patients who are not operative candidates or have solitary kidneys, multiple medical problems, or unresectable tumors. Indications for RF ablation include renal cell carcinoma in patients with comorbidities that preclude surgery, a solitary kidney, or a minimally functioning of contralateral kidney or comorbidities that preclude surgery. Since the kidney is surrounded by fat, which has limited blood supply for cooling, the effectiveness of RF ablation for exophytic tumors is high. Since its first application in 1977 [166], many investigators have suggested that RF ablation could represent a promising, safe, and well-tolerated treatment for renal tumors [49,113,167,168].

Breast

RF ablation is considered to be the most promising treatment for breast cancer because of its effective destruction of cancer cells and having a low complication rate [169,170]. One feasibility series on RF ablation for breast cancer in five patients suggests that it might play a role in select patient populations, although this is experimental. It is too early to say that RF ablation is the therapy of choice for breast cancer. It is most likely that different techniques are necessary for different patients. Each of these techniques holds tremendous potential, and continued research is crucial. Currently, most of the ongoing trials consist of *in situ* ablation followed by standard surgical resection. The barrier to the widespread use of RF ablation in the breast at present is the lack of surgical excision data whereby the tumors are graded histologically and the margins are analyzed [79]. Finally, Bansal [171] described a successful clinical trial of RF ablation for breast cancer treatment.

Other Cancers

RF ablation may provide a safer option for removing abnormal prostate tissue [172], as well as predictably destroying the entire gland with a low complication rate to the adjacent rectum, sphincter, bladder base, and urethra [78,173].

RF ablation can be the treatment of choice for the majority of patients suffering with a benign but painful bone tumor known as osteoid osteoma [25,59,174]. Osteoid osteomas predominantly occur in the pediatric age group and arise within the cortex of long bones [48].

Ablation of nerve and nerve ganglia continues to be used safely and effectively in the treatment of multiple pain syndromes, including trigeminal neuralgia, cluster headaches, chronic segmental thoracic pain, cervicobrachialgia, and plantar fasciitis [175–179].

Patients with functional or tumorous disorders of the brain, such as Parkinson's disease, and benign or malignant lesions may also be candidates for RF ablation [180]. Recently, therapeutic efficacy of RF thermal ablation on primary pleural synovial sarcoma has been reported [181].

A venue in which RF ablation may hold promise is the treatment of recurrent head and neck tumors. Many patients may not be surgical candidates for tumor resection because of the location and extent of tumor, concomitant debilitating medical conditions, or a history of multiple surgeries. These patients may be safely treated with RF ablation because the procedure is performed almost exclusively in the outpatient setting with local anesthesia and intravenous conscious sedation [48].

10.3.2.2 Cardiac Diseases

RF ablation is increasingly being used for intraoperative treatment for arrhythmias such as AF, AV nodal reentrant tachycardia, and Wolf Parkinson White syndrome. A major drawback of these procedures, especially those that necessitate ablation close to the atriocentriclar node, is the risk of inadvertent AV block. In the cardiac ablation literature, 47°C is generally accepted as the onset of tissue damage [155].

McRury and Haines [67] discussed the role of electrical ablation, especially RF ablation, as a treatment for SVTs and reviewed the engineering principles and biological responses to ablation. The authors stated that RF catheter ablation is a successful technique in clinical arrhythmia management, with reported success rates of greater than 95% in many series. The indications for clinical RF catheter ablation continue to broaden.

Different electrode designs for cardiac RF ablation, such as handheld probes [182–185], catheters [186–188], and irrigated-tip probes [126,189] have been experimentally and clinically used. Several models of percutaneous RF cardiac ablation have been proposed and a few experimentally validated [190,191].

Intensive research is currently ongoing in this area in both animal models and in clinical trials. The literature shows that RF ablation as an adjunctive procedure is a feasible, safe, time-sparing, and effective means to cure cardiac diseases with negligble technical and time requirements [183,192–204].

Early reports of RF ablation for AF suggested that a limited right atrial linear ablation procedure might be able to terminate and prevent its recurrence [187,205,206]. However, right atrial ablation is not uniformly effective in preventing recurrence of AF. Accordingly, additional studies have been done combining right and left atrial linear ablation [186].

Most electrophysiology laboratories working on catheter ablation for paroxysmal AF target pulmonary veins using a transseptal approach. The aim of the procedure is to achieve complete disconnection of the pulmonary veins, demonstrated by the disappearance or dissociation of their potentials. This is clearly facilitated by the use of a circular catheter dedicated to the mapping of the pulmonary vein ostia, which allows the identification of the connections from the atrium to the vein. Using this approach in targeting all four pulmonary veins, 70% of patients are cured without the need for antiarrhythmic drugs. However, some complications have been described, including tamponade, embolic events, and pulmonary vein stenosis [207].

10.3.2.3   Snoring and Obstructive Sleep Apnea (OSA)

Snoring is a common affliction affecting persons of all ages but particularly middle-aged and elderly men and women who are overweight. OSA is a disorder in which the sufferer's upper airway becomes intermittently blocked during sleep, creating an interruption in normal breathing. Although not all snorers have sleep apnea, snoring is a cardinal symptom of OSA and may by this mechanism be associated with increased morbidity [208]. Treatment of snoring and OSA is directed at the upper airway and the therapeutic approach depends upon the frequency and severity of the symptoms. Dental appliances and ventilators have both been effective at maintaining airway patency. However, these therapies are uncomfortable and suffer from low patient compliance rates (40–70%). Cure rates using surgical interventions have been between 30 and 75% [209].

RF ablation of the soft palate aims to reduce the volume of the palate tissue and to improve the texture of the remaining palate for snoring so that it becomes more dynamically stable. It is usually an outpatient procedure, which involves the use of a topical local anesthetic [210]. RF systems (somnoplasty) that used needle electrodes to create precise regions of submucosal tissue coagulation have been developed. Therefore, both the tissue volume and its resulting airway obstruction are reduced. Applicator probes have been developed to target specific tissues, including the base of the tongue [63].

The National Institute for Clinical Excellence (NICE) [210] presented an overview of the subject based on medical literature and specialist opinion: 6 studies, 1 randomized controlled study, 2 comparative studies, and 3 case studies. This overview was prepared to assist members of the Interventional Procedures Advisory Committee in making recommendations about the safety and efficacy of this interventional procedure. No existing systematic reviews or guidelines on this topic were identified during the literature search. The overview concluded that most studies use a carefully selected patient population, whose snoring has been determined to be attributable to the soft palate. Also, RF ablation was found to be less painful than other invasive alternatives.

10.3.3 LIMITATIONS

The limitation of the RF method can be traced to the physics of its operation. In particular, current flow away from the electrode is virtually omnidirectional, creating a time-average power deposition decay rate $P \sim 1/r^4$, where r is the radial distance from the electrode [211]. A fundamental understanding of RF principles is necessary to ensure maximum performance safety when performing this procedure in clinical practice.

RF ablation is a highly complex procedure that mandates appropriate and adequate training, operator skill, and dedicated clinical resources. Accordingly, the safety (and efficacy) of the RF ablation procedure will be highly dependent on the degree of operator experience and familiarity with RF ablation procedures [48].

One of the major limitations of RF ablation is the extent of induced necrosis. The size of potentially treatable tumors is limited because the volume of active heating caused by this technique is limited to a few millimeters from the active element, with the remainder of tissue being heated by thermal conduction [212]. In addition, the diameter of the ablation zone usually does not exceed 4 cm unless the ablation probe is repositioned for a second ablation to obtain complete tumor necrosis [213]. Often tumor cells survive, which leads to high recurrence rates [77,133,214]. Several techniques have been investigated for increasing lesion size and improving efficacy, including cooled probes [6], pulsed RF [98], and saline-enhanced RF [94,101].

Unpredictable electrical current paths between the ablation electrode and the grounding pad may lead to heterogeneous energy deposition and, thus, to eccentric ablation zones or even collateral damage. Skin burns at the grounding pad have been reported in a few instances [215]. Criticism of RF ablation has focused on the potential for incomplete ablation near blood vessels because of the heat-sink effect of local blood flow [216]. If a tumor is near large vessels (for example, >1–2 mm, or the vessels are visible by CT), it is unlikely that all the malignant cells adjacent to the vessel will be completely eradicated as a result of the previously described perfusion-mediated tissue cooling [10]. That does not mean such areas cannot undergo repeat treatment; a single RF ablation session is unlikely to adequately treat these lesions [48].

Strategies are being pursued to improve RF ablation efficacy by altering the physiologic characteristics of the tumor, including tissue ionic conductivity and blood flow. Several investigators have been able to increase RF-induced necrosis by occluding blood flow to the liver during ablation procedures [136,167,217,218].

10.3.4 COMPLICATIONS

RF ablation has a low complication rate (0–12%) [87,219]. Like all other ablation procedures, RF ablation involves some element of risk. The main criticisms of RF ablation have focused on (1) high local recurrence rates, particularly in the treatment of masses larger than 3 cm in diameter, (2) potential for incomplete tumor ablation near blood vessels because of the heat sink effect of local blood flow, (3) difficulty in imaging of RF lesions, and (4) evidence of surveying tumor cells even within RF lesions [45]. Varying degrees of complications can be expected, depending on factors such as the organ site and the aggressiveness of the procedure [220]. These complications range from reversible problems such as bleeding, damage to the arteries or veins and blood clots, to potentially life-threatening complications such as cardiac perforation, valve trauma, and stroke. In addition to well-known complications [221], two broad categories of complications specific to methods of thermal ablation therapy, grounding pad burns [222] and thermal damage to adjacent organs [223], need to be fully addressed. The use of high-current RF technique has increased the risk of one significant potential complication: burns at the grounding pad site. Deleterious heating has been encountered at grounding pad sites in several cases in which high-current RF has been used [223]. Goldberg et al. [222] have recently determined which factors promote inappropriate thermal deposition at the grounding pad site during RF ablation. Temperatures were found not to be uniform underneath the entire grounding pad surface, with the greatest heating at the edges of the pad. Third-degree burns were observed when inappropriate grounding was used. Grounding pad construction was also found to influence the formation of skin burns, with lower temperatures achieved with use of foil pads than with mesh pads.

Initial reported success with RF ablation in liver tumors is coupled with its very low complication rate [134,135,223]. The most common reported complications in liver tumor ablation are focal pain, pleural effusion, and regional hemorrhage, with most requiring no surgical intervention. Mulier et al. [152] reported 10 treatment-related deaths in their review of 1931 patients treated with RF ablation. Major complications occurred in 137 patients (7%) and the most common complications were impairment of hepatic function, hemorrhage, and infection [83].

According to the multicenter (1139 patients in 11 institutions) survey data of the Korean Study Group of Radiofrequency Ablation, a spectrum of complications occurred after RF ablation of hepatic tumors. The prevalence of major complications was 2.43%. The most common complications were hepatic abscess (0.66%), peritoneal hemorrhage (0.46%), biloma (0.20%), ground pad burn (0.20%), pneumothorax (0.20%), and vasovagal reflex (0.13%). Other complications were biliary stricture, diaphragmatic injury, gastric ulcer, hemothorax, hepatic failure, hepatic infarction, renal infarction, sepsis, and transient ischemic attack. One procedure-related death (0.09%) occurred (due to peritoneal hemorrhage) [224].

Buscarini and Buscarini [225] conducted a study to describe type and rate of complications in a series of patients with liver tumors treated by the RF ablation. A total of 166 patients, 114 with HCC and 52 with liver metastasis, were treated by the percutaneous RF expandable system. Among 151 patients followed, there were 7 (4.6%) early major complications, severe pain with session interruption in 3 cases, capsular necrosis in 1 case, 1 abdominal wall necrosis, 1 dorsal burning, 1 peritoneal hemorrhage, and 3 (1.9%) delayed major complications: sterile fluid collection at the site of the treated tumor in 2 cases and coetaneous seeding in 1 case. There were 49 (32.5%) minor complications. The complication rate is similar to that observed after percutaneous alcohol injection.

A team from the Netherlands evaluated the complication rates encountered in 122 patients after treatment of 143 liver tumors with RF ablation between June 1999 and November 2003. Death occurred in two cases. In both, RF ablation was combined with partial hepatectomy. The team found 19 major complications, including biliary tract damage, liver failure, hepatic abscess, peritoneal infection, intrahepatic hematoma, hepatic artery aneurysm, and pulmonary embolism, and 24 minor complications related to concomitant partial hepatectomy or laparotomy. The overall complication rate was 20.3%, and the rate of complications related directly to RF ablation was 9.8%. The team recommended that RF ablation be performed only by an experienced team comprising a hepatobiliary surgeon, gastroenterologist, hepatologist, and interventional radiologist [226].

A Japanese research team detailed the types of complications found over 5 years of experience performing RF ablation for the treatment of unresectable HCC. Complications are classified in three groups: vascular (e.g., portal vein thrombosis, hepatic vein thrombosis with partial hepatic congestion, hepatic infarction, and subcapsular hematoma), biliary (e.g., bile duct stenosis and biloma, abscess, and hemobilia), and extrahepatic (e.g., injury to the gastrointestinal tract, injury to the gallbladder, pneumothorax and hemothorax, and tumor seeding). The team concluded that most complications can be managed with conservative treatment, percutaneous or endoscopic drainage, or surgical repair [227].

While controlled, long-term studies of RF ablation have not been done, survival rates are likely to be similar to those of patients undergoing surgery [127,134,135,223]. Sutherland et al. [43] conducted a systematic review of RF ablation for treating liver tumors. They compared RF ablation with other therapies for 13 cases of HCC and 13 cases for CLM. There did not seem to be any distinct differences in the complication rates between RF ablation and any of the other procedures for treatment of HCC.

Finally, three important strategies for decreasing the rate of complications are prevention, early detection, and proper management. A physician who performs RF ablation of hepatic malignancies should be aware of the broad spectrum of major complications so that these strategies can be used [224].

10.4   MICROWAVE ABLATION

Microwave ablation is the most recent development in the field of tumor ablation. The technique allows for flexible approaches to treatment, including percutaneous, laparoscopic, and open surgical access [45]. RF heating techniques use frequencies in the RF band where a quasi-static condition applies. In the microwave frequency range, energy is coupled into tissues through waveguides or antennas (applicators) that emit microwaves (typically 915 MHz or 2.45 GHz). The shorter wavelengths of microwaves, as compared to RF, provide the capability to direct and focus the energy into tissues by direct radiation from a small applicator.

There is an increasing number of relevant scientific articles published in high-ranked journals that provide a good review on physical background, technical realization, and clinical trials of RF ablation [45,228–231].

10.4.1   TECHNICAL CONSIDERATIONS

10.4.1.1   Mechanisms

Microwave energy is known for its potential for creating larger and more effective lesions (up to 2.6 cm in diameter) at greater depth, resulting in shorter application times (typically 1–5 min) than RF devices [128]. Compared with RF, microwaves have a much broader field of power density (up to 2 cm surrounding the antenna), with a correspondingly larger zone of active heating [232]. This may allow for more uniform tumor kill both within a targeted zone and next to vessels. Since microwave power deposition inside tissues decays with distance following a second power law as compared to the fourth-power dependence of RF ablation, deeper lesions can be obtained [233]. Unlike RF ablation, the volume heating due to microwave energy is dielectric, not resistive. Heating by microwave energy is determined by the permittivity of tissue. Microwave produces EM radiation, which stimulates oscillation of dipoles such as water molecules, resulting in kinetic energy (heat). Also in contrast to RF ablation, increasing the applied microwave power results in a significant increase in the volume of lesions, without causing charring [234]. The lesion dimensions are proportional to the power and duration of energy delivery. Poor dielectric properties and improper impedance matching result in power reflection and energy dissipation within the catheter transmission line and antenna, and inadequate lesion formation. Hines-Peralta et al. [235] characterized the relationship between applied power and treatment duration in their effect on extent of coagulation produced with a 2.45-GHz microwave applicator in both an *ex vivo* and a perfused *in vivo* liver model. Large zones of ablation were achieved. For higher-power ablations, larger zones of coagulation were achieved for *in vivo* liver than for *ex vivo* liver with short energy applications.

Currently, RF ablation devices are more technically advanced than microwave ablation devices, likely because they of their effectiveness, safety in both percutaneous and surgical settings, and relative ease of use. However, RF ablation is fundamentally restricted by the need to conduct electric energy into the body [236]. Microwave ablation devices, while not yet commercially available in the United States, have the potential to become the superior treatment modality if they receive more attention from the research community. These devices still use comparatively simple control algorithms (i.e., constant power) without any sort of feedback to adjust power according to requirements, compared with temperature or impedance feedback used in RF devices [90].

According to Simon et al. [45], the main advantages of microwave technology, when compared with existing thermoablative technologies, include consistently higher intratumoral temperatures, larger tumor ablation volumes, faster ablation times, and an improved convection profile.

10.4.1.2 Antenna Designs

Microwave antennas are the critical elements in the microwave ablation procedure, as the generation of continuous linear transmural lesions depends on the control of radiation characteristics of the antrenna [237]. Most ablation antennas are fed by coaxial lines, which have an unbalanced design that allows return current flow on the outer conductor. These currents restrict impedance matching. If the antenna's input impedance is not matched to the feed line, too much of the applied power is reflected from the antenna and, hence, not deposited in the tissue [212]. Poor dielectric and impedance matching results in power reflection and energy dissipation within the transmission line and antenna, and accordingly leads to improper lesion formation. Recent engineering advances have allowed the design of microwave antennae that are tuned to the dielectric properties of tissues, reducing feedback and increasing the amount of energy deposited into the surrounding tissue. This new microwave ablation system (Vivant Medical, Inc., Mountain View, CA) has the potential to create larger, hotter lesions than previously possible. Additionally, the prototype microwave generator has the capacity to drive up to eight antennas at one time [238].

Numerous antenna designs have been presented in the literature for microwave ablation [17,111,211,212,235,237,239–250]. Several of the designs are targeted for cancer treatment and others for cardiac ablation. Antennas are grouped into three categories: the monopolar antennas, dipole antennas, and helical coil antennas. With the exception of the split-tip dipole, each type radiates in the normal mode, with waves propagating perpendicular to the axis of the helix [234]. In general, microwave catheter antennas can broadly be categorized into two types: those antennas that are designed to produce radiation mainly around the antenna tip [241–243] and those that produce radiation normal to the antenna axis [211,242].

Nevels et al. [211] observed that coating the catheter with a Teflon sheath prevents a radiation "hot spot" at the feed line/antenna junction and antenna tip. It was shown that a disk placed at the end of the antenna probe forces the radiated power forward, toward the probe tip, which is the part of the antenna in closest contact with the heart tissue. The terminating disk provides an additional benefit by halving the length of the antenna at the 2.45 GHz frequency, which is an advantage in the confined space of the heart cavity. Gu et al. [243] reported on a wide aperture microwave spiral antenna for cardiac ablation, which created lesions that are too wide for ablation in the atrium, where the available cardiac tissue is limited. The antenna reported by Pisa et al. [244] has shown increased radiation along the antenna length as well as around the tip. The enhanced radiation around the tip of the antenna can be problematic when the antenna is placed near the valves as it may cause unintentional valvular damage due to EM radiation. Chiu et al. [237] proposed a novel expanded tip wire (ETW) catheter antenna for the treatment of atrial fibrillation. The antenna is designed as an integral part of coaxial cable so that it can be inserted via a catheter. Both numerical modeling and *in vitro* experimentation show that the proposed ETW antenna produces a well-defined electric field distribution that provides continuous long and linear lesions for the treatment of AF. Rappaport [19] described a novel catheter-based unfurling wide aperture antenna. This antenna consists of the center conductor of a coaxial line, shaped into a spiral and insulated from blood and tissue by a nonconductive fluid-filled balloon. Initially stretched straight inside a catheter for transluminal guiding, once in place at the cardiac target, the coiled spiral antenna is advanced into the inflated balloon. Power is applied in the range of 50–150 W at the reserved ISM frequency of 915 MHz for 30–90 s to create an irreversible lesion. Yang et al. [250] reported a novel coaxial antenna operating at 2.45 GHz for hepatic microwave ablation. This device uses a floating sleeve, that is, a metal conductor electrically isolated from the outer connector of the antenna coaxial body, to achieve a highly localized SAR that is independent of insertion length.

10.4.1.3 Multiple Insertions and Multiple Antennas

Similar to current clinical practice in RF ablation, multiple sequential insertions are typically used to treat large tumors by microwave ablation [251,252]. Due to the limited size of the ablation zone, this practice can require a large number of applications. For example, Sato et al. [128] used 46 antenna insertions for treatment of HCC. Three different methods have been described in the literature that allow simultaneous use of multiple microwave antennas: coherent, incoherent, and phase modulated [90]. Wright et al. [238] found that simultaneous three-probe microwave ablation lesions were three times larger than sequential lesions and nearly six times greater in volume than single-probe lesions. Additionally, simultaneous multiple-probe ablation resulted in qualitatively better lesions, with more uniform coagulation and better performance near blood vessels. The investigators found also that simultaneous multiple-probe ablation may decrease inadequate treatment of large tumors and decrease recurrence rates after tumor ablation. Yu et al. [249] evaluated the clinical implementation of triangular and spherical designs for simultaneous multiple-antenna ablation of human HCC with a recently engineered microwave coagulation system. The triple-loop configuration yielded the most uniformly round ablation shape. Simultaneous activation of multiple straight or loop antennae is a potentially promising technique for rapid and effective treatment of large HCCs.

Using a different microwave system, Sato et al. [253] described their experience with multiple-probe microwave ablation in a small clinical series. Using a disk-shaped introducer to guide placement of seven antennae, they were able to create lesions from 5 to 6 cm in diameter, successfully treating 3 of 6 tumors. However, in this instance, the multiple antenna system was activated sequentially, rather than simultaneously. Similarly, Lu et al. [252] used sequential multiple-probe ablation to treat tumors >2 cm in 61 patients with a 92% technical success rate and 8% recurrence after a mean 18-month follow-up.

With continuing technical advances in microwave medical technology, minimally invasive treatments have emerged to treat common medical conditions. One such advance is the transurethral microwave thermotherapy (TUMT) to treat BPH or the enlarged prostate. TUMT uses a catheter with microwave antenna built in just below the balloon. The balloon at the tip localizes the antenna at the correct position in the object area. Thermosensors on the catheter and in the surrounding area autoregulate power output to optimally heat the object. Different types of microwave antennas are used for TUMT including helical, dipole, and whip designs [70].

10.4.2 CLINICAL ADVANTAGES AND APPLICATIONS

10.4.2.1 Treating Cancer

Clinical applications of microwave ablation include treatment of liver tumors, lung tumors, renal and adrenal disease, and bone metastases. In several clinical studies, microwave tissue coagulation has been performed by using both percutaneous and laparoscopic techniques. The technology is still in its infancy, and future developments and clinical implementation will help improve the care of patients with cancer [45].

Clinical use of microwave ablation has been most prevalent in Asia to date, where a number of case series have shown it to be effective in local control of both HCC and metastatic colorectal carcinoma [39,254–257]. Currently, there are no FDA approved commercial microwave ablation devices available in the USA [90].

Liver
The first clinical report of microwave therapy in Asia was made by Seki et al. [258]. They evaluated the efficacy of this technique in 18 patients with single unresectable HCCs, all of which were 2 cm in diameter or smaller. Microwaves at 60 W for 120 s were used to irradiate the tumor and surrounding area. They used a 1450-MHz generator and a 15 gauge coaxial electrode. No recurrences were noted at the treated sites during 11–33 months of follow-up. Three patients developed new tumors in sites remote from the treated sites. No serious complications were encountered. The investigators treated a total of 650 patients from 1992. Five-year survival rates were 70% in tumors <2 cm and 52% in tumors measuring 2–3 cm. More promising clinical results for the treatment of liver tumors were reported in the following years with low complication rates [107,129,130,252,254,259–266].

Prostate
One of the most prolific areas of development of microwave ablation technology is for treating disease of the prostate. To date, few examples of clinical trials have demonstrated durability and efficacy [267–269].

Other Tumors
A new therapeutic modality called electrochemotherapy is starting to be used to treat a variety of cutaneous tumors, including head and neck tumors, superficial breast cancer lesions, etc. In this therapy, the resistance of malignant cells to penetration by certain chemotherapeutic agents is temporarily lowered by creating temporary pores in the membranes of the malignant cells by the application of short DC pulses that generate electric fields of several kilovolts per centimeter. Once the cells are porated, the chemotherapeutic agents can enter the malignant cells and destroy them. Electrochemotherapy can not only increase the efficacy of certain chemotherapeutic agents, but also can reduce side effects because malignant cells can be destroyed with much lower doses of chemotherapeutic agents than with conventional chemotherapy [228].

Furukawa et al. [270] evaluated the use of microwave coagulation therapy, which has been used successfully for coagulation of hepatic tumors, in normal canine lung tissue to evaluate its efficacy and safety. Measurements of thermal response and coagulation area and histological examinations after microwave coagulation were performed in normal canine lung tissue. The temperature in normal canine lung tissue increased to 90–100°C at 5 mm from the electrode after 60 s and 70–80°C at 10 mm after 90 s at 40 or 60 W. The coagulation area was approximately 20 mm in diameter at 40 W and 60 W. Histological analysis demonstrated thickening of collagen fiber shortly after coagulation, stromal edema and granulation of tissue after 3 months, and, finally, scar tissue was seen after 6 months.

10.4.2.2 Cardiac Diseases

Microwave Balloon Angioplasty (MBA)
New approaches are steadily emerging in the fast-paced progress of treating cardiac diseases using microwave energy. For example, balloon angioplasty is a surgical repair of a blood vessel by inserting a balloon-tipped catheter to unblock it. Balloons can be produced with diameters from 0.5 to 50 mm or more, in any working length,

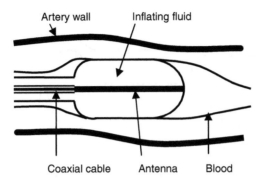

FIGURE 10.2 A schematic view of a MBA.

with very thin walls. They can be custom designed with varying diameters. The process employs a narrow balloon catheter that is advanced to the site of arterial stenosis through an incision in the neck or leg and fed through blood vessels. Fluid is then pumped into the balloon, inflating it to several times its normal diameter. The enlarged tip quickly compresses the layer of plaque which is clogging the artery, leaving a much wider opening for blood flow. The balloon is then deflated and it is withdrawn with the catheter. The procedure avoids cardiac bypass surgery. An alternative process to deposit power is microwave irradiation. MBA takes advantage of the volume heating property of microwave irradiation. MBA devices were first reported by Rosen et al. [231] and clinically tested by Smith et al. [271] and Nardone et al. [272]. These devices used a variety of narrow antennas incorporated within and surrounding a catheter balloon. The design of the antenna is the key to the success of the MBA. A cable-antenna assembly is threaded through the catheter, with the antenna centered in the balloon portion of the catheter. The first MBA devices employed dipoles and small helical antennas. Although the healthy tissue may still be heated less than the inner plaque surface, it is important to avoid overheating the artery wall, if possible [273]. Figure 10.2 shows a schematic view of an MBA.

Microwave Ablation Catheter
Another application of microwaves is the treatment of abnormal heart rhythm or some cardiac arrhythmias such as AV node reentrant tachycardias, accessory pathways, ventricular tachycardias, SVTs, AF, and atrial flutter. Cardiac ablation reached a successful rate of about 75–95% depending on the heart rhythm disorders [64,69,274]. The procedure involves having catheters threaded through veins or arteries to the site of the abnormal electrical pathway responsible for the arrhythmia. Catheter ablation is usually performed in conjunction with an invasive diagnostic electrophysiology study, which will identify the origin of abnormal impulse formation. RF ablation operating at frequencies between 100 kHz and 10 MHz has a high success rate in treating a wide range of cardiac arrhythmias. An electric current is applied between the catheter electrode (~2.6 mm in diameter) in contact with the endocardium and a rectangular (~15 cm × 9 cm) dispersive electrode attached at the back of the patient. Microwave power is also used to treat abnormal heart rhythm, especially ventricular tachycardia. Microwave power can ablate tissues at greater depth and across a larger

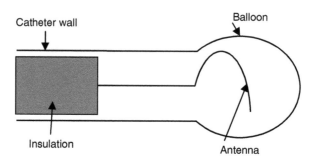

FIGURE 10.3   A schematic view of a microwave ablation catheter.

volume heating than RF ablation by using monopole and helical antennas [273]. Figure 10.3 shows a schematic view of a microwave ablation catheter.

In the literature, several investigators confirm that microwave ablation is a satisfactory and safe method of cardiac ablation and it can be added to surgical procedures without undue risk to the patient [275–280]. The use of microwave energy for cardiac ablation was also successfully examined in open-chest dogs [281] and domestic pigs [282]. Rappaport [19] reviewed the recent state of the art in microwave cardiac ablation and described a novel catheter-based unfurling wide aperture antenna.

10.4.2.3   Microwave Endometrial Ablation (MEA)

MEA is an effective treatment for dysfunctional uterine bleeding. Patients with leiomyomata, including submucosal leiomyomata up to 3 cm, may also be treated with microwave endometrial ablation. Goldberg et al. [1] conducted a microwave endometrial ablation on a 46-year-old woman with multiple leiomyomata and menometrorrhagia. Two months after microwave endometrial ablation, she developed signs of peritoneal irritation. A negative laparoscopy excluded a thermal bowel injury. Imaging and clinical examination ultimately determined that her symptoms were due to leiomyoma degeneration. A 38-year-old woman with menometrorrhagia and leiomyomata underwent microwave endometrial ablation. Fifteen days after microwave endometrial ablation, she developed signs of peritoneal irritation. With a presumptive clinical diagnosis of microwave endometrial ablation degeneration, the patient was expectantly managed with pain medications and observation.

Jack and Cooper [283] reviewed the scientific basis, clinical research, safety, and clinical applications of endometrial ablative technique. The investigators concluded that this technology is suitable for the majority of women who present with the complaint of excessive menstrual bleeding. The treatment is effective and acceptable to patients giving high levels of reported satisfaction. Randomized evidence supports its use in a variety of clinical situations using general or local anesthesia, with or without drug preparation, in theater or outpatient environment, without loss of clinical or economic effectiveness.

In 2002, the NICE requested that the effectiveness of MEA and thermal balloon endometrial ablation (TBEA) be systematically reviewed. MEA and TBEA were identified as the most commonly used second generation techniques in the UK. Garside et al. [229] reviewed two randomized controlled trials of MEA and eight trials (six randomized controlled trials) of TBEA. Both techniques had significantly shorter operating and theatre times than first generation techniques (transcervical resection, rollerball ablation and laser ablation). Adverse effects were few with all techniques, but there were fewer postoperative adverse effects with the second generation techniques. The investigators concluded that MEA and TBEA are effective alternatives in the surgical treatment of women with heavy menstrual bleeding.

Downes and O'Donovan [284] described the status of microwave endometrial ablation, its clinical efficacy, its safety profile, and future development. According to Jameel et al. [285], MEA is regarded as an effective nonsurgical option for managing dysfunctional uterine bleeding. It is believed to be safe, quick, and easy to perform. According to the investigators, there has been only one reported case of a serious complication of a bowel injury during MEA.

10.4.3 LIMITATIONS

Microwave ablation offers many of the benefits of RF but has several theoretical advantages that may result in improved performance, especially near blood vessels. During RF ablation, the zone of active tissue heating is limited to a few millimeters surrounding the active electrode, with the remainder of the ablation zone being heated via thermal conduction [232]. Due to the much broader field of power density (up to 2 cm surrounding the antenna), microwave ablation results in a much larger zone of active heating [286]. This larger heating zone has the potential to allow for a more uniform tumor kill in the ablation zone, but within the targeted zone and next to blood vessels.

In spite of significant success in the clinical application of microwave ablation, as with other thermal-based therapies, tumor size continues to limit overall complete response rates. Perfusion-mediated vascular cooling appears to produce a heat-sink effect that prevents greater volumes of coagulation. In addition, the application of microwave energy by means of single electrode insertions results in necrosis measuring 2.5 cm in diameter. Although the use of multisession or multiple electrodes to achieve greater coagulation has been attempted, limitations with this practice center on the impracticality of multiple puncture wounds within a small area in the tumor. There is also reduced penetration with microwave energy compared with several other thermoablative strategies, which makes this particular thermal ablative strategy less suitable for deeply placed tumors.

Practical problems remain to be solved before microwaves can become a useful energy source. These problems include (1) power loss in the coaxial cable; (2) resultant heating of the coaxial cable during power delivery that may lead to breakdown in the dielectric and catheter material; (3) lack of a unidirectional antenna that can radiate energy into tissue and not the circulating blood pool, a condition which prevents proper catheter operation over the range of dielectric properties of human blood and heart tissue [63,211]. An important limitation of microwave ablation is the complexity of microwave antenna design, which limits the antenna to specific lengths corresponding to the microwave generator waveform. This differs from RF and laser ablation, in which a more variable length of tissue can be subject to treatment. Even greater limitations in lesion geometry are imposed when microwave arrays are used

[287]. So far, microwave antenna designs have not achieved efficient energy transfer into the object. Poor dielectric and impedance matching have resulted in power reflection and energy dissipation within the catheter transmission line and antenna, and inadequate lesion formation [67].

10.4.4 COMPLICATIONS

Although complication rates for microwave ablation are lower than those for surgical resection, clinical studies in which microwave ablation has been used to treat HCC have reported relatively higher complication rates compared with other thermal ablation strategies.

Murakami et al. [259] reported clinical results of microwave ablation in nine patients with HCCs greater than 3 cm in diameter. Three to twelve ablations were performed per tumor. Four of nine patients developed recurrent tumors within 6 months of the treatment. No major complications were noted. Matsukawa et al. [251] examined postprocedural complications in 20 patients with HCC. Their patients experienced slight pain (24%), fever (20%), and subcutaneous hematomas (8%) after microwave ablation sessions. Beppu et al. [260] reported a 12% complication rate when using microwave ablation to treat 84 patients with HCC. Shimada et al. [254] reported a 14.2% complication rate in 42 patients with HCC. Complications included abscesses, a biloma, bleeding, hepatic failure, and tumor seeding in the microwave needle track. Significantly higher complication rates were seen in patients with higher clinical stages of disease and larger tumor size (diameter greater than 4.0 cm). Although abscesses and bleeding were treated without incident, other serious complications were unsuccessfully treated after they developed. The authors recommended several prophylactic measures to reduce the incidence of complications, including transcatheter cooling of the intrahepatic bile duct and administration of an anticancer agent in the abdominal cavity to prevent bilomas and tumor dissemination. Shibata et al. [266] evaluated the effectiveness of percutaneous RF ablation and microwave ablation for treatment of HCC in 72 patients with 94 HCC nodules. Complete therapeutic effect was achieved in 46 (96%) of 48 nodules treated with RF ablation and 41 (89%) of 46 nodules treated with microwave ablation. Major complications occurred in one patient treated with RF ablation and in four patients treated with microwave ablation.

10.5 TRENDS AND FUTURE RESEARCH

The most important issues regarding thermal ablation are the safety, true efficacy, and survival benefits of the ablation techniques. None of the five thermal ablative techniques discussed in this article are directly comparable, since the patient populations, extent of disease, and other factors are relatively different. In addition, so far there have been no prospective comparative studies in this regard.

10.5.1 IMPROVED TECHNIQUES

Thermal ablation is relatively a new technique and the technology has evolved rapidly. There certainly will be a room for continued developments so that ablation may

TABLE 10.1

Comparison of Radiofrequency and Microwave Ablation Techniques

Type of Ablation	Mechanism	Advantages	Disadvantages
Radiofrequency	Resistive heating by RF current	Simple system design, proven effective, and worldwide availability The complication profile is acceptable Ability to treat different tumor types	Limited extent of induced necrosis Ablation zones do not exceed 4 cm unless the ablation probe is repositioned for a second ablation Necrosis incomplete in ablation near blood vessels
Microwaves	Heating by propagating EM waves	High temperature available Limited use (Asia) Larger zone of active heating compared to RF ablation	Complications include pleural effusion, hemorrhage, and abscess

be created more rapidly, of a large volume of tumors, and with precise monitoring when sufficient cell kill with adequate margins has been obtained. Currently, many ablation devices are being studied with multiple commercial devices now becoming available. Given the rapid pace of evolution in the state of the art for ablation technologies, we cannot confidently predict which method, if any, will prove dominant for any given clinical application. Competitive technologies must be able to ablate the desired volume of tissue in a reproducible and predictable fashion. However, other factors, including ease of clinical use and cost, will play a role in determining which of these technologies will receive the greatest attention. Table 10.1 compares the five ablation techniques considered in this article.

Among EM ablation techniques, RF ablation devices are more technically advanced than microwave devices, in part because they have received more attention. Microwave ablation devices, while not yet commercially available in the United States, have the potential to become the superior treatment modality if they receive more attention from the research community. Microwaves provide deeper tissue heating compared with RF and multiple antenna arrays provide the advantage of constructive interference in between antennas. This may eventually enable more rapid creation of large ablation zones and more effective treatment of tumors located close to vessels [90].

10.5.2 ABLATION IN CLINICAL PRACTICE

Currently, there is more enthusiasm for RF ablation. The low complication (0–12%) and mortality rate (0–1%), and the ability of RF ablation to ablate large tumors are the main advantages [37]. Microwave ablation, however, has a low complication rate too (11–14%), as reported in many studies [254,263].

The relative risks and benefits of ablation must be measured rigorously to better define its role in clinical practice. Future improvements in patient survival will require multidisciplinary treatment approaches that include cytoxic and novel agents to prevent tumor recurrence. Well-designed and controlled multicenter clinical trials are required to find out and measure the extent of benefit provided by ablation techniques for any given indication. The results from single-center or retrospective studies vary significantly from report to report. Therefore, good communication between centers will be required to assist the rapid diffusion of the many new ways in which thermal ablation is being used to help individual patients, especially the approach in which the role of thermal ablation will likely be developed to include additional organ sites.

Given the high likelihood of incomplete treatment by heat-based techniques alone, the case for combining thermal ablation with other therapies such as radiotherapy, chemotherapy, or chemoembolization cannot be overstated. A similar multidisciplinary approach including surgery, radiation, and chemotherapy is used for the treatment of most solid tumors.

10.5.3 FUTURE RESEARCH

The ultimate goal of current research on ablation techniques is to develop technologies to increase induced coagulation volume while reducing the treatment time associated with the ablation technique. However, clinical research focuses on the implementation of ablation in clinical practice and patient outcomes. The desired advances include improvements in image guidance for targeting tumors to be ablated, better detection of residual disease, and making the therapy more straightforward by reducing device complexity and the overall time required to ablate a given tumor.

Research should be based on developing rational and reasonably sized lesions that do not require inordinate amounts of time to create. However, bigger is not always better, because injury to surrounding tissues and organs may be more likely [132]. The use of multiple applicators is one way to reach this target, which may help decrease the number of local tumor progressions that result when treating a large tumor with overlapping sequential ablations. In addition, multiple tumors could be treated simultaneously with multiple applicator devices and treatment time, and anesthetic complications and costs could potentially be decreased [90].

Over the next several years, we expect more substantial research efforts combining various ablation techniques with adjunctive therapies such as chemotherapy to improve overall tumor destruction [132]. To study, investigate, and develop new techniques and to improve those currently employed, research can make use of clinical and experimental studies, phantoms, and theoretical models. The latter are a powerful tool in this kind of investigation, since they rapidly and economically provide an understanding of the electrical and thermal behavior involved in ablation [115]. Much of the future success will be based on (1) accurate modeling of the electrical and thermal characteristics of biological tissues, (2) realistic modeling of the cooling effect of large and medium blood vessels, (3) determining the parameters (frequency factor and energy) of the thermal damage function for different types of tissues (hepatic, breast, cardiac, etc.), (4) technological advances in electrode and generator design, (5) better understanding of methods to ensure adequacy of tumor necrosis, and (6) conducting research on new histological markers of thermal injury.

Furthermore, successful ablation of all tumors may be improved in the future using fast computer simulation and accurate imaging and mapping techniques such as real-time MRI, thermal mapping, or ultrasonographic contrast agents to determine the adequacy of complete thermal coagulation.

REFERENCES

1. Goldberg SN, Grassi CJ, Cardella JF, Charboneau JW, Dodd GD, Dupuy DE, Gervais D, Gillams AR, Kane RA, Lee FT, Livraghi T, McGahan J, Phillips DA, Rhim H, Silverman SG. Image-guided tumor ablation: standardization of terminology and reporting criteria. *J Vasc Interv Radiol* 2005; 16: 765–778.
2. Hines-Peralta A, Liu Z-J, Horkan C, Solazzo S, Goldberg SN. Chemical tumor ablation with use of a novel multiple-tine infusion system in a canine sarcoma model. *J Vasc Interv Radiol* 2006; 17: 351–358.
3. Ahmed M, Goldberg SN. Thermal ablation therapy for hepatocellular carcinoma. *J Vasc Interv Radiol* 2002; 13: S231–S244.
4. Pennes HH. Analysis of tissue and arterial blood temperatures in the resting human arm. *J Appl Physiol* 1948; 1: 93–122.
5. Goldberg SN, Gazelle GS, Mueller PR. Thermal ablation therapy for focal malignancy: a unified approach to underlying principles, techniques, and diagnostic imaging guidance. *AJR Am J Roentgenol* 2000; 174: 323–331.
6. Goldberg SN, Gazelle GS, Solbiati L, Rittman WJ, Mueller PR. Radiofrequency tissue ablation: increased lesion diameter with a perfusion electrode. *Acad Radiol* 1996; 3: 636–644.
7. Goldberg SN, Gazelle GS, Dawson SL, Rittman WJ, Mueller PR, Rosenthal DI. Tissue ablation with radiofrequency: effect of probe size, gauge, duration, and temperature on lesion volume. *Acad Radiol* 1996; 3: 212–218.
8. Lorentzen T, Christensen NE, Nolsoe CP, Torp-Pedersen ST. Radiofrequency tissue ablation with a cooled needle in vitro: ultrasonography, dose response, and lesion temperature. *Acad Radiol* 1997; 4: 292–297.
9. Goldberg SN, Hahn PF, Halpern E, Fogle R, Gazelle GS. Radiofrequency tissue ablation: effect of pharmacologic modulation of blood flow on coagulation diameter. *Radiology* 1998; 209: 761–769.
10. Patterson EJ, Scudamore CH, Owen DA, Nagy AG, Buczkowski AK. Radiofrequency ablation of porcine liver in vivo: effects of blood flow and treatment time on lesion size. *Ann Surg* 1998; 227: 559–565.
11. Vierra M. Minimally invasive surgery. *Annu Rev Med* 1995; 46: 147–158.
12. Siperstein A, Garland A, Engle K, Rogers S, Berber E, String A, Foroutani A, Ryan T. Laparoscopic radiofrequency ablation of primary and metastatic liver tumors. Technical considerations. *Surg Endosc* 2000; 14: 400–405.
13. Curley SA, Izzo F, Ellis LM, Nicolas Vauthey J, Vallone P. Radiofrequency ablation of hepatocellular cancer in 110 patients with cirrhosis. *Ann Surg* 2000; 232: 381–391.
14. Siperstein AE, Rogers SJ, Hansen PD, Gitomirsky A. Laparoscopic thermal ablation of hepatic neuroendocrine tumor metastases. *Surgery* 1997; 122: 1147–1155.
15. Dodd GD, Soulen MC, Kane RA, Livraghi T, Lees WR, Yamashita Y, Gillams AR, Karahan OI, Rhim H. Minimally invasive treatment of malignant hepatic tumors: at the threshold of a major breakthrough. *RadioGraphics* 2000; 20: 9–27.
16. Goldberg SN. Comparison of techniques for image-guided ablation of focal liver tumors. *Radiology* 2002; 223: 304–307.
17. Williams MR, Garrido M, Oz MC, Argenziano M. Alternative energy sources for surgical atrial ablation. *J Card Surg* 2004; 19: 201–206.

18. Haemmerich D, Laeseke PF. Thermal tumour ablation: devices, clinical applications and future directions. *Int J Hyperthermia* 2005; 21: 755–760.
19. Rappaport C. Cardiac tissue ablation with catheter-based microwave heating. *Int J Hyperthermia* 2004; 20: 769–780.
20. Woo EJ, Tungjitkusolmun S, Cao H, Tsai JZ, Webster JG, Vorperian VR, Will JA. A new catheter design using needle electrode for subendocardial RF ablation of ventricular muscles: finite element analysis and in vitro experiments. *IEEE Trans Biomed Eng* 2000; 47: 23–31.
21. De Sanctis JT, Goldberg SN, Mueller PR. Percutaneous treatment of hepatic neoplasms: a review of current techniques. *Cardiovasc Interv Radiol* 1998; 21: 273–296.
22. Van Rhoon GC, Wust P. Introduction: non-invasive thermometry for thermotherapy. *Int J Hyperthermia* 2005; 21: 489–495.
23. Stauffer PR, Goldberg SN. Introduction: thermal ablation therapy. *Int J Hyperthermia* 2004; 20: 671–677.
24. Tillotson CL, Rosenberg AE, Rosenthal DI. Controlled thermal injury of bone. Report of a percutaneous technique using radiofrequency electrode and generator. *Invest Radiol* 1989; 24: 888–892.
25. Rosenthal DI, Hornicek FJ, Torriani M, Gebhardt MC, Mankin HJ. Osteoid osteoma: percutaneous treatment with radiofrequency energy. *Vasc Interv Radiol* 2003; 229: 171–175.
26. McGahan JP, Dodd GD. Radiofrequency ablation of the liver. *Am J Roentgenol* 2001; 176: 3–16.
27. Lau WY. Primary hepatocellular carcinoma. In: Blumgart LH, Fong Y, Editors. *Surgery of Liver and Biliary Tract.* Vol. II, 3rd ed. London, UK: WB Saunders, pp. 1423–1450, 2000.
28. Nagorney DM, van Heerden JA, Ilstrup D, Adson MA. Primary hepatic malignancy: surgical management and determinants of survival. *Surgery* 1989; 106: 740–748.
29. Framer DG, Rosove MH, Shaked A, Busuttil RW. Current treatment modalities for hepatocellular carcinomas. *Ann Surg* 1994; 219: 236–247.
30. Fong Y, Kemedy N, Paty P, Blumgart LH, Cohen AM. Treatment of colorectal cancer: hepatic metastases. *Semin Surg Oncol* 1996; 12: 219–252.
31. Badvie S. Hepatocellular carcinoma. *Postgrad Med J* 2000; 76: 4–11.
32. Hardie D, Sangster AJ, Cronin NJ. Coupled field analysis of heat flow in the near field of a microwave applicator for tumor ablation. *Electromagn Bio Med* 2006; 25: 29–43.
33. Krishnamurthy VN, Casillas J, Latorre L. Radiofrequency ablation of hepatic lesions: a review. *Appl Radiol* 2003; 32: 11–26.
34. Scudamore CH, Patterson EJ, Shapiro J, Buczkowski AK. Liver tumor ablation techniques. *J Invest Surg* 1997; 10: 157–164.
35. Poon RT, Fan ST, Tsang FH, Wong J. Locoregional therapies for hepatocellular carcinoma: a critical review from the surgeon's perspective. *Ann Surg* 2002; 235: 466–486.
36. Garsea G, Lloyd TD, Aylott C, Maddern, G, Berry DP. The emergent role of focal liver ablation techniques in the treatment of primary and secondary liver tumors. *Eur J Cancer* 2003; 39: 2150–2164.
37. Ng KK, Lam CM, Poon RT, Ai V, Tso WK, Fan ST. Thermal ablative therapy for malignant liver tumors: a critical appraisal. *J Gastroenterol Hepatol* 2003; 18: 616–629.
38. Lau WY, Leung TW, Yu SC, Ho SK. Percutaneous local ablative therapy for hepatocellular carcinoma: a review and look into the future. *Ann Surg* 2003; 237: 171–179.
39. Rhim H. Review of Asian experience of thermal ablation techniques and clinical practice. *Int J Hyperthermia* 2004; 20: 699–712.
40. Ng KK-C, Poon RT-P. Role of radiofrequency ablation for liver malignancies. *Surg Pract* 2005; 9: 94–103.

41. Buscarini E, Savoia A, Brambilla G, Menozzi F, Reduzzi L, Strobel D, Hänsler J, Buscarini L, Gaiti L, Zambelli A. Radiofrequency thermal ablation of liver tumors. *Eur Urol* 2005; 15: 884–894.
42. Lencioni R. Image-guided radiofrequency ablation of hepatocellular carcinoma and colorectal Hepatic metastases—long-term survival outcomes. *US Oncol Rev* 2006; 1–4.
43. Sutherland LM, Williams JAR, Padbury RTA, Gotley DC, Stokes B, Maddern GJ. Radiofrequency ablation of liver tumors. *Arch Surg* 2006; 141: 181–190.
44. Steinke K, Sewell PE, Dupuy D, Lencioni R, Helmberger T, Kee ST, Jacob AL, Glenn DW, King J, Morris DL. Pulmonary radiofrequency ablation—an international study survey. *Anticancer Res* 2004; 24: 339–343.
45. Simon CJ, Dupuy DE, Mayo-Smith WW. Microwave ablation: principles and applications. *RadioGraphics* 2005; 25: S69–S83.
46. Berry SJ, Coffey DS, Walsh PC, Ewing LL. The development of human benign prostatic hyperplasia with age. *J Urol* 1984; 132: 474–479.
47. Shinohara K. Thermal ablation of prostate diseases: advantages and limitations. *Int J Hyperthermia* 2004; 20: 679–697.
48. Dupuy DE, Goldberg SN. Image-guided radiofrequency tumor ablation: challenges and opportunities—Part II. *J Vasc Interv Radiol* 2001; 12: 1135–1148.
49. Gervais DA, McGovern FJ, Arellano RS, McDougal WS, Mueller PR. Radiofrequency ablation of renal cell carcinoma. Part 1: Indications, results, and role in patient management over a 6-year period and ablation of 100 tumors. *Am J Roentgenol* 2005; 185: 64–71.
50. Murphy DP, Gill IS. Energy-based renal tumor ablation: a review. *Semin Urol Oncol* 2001; 19: 133–140.
51. Trabulsi EJ, Kalra P, Gomella LG. New approaches to the minimally invasive treatment of kidney tumors. *Cancer J* 2005; 1: 57–63.
52. Kricker A, Armstrong B. Surgery and outcomes of ductal carcinoma in situ of the breast: a population-based study in Australia. *Eur J Cancer* 2004; 40: 2396–2402.
53. Solin LJ, Fourquet A, Vicini FA, Taylor M, Olivotto IA, Haffty B, Strom EA, Pierce LJ, Marks LB, Bartelink H, McNeese MD, Jhingran A, Wai E, Bijker N, Campana F, Hwang WT. Long-term outcome after breast-conservation treatment with radiation for mammographically detected ductal carcinoma in situ of the breast. *Cancer* 2005; 103: 1137–1146.
54. Gazelle GS, Goldberg SN, Solbiati L, Livraghi T. Tumor ablation with radio-frequency energy. *Radiology* 2000; 217: 633–646.
55. Singletary S. Minimally invasive techniques in breast cancer treatment. *Semin Surg Oncol* 2001; 20: 246–250.
56. Hall-Craggs MA, Vaidya JS. Minimally invasive therapy for the treatment of breast tumours. *Eur J Radiol* 2002; 42: 52–57.
57. Ekstrand V, Wiksell H, Schultz I, Sandstedt B, Rotstein S, Eriksson A. Influence of electrical and thermal properties on RF ablation of breast cancer: is the tumour preferentially heated? *Biomed Eng Online* 2005; 4: 41.
58. Cioni R, Armillota N, Bargellina I, Zampa V, Capelli C, Vagli P, Boni G, Marchetti S, Consoli V, Bartolozzi C. CT-guided radiofrequency ablation of osteoid osteoma: long-term results. *Eur Radiol* 2004; 14: 1203–1208.
59. Goetz MP, Callstrom MR, Charboneau JW, Farrell MA, Maus TP, Welch TJ, Wong GY, Sloan JA, Novotny PJ, Petersen IA, Beres RA, Regge D, Capanna R, Saker MB, Gronemeyer DHW, Gevargez A, Ahrar K, Choti MA, de Baere TJ, Rubin J. Percutaneous image-guided radiofrequency ablation of painful metastases involving bone: a multicenter study. *J Clin Oncol* 2004; 22: 300–306.

60. Greenspon AJ, Walinsky P, Rosen A. Catheter ablation for the treatment of cardiac arrhythmias. In: Rosen A, Rosen HD, Editors. *New Frontiers in Medical Device Technology.* Vol. 2. New York: Wiley, pp. 61–77, 1995.
61. Lin JC. Studies on microwaves in medicine and biology: from snails to humans. *Bioelectromagnetics* 2004; 25: 146–159.
62. Jordan PN, Christini DJ. Therapies for ventricular cardiac arrhythmias. *Crit Rev Biomed Eng* 2005; 33: 557–604.
63. Rosen A, Stuchly MA, Vorst AV. Applications of RF/microwaves in medicine. *IEEE Trans Microw Theory Tech* 2002; 50: 963–974.
64. Huang SKS, Wilber DJ, Editors. *Radiofrequency Catheter Ablation of Cardiac Arrhythmias: Basic Concepts and Clinical Applications.* New York: Blackwell Publishing, 2000.
65. Lin JC. Biophysics of radiofrequency ablation. In: Huang SKS, Wilber DJ, Editors. *Radiofrequency Catheter Ablation of Cardiac Arhhythmias: Basic Concepts and Clinical Applications.* New York: Blackwell Publishing, pp. 13–24, 2000.
66. Schumacher B, Lüderitz B. Catheter ablation of atrial fibrillation: what did we learn? *Herzschrittmachertherapie und Elektrophysiologie* 1999; 10: S039–S046.
67. McRury ID, Haines DE. Ablation for the treatment of arrhythmias. *Proc IEEE* 1996; 84: 404–416.
68. Spitzer SG, Richter P, Knaut M, Schuler S. Treatment of atrial fibrillation in open heart surgery—the potential role of microwave energy. *Thorac Cardiovasc Surg* 1999; 47: 374–378.
69. Zipes DP. *Catheter Ablation of Arrhythmias.* New York: Blackwell Publishing, 2001.
70. Keane D. New catheter ablation techniques for the treatment of cardiac arrhythmias. *Card Electrophysiol Rev* 2002; 6: 341–348.
71. Gillinov AM, Blackstone EH, McCarthy PM. Atrial fibrillation: current surgical options and their assessment. *Ann Thorac Surg* 2002; 74: 2210–2217.
72. Geidel S, Lass M, Boczor S, Kuck K-H, Ostermeyer J. Surgical treatment of permanent atrial fibrillation during heart valve surgery. *Interact Cardiovas Thorac Surg* 2003; 2: 160–165.
73. Benussi S. Treatment of atrial fibrillation. *Eur J Cardiothorac Surg* 2004; 26: S39–S41.
74. Francis J, Fontaine G. Role of catheter ablation in arrhythmogenic right ventricular dysplasia. *Indian Pacing Electrophysiol J* 2005; 5: 81–85.
75. Gillinov AM. Ablation of atrial fibrillation with mitral valve surgery. *Curr Opin Cardiol* 2005; 20: 107–114.
76. Lencioni R, Goletti O, Armillotta N, Paolicchi A, Moretti M, Cioni D, Donati F, Cicorelli A, Ricci S, Carrai M, Conte PF, Cavina E, Bartolozzi C. Radio-frequency thermal ablation of liver metastases with a cooled-tip electrode needle: results of a pilot clinical trial. *Eur Radiol* 1998; 8: 1205–1211.
77. Curley SA, Izzo F, Delrio P. Radiofrequency ablation of unresectable primary and metastatic hepatic malignancies: results in 123 patients. *Ann Surg* 1999; 230: 1–8.
78. Zlotta AR, Djavan B, Matos C, Noel JC, Peny MO, Silverman DE, Marberger M, Schulman CC. Percutaneous transperineal radiofrequency ablation of prostate tumour: safety, feasibility and pathological effect on human prostate cancer. *Br J Urol* 1998; 81: 265–275.
79. Jeffrey SS, Birdwell RL, Ikeda DM, Daniel BL, Nowels KW, Dirbas FM, Griffey SM. Radiofrequency ablation of breast cancer: first report of an emerging technology. *Arch Surg* 1999; 134: 1064–1068.
80. Dupuy DE, Mayo-Smith WW, Abbott GF, DiPetrillo T. Clinical applications of radio-frequency tumor ablation in the thorax. *Radiographics* 2002; 22: S259–S269.
81. Sackenheim MM. Radio frequency ablation. *J Diagn Med Sonography* 2003; 19: 88–92.

82. Hines-Peralta A, Goldberg SN. Review of radiofrequency ablation for renal cell carcinoma. *Clin Cancer Res* 2004; 10: 6328S–6334S.
83. Decadt B, Siriwardena AK. Radiofrequency ablation of liver tumours: systematic review. *Lancet Oncol* 2004; 5: 550–560.
84. Mahnken AH, Gunter RW, Tacke J. Radiofrequency ablation of renal tumors. *Eur Radiol* 2004; 14: 1449–1455.
85. Brown DB. Concepts, considerations, and concerns on the cutting edge of radiofrequency ablation. *J Vasc Interv Radiol* 2005; 16: 597–613.
86. Wagner AA, Solomon SB, Su L-M. Treatment of renal tumors with radiofrequency ablation. *J Endourol* 2005; 19: 643–653.
87. Gillams AR. The use of radiofrequency in cancer. *Br J Cancer* 2005; 92: 1825–1829.
88. Rose SC, Thistlethwaite PA, Sewell PE, Vance RB. Lung cancer and radiofrequency ablation. *J Vasc Interv Radiol* 2006; 17: 927–951.
89. Lucey BC. Radiofrequency ablation: the future is now. *Am J Roentgenol* 2006; 186: S237–S240.
90. Haemmerich D, Lee FT Jr. Multiple applicator approaches for radiofrequency and microwave ablation. *Int J Hyperthermia* 2005; 21: 93–106.
91. Scudamore C. Volumetric radiofrequency ablation: technical considerations. *Cancer J* 2000; 6: S316–S318.
92. Issa MM, Myrick SE, Symbas NP. The TUNA procedure for BPH—review of technology. *Infect Urol* 1998; 11: 104–111.
93. Livraghi T, Goldberg SN, Lazzaroni S, Meloni F, Pellicano S, Solbiati L, Gazelle GS. Saline-enhanced radiofrequency tissue ablation in the treatment of liver metastases. *Radiology* 1997; 202: 205–210.
94. Miao Y, Ni Y, Mulier S, Wang K, Hoey MF, Mulier P, Penninckx F, Yu J, De Scheerder I, Baert AL, Marchal G. Ex vivo experiment on radiofrequency liver ablation with saline infusion through a screw-tip cannulated electrode. *J Surg Res* 1997; 71: 19–24.
95. Rossi S, Garbagnati F, De Francesco I, Accocella F, Leonardi L, Quaretti P, Zangrandi A, Paties C, Lencioni R. Relationship between the shape and size of radiofrequency induced thermal lesions and hepatic vascularization. *Tumori* 1999; 85: 128–132.
96. Chinn SB, Lee FT Jr., Kennedy GD, Chinn C, Johnson CD, Winter III TC, Warner TF, Mahvi DM. Effect of vascular occlusion on radiofrequency ablation of the liver: results in a porcine model. *Am J Roentgenol* 2001; 176: 789–795.
97. McGahan JP, Browning PD, Brock JM, Tesluk H. Hepatic ablation using radiofrequency elektrocautery. *Invest Radiol* 1990; 25: 267–270.
98. Goldberg SN, Stein MC, Gazelle GS, Sheiman RG, Kruskal JB, Clouse ME. Percutaneous radiofrequency tissue ablation: optimization of pulsed-radiofrequency technique to increase coagulation necrosis. *J Vasc Interv Radiol* 1999; 10: 907–916.
99. Goldberg SN, Ahmed M, Gazelle GS, Kruskal JB, Huertas JC, Halpern EF, Oliver BS, Lenkinski RE. Radiofrequency thermal ablation with adjuvant saline injection: effect of electrical conductivity on tissue heating and coagulation. *Radiology* 2001; 219: 157–165.
100. McGahan JP, Gu WZ, Brock JM, Tesluk H, Jones CD. Hepatic ablation using bipolar radiofrequency electrocautery. *Acad Radiol* 1996; 3: 418–422.
101. Burdio F, Guemes A, Burdio JM, Castiella T, De Gregorio MA, Lozano R, Livraghi T. Hepatic lesion ablation with bipolar saline-enhanced radiofrequency in the audible spectrum. *Acad Radiol* 1999; 6: 680–686.
102. Burdio F, Guemes A, Burdio JM, Navarro A, Sousa R, Castiella T, Cruz I, Burzaco O, Guirao X, Lozano R. Large hepatic ablation with bipolar saline-enhanced radiofrequency: an experimental study in in vivo porcine liver with a novel approach. *J Surg Res* 2003; 110: 193–201.

103. Haemmerich D, Staelin ST, Tungjitkusolmun S, Lee FT Jr., Mahvi DM, Webster JG. Hepatic bipolar radiofrequency ablation between separated multiprong electrodes. *IEEE Trans Biomed Eng* 2001; 48: 1145–1152.
104. Haemmerich D, Lee FT Jr., Schutt DJ, Sampson LA, Webster JG, Fine JP, Mahvi DM. Large-volume radiofrequency ablation of ex vivo bovine liver with multiple cooled cluster electrodes. *Radiology* 2005; 234: 563–568.
105. Tacke J, Mahnken A, Roggan A, Gunther RW. Multipolar radiofrequency ablation: first clinical results. *Rofo* 2004; 176: 324–329.
106. Frericks BB, Ritz JP, Roggan A, Wolf K-J, Albrecht T. Multipolar radiofrequency ablation of hepatic tumors: initial experience. *Radiology* 2005; 237: 1056–1062.
107. Clasen S, Schmidt D, Boss A, Dietz K, Kröber SM, Claussen CD, Pereira PL. Multipolar radiofrequency ablation with internally cooled electrodes: experimental study in ex vivo bovine liver with mathematic modeling. *Radiology* 2006; 238: 881–890.
108. Shibata T, Shibata T, Maetani Y, Isoda H, Hiraoka, M. Radiofrequency ablation for small hepatocellular carcinoma: prospective comparison of internally cooled electrode and expandable electrode. *Vasc Interv Radiol* 2006; 238: 346–353.
109. Lee FT, Haemmerich D, Wright AS, Mahvi DM, Sampson LA, Webster JG. Multiple probe radiofrequency ablation: pilot study in an animal model. *J Vasc Interv Radiol* 2003; 14: 1437–1442.
110. Dodd GD, Frank MS, Aribandi M, Chopra S, Chintapalli KN. Radiofrequency thermal ablation: computer analysis of the size of the thermal injury created by overlapping ablation. *Am J Roentgenol* 2001; 177: 777–782.
111. Laeseke PF, Sampson LA, Haemmerich D, Brace CL, Fine JP, Frey TM, Winter TC, Lee FT Jr. Multiple-electrode radiofrequency ablation: simultaneous production of separate zones of coagulation in an in vivo porcine liver model. *J Vasc Interv Radiol* 2005; 16: 1727–1735.
112. Siperstein A, Garland A, Engle K, Rogers S, Berber E, Foroutani A, String A, Ryan T, Ituarte P. Local recurrence after laparoscopic radiofrequency thermal ablation of hepatic tumors. *Ann Surg Oncol* 2000; 7: 106–113.
113. Wood BJ, Bates J. Radiofrequency thermal ablation of a splenic metastasis. *J Vasc Interv Radiol* 2001; 12: 261–263.
114. Reithmann C, Hoffmann E, Dorwarth U, Remp T, Steinbeck G. Electroanatomical mapping for visualization of atrial activation in patients with incisional atrial tachycardias. *Eur Heart Journal* 2001; 22: 237–246.
115. Berjano EJ. Theoretical modeling for radiofrequency ablation: state-of-the-art and challenges for the future. *Biomed Eng Online* 2006; 5: 24.
116. Chang IA, Nguyen UD. Thermal modeling of lesion growth with radiofrequency ablation devices. *Biomed Eng Online* 2004; 3: 27–46.
117. Labonte S. A computer simulation of radio-frequency ablation of the endocardium. *IEEE Trans Biomed Eng* 1994; 41: 883–890.
118. Yeung CJ, Atalar E. A green's function approach to local RF heating in interventional MRI. *Med Phys* 2001; 28: 826–832.
119. Haemmerich D, Tungjitkusolmun S, Staelin ST, Lee FT, Mahvi DM, Webster JG. Finite-element analysis of hepatic multiple probe radio-frequency ablation. *IEEE Trans Biomed Eng* 2002; 49: 836–842.
120. Tungjitkusolmun S, Woo EJ, Cao H, Tsai JZ, Vorperian VR, Webster JG. Thermal-electrical finite element modelling for radio frequency cardiac ablation: effects of changes in myocardial properties. *Med Biol Eng Comput* 2000; 38: 562–568.
121. Tungjitkusolmun S, Woo EJ, Cao H, Tsai JZ, Vorperian VR, Webster JG. Finite element analyses of uniform current density electrodes for radio frequency cardiac ablation. *IEEE Trans Biomed Eng* 2000; 47: 32–40.

122. Tungjitkusolmun S, Staelin ST, Haemmerich D, Tsai JZ, Webster JG, Lee FT Jr, Mahvi DM, Vorperian VR. Three-dimensional finite element analyses for radio-frequency hepatic tumor ablation. *IEEE Trans Biomed Eng* 2002; 49: 3–9.

123. Chang I. Finite element analysis of hepatic radiofrequency ablation probes using temperature-dependent electrical conductivity. *Biomed Eng Online* 2003; 2: 12.

124. Shahidi AV, Savard P. A finite element model for radiofrequency ablation of the myocardium. *IEEE Trans Biomed Eng* 1994; 41: 963–968.

125. Gopalakrishnan J. A mathematical model for irrigated epicardial radiofrequency ablation. *Ann Biomed Eng* 2002; 30: 884–893.

126. Caccitolo JA, Stulak JM, Schaff HV, Francischelli D, Jensen DN, Mehra R. Open-heart endocardial radiofrequency ablation: an alternative to incisions in maze surgery. *J Surg Res* 2001; 97: 27–33.

127. Livraghi T, Lazzaroni S, Meloni F. Radiofrequency thermal ablation of hepatocellular carcinoma. *Eur J Ultrasound* 2001; 13: 159–166.

128. Sato M, Watanabe Y, Ueda S, Iseki S, Abe Y, Sato N, Kimura S, Okubo K, Onji M. Microwave coagulation therapy for hepatocellular carcinoma. *Gastroenterology* 1996; 110: 1507–1514.

129. Abe T, Shinzawa H, Wakabayashi H, Aoki M, Sugahara K, Iwaba A, Haga H, Miyano S, Terui Y, Mitsuhashi H, Watanabe H, Matsuo T, Saito K, Saito T, Togashi H, Takahashi T. Value of laparoscopic microwave coagulation therapy for hepatocellular carcinoma in relation to tumor size and location. *Endoscopy* 2000; 32: 598–603.

130. Seki T, Wakabayashi M, Nakagawa T, Imamura M, Tamai T, Nishimura A, Yamashiki N, Okamura A, Inoue K. Percutaneous microwave coagulation therapy for patients with small hepatocellular carcinoma: comparison with percutaneous ethanol injection therapy. *Cancer* 1999; 85: 1694–1702.

131. Geoghegan JG, Scheele J. Treatment of colorectal liver metastases. *Br J Surg* 1999; 86: 158–169.

132. Tanabe KK, Curley SA, Dodd GD, Siperstein AE, Goldberg SN. Radiofrequency abla-tion: the experts weigh in. *Cancer* 2003; 100: 641–650.

133. Rossi S, Buscarini E, Garbagnati F. Percutaneous treatment of small hepatic tumors by an expandable RF needle electrode. *Am J Roentgenol* 1998; 170: 1015–1022.

134. Livraghi T, Goldberg SN, Lazzaroni S, Meloni F, Solbiati L, Gazelle GS. Small hepa-tocellular carcinoma: treatment with radio-frequency ablation versus ethanol injection. *Radiology* 1999; 210: 655–661.

135. Livraghi T, Goldberg SN, Meloni F, Solbiati L, Gazelle GS. Hepatocellular carcinoma: comparison of efficacy between percutaneous ethanol instillation and radiofrequency. *Radiology* 1999; 210: 655–663.

136. Aschoff AJ, Merkle EM, Wong V, Zhang Q, Mendez MM, Duerk JL, Lewin JS. How does alteration of hepatic blood flow affect liver perfusion and radiofrequency-induced thermal lesion size in rabbit liver? *J Magn Reson Imaging* 2001; 13: 57–63.

137. Buscarini L, Buscarini E, Di Stasi M, Vallisa D, Quaretti P, Rocca A. Percutaneous radiofrequency ablation of small hepatocellular carcinoma: long-term results. *Eur Radiol* 2001; 11: 914–921.

138. Shiina S, Teratani T, Obi S, Hamamura K, Koike Y, Omata M. Nonsurgical treatment of hepatocellular carcinoma: from percutaneous ethanol injection therapy and percu-taneous microwave coagulation therapy to radiofrequency ablation. *Oncology* 2002; 62: 64–68.

139. De Baere T, Risse O, Kuoch V, Dromain C, Sengel C, Smayra T, Din MGE, Letoublon C, Elias D. Adverse events during radiofrequency treatment of 582 hepatic tumors. *Am J Roentgenol* 2003; 181: 695–700.

140. Curley SA. Radiofrequency ablation of malignant liver tumors. *Ann Surg Oncol* 2003; 10: 338–347.

141. Livraghi T, Solbiati L, Meloni MF, Gazelle GS, Halpern EF, Goldberg SN. Treatment of focal liver tumors with percutaneous radio-frequency ablation: complications encountered in a multicenter study. *Radiology* 2003; 226: 441–451.

142. Gazelle GS, McMahon PM, Beinfeld MT, Halpern EF, Weinstein MC. Metastatic colorectal carcinoma: cost-effectiveness of percutaneous radiofrequency ablation versus that of hepatic resection. *Radiology* 2004; 233: 729–739.

143. Chen M-H, Yang W, Yan K, Zou M-W, Solbiati L, Liu J-B, Dai Y. Large liver tumors: protocol for radiofrequency ablation and its clinical application in 110 patients— mathematic model, overlapping mode, and electrode placement process. *Radiology* 2004; 232: 260–271.

144. Chen MH, Wei Y, Yan K, Gao W, Dai Y, Huo L, Yin SS, Zhang H, Poon RTP. Treatment strategy to optimize radiofrequency ablation for liver malignancies. *J Vasc Interv Radiol* 2006; 17: 671–683.

145. Seror O, Haddar D, N'Kontchou G, Ajavon Y, Trinchet J-C, Beaugrand M, Sellier N. Radiofrequency ablation for the treatment of liver tumors in the caudate lobe. *J Vasc Interv Radiol* 2005; 16: 981–990.

146. Ruers TJM, de Jong KP, Ijzermans JNM. Radiofrequency for the treatment of liver tumours. *Dig Surg* 2005; 22: 245–253.

147. Han JK, Lee JM, Kim SH, Lee JY, Park HS, Eo H, Choi BI. Radiofrequency ablation in the liver using two cooled-wet electrodes in the bipolar mode. *Eur Radiol* 2005; 15: 2163–2170.

148. Yang W, Chen MH, Yin SS, Yan K, Gao W, Wang YB, Huo L, Zhang XP, Xing BC. Radiofrequency ablation of recurrent hepatocellular carcinoma after hepatectomy: therapeutic efficacy on early- and late-phase recurrence. *Am J Roentgenol* 2006; 186: S275–S283.

149. Cabassa P, Donato F, Simeone F, Grazioli L, Romanini L. Radiofrequency ablation of hepatocellular carcinoma: long-term experience with expandable needle electrodes. *Am J Roentgenol* 2006; 186: S316–S321.

150. Aloia TA, Vauthey J-N, Loyer EM, Ribero D, Pawlik TM, Wei SH, Curley SA, Zorzi D, Abdalla EK. Solitary colorectal liver metastasis: resection determines outcome. *Arch Surg* 2006; 141: 460–467.

151. Allgaier H-P, Galandi D, Zuber I, Blum HE. Radiofrequency thermal ablation of hepatocellular carcinoma. *Dig Dis Crit Rev* 2001; 19: 301–310.

152. Mulier S, Mulier P, Ni Y, Miao Y, Dupas B, Marchal G, De Wever I, Michel L. Complications of radiofrequency coagulation of liver tumours. *Br J Surg* 2002; 89: 1206–1222.

153. Mulier S, Miao Y, Michel L, Marchal G. A review of the general aspects of radiofrequency ablation. *Abdom Imaging* 2005; 30: 381–400.

154. Dupuy DE, Zagoria RJ, Akerley W, Mayo-Smith WW, Kavanagh PV, Safran H. Percutaneous radiofrequency ablation of malignancies in the lung. *Am J Roentgenol* 2000; 174: 57–59.

155. Steinke K, Arnold C, Wulf S, Morris DL. Safety of radiofrequency ablation of myocardium and lung adjacent to the heart: an animal study. *J Surg Res* 2003; 114: 140–145.

156. Steinke K, Glenn D, Franczr, King J, Morris DL. Percutaneous pulmonary radiofrequency ablation: difficulty achieving complete ablations in big lung lesions. *Br J Radiol* 2003; 76: 742–745.

157. Steinke K, King J, Glenn DW, Morris DL. Percutaneous radiofrequency ablation of lung tumors with expandable needle electrodes: tips from preliminary experience. *Am J Roentgenol* 2004; 183: 605–611.

158. Belfiore G, Moggio G, Tedeschi E, Greco M, Cioffi R, Cincotti F, Rossi R. CT-guided radiofrequency ablation: a potential complementary therapy for patients with unresectable primary lung cancer—a preliminary report of 33 patients. *Am J Roentgenol* 2004; 183: 1003–1011.

159. Gadaleta C, Catino A, Ranieri G, Armenise F, Colucci G, Lorusso V, Cramarossa A, Fiorentini G, Mattioli V. Radiofrequency thermal ablation of 69 lung neoplasms. *J Chemother* 2004; 16: 86–89.

160. Jin GY, Lee JM, Lee YC, Han YM, Lim YS. Primary and secondary lung malignancies treated with percutaneous radiofrequency ablation: evaluation with follow-up helical CT. *Am J Roentgen* 2005; 183: 1013–1020.

161. Tominaga J, Miyachi H, Takase K, Matsuhashi T, Yamada T, Sato A, Saito H, Ishibashi T, Endoh M, Higano S, Takahashi S. Time-related changes in computed tomographic appearance and pathologic findings after radiofrequency ablation of the rabbit lung: preliminary experimental study. *J Vasc Interv Radiol* 2005; 16: 1719–726.

162. Nguyen CL, Scott WJ, Young NA, Rader T, Giles LR, Goldberg M. Radiofrequency ablation of primary lung cancer. *Chest* 2005; 128: 3507–3511.

163. Rossi S, Dore R, Cascina A, Vespro V, Garbagnati F, Rosa L, Ravetta V, Azzaretti A, Di Tolla P, Orlandoni G, Pozzi E. Percutaneous computed tomography-guided radiofrequency thermal ablation of small unresectable lung tumours. *Eur Respir J* 2006; 27: 556–563.

164. Ambrogi MC, Fontanini G, Cioni R, Faviana P, Fanucchi O, Mussi A. Biologic effects of radiofrequency thermal ablation on non-small cell lung cancer: results of a pilot study. *J Thorac Cardiovasc Surg* 2006; 131: 1002–1006.

165. Grieco CA, Simon CJ, Mayo-Smith WW, DiPetrillo TA, Ready NE, Dupuy DE. Percutaneous image-guided thermal ablation and radiation therapy: outcomes of combined treatment for 41 patients with inoperable stage I/II non–small-cell lung cancer. *J Vasc Interv Radiol* 2006; 17: 1117–1124.

166. Zlotta AR, Wildschutz T, Raviv G, Peny MO, Van Gansbeke D, Noel JC, Schulman CC. Radiofrequency interstitial tumor ablation (RITA) is a possible new modality for treatment of renal cancer: ex vivo and in vivo experience. *J Endourol* 1997; 11: 251–258.

167. Aschoff AJ, Wendt M, Merkle EM, Shankaranarayanan A, Chung Y, Duerk JL, Lewin JS. Perfusion-modulated MR imaging-guided radiofrequency ablation of the kidney in a procine model. *Am J Roentgenol* 2001; 177: 151–158.

168. Zagoria RJ, Hawkins AD, Clark PE, Hall MC, Matlaga BR, Dyer RB, Chen MY. Percutaneous CT-guided radiofrequency ablation of renal neoplasms: factors influencing success. *Am J Roentgenol* 2004; 183: 201–207.

169. Noguchi M. Minimally invasive surgery for small breast cancer. *J Surg Oncol* 2003; 84: 94–101.

170. Singletary ES. Feasibility of radiofrequency ablation for primary breast cancer. *Breast Cancer* 2003; 10: 4–9.

171. Bansal R. Coming soon to a hospital near you! [biomedical applications of RF/microwaves]. *IEEE Microw Mag* 2002; 3: 34–36.

172. Schulman CC, Zlotta AR, Rasor JS, Hourriez L, Noel JC, Edwards SD. Transurethral needle ablation (TUNA): safety, feasibility, and tolerance of a new office procedure for treatment of benign prostatic hyperplasia. *Eur Urol* 1993; 24: 415–423.

173. Djavan B, Zlotta AR, Susani M, Heinz G, Shariat S, Silverman DE, Schulman CC, Marberger M. Transperineal radiofrequency interstitial tumor ablation of the prostate: correlation of magnetic resonance imaging with histopathologic examination. *Urology* 1997; 50: 986–993.

174. Woertler K, Vestring T, Boettner F, Winkelmann W, Heindel W, Lindner N. Osteoid osteoma: CT-guided percutaneous radiofrequency ablation and follow-up in 47 patients. *J Vasc Interv Radiol* 2001; 12: 717–722.

175. Stolker RJ, Vervest AC, Groen GJ. The treatment of chronic thoracic segmental pain by radiofrequency percutaneous partial rhizotomy. *J Neurosurg* 1994; 80: 986–992.

176. Oturai AB, Jensen K, Eriksen J, Madsen F. Neurosurgery for trigeminal neuralgia: comparison of alcohol block, neurectomy, and radiofrequency coagulation. *Clin J Pain* 1996; 12: 311–315.

177. Slappendel R, Crul BJ, Braak GJ, Geurts JW, Booij LH, Voerman VF, de Boo T. The efficacy of radiofrequency lesioning of the cervical spinal dorsal root ganglion in a double blinded randomized study: no difference between 40 degrees C and 67 degrees C treatments. *Pain* 1997; 73: 159–163.

178. Sanders M, Suurmond WW. Efficacy of sphenopalatine ganglion blockage in 66 patients suffering from cluster headache: a 12–70 month follow-up evaluation. *J Neurosurg* 1997; 87: 876–880.

179. Sollitto RJ, Plotkin EL, Klein PG, Mullin P. Early clinical results of the use of radio-frequency lesioning in the treatment of plantar fasciitis. *J Foot Ankle Surg* 1997; 36: 215–219.

180. De Salles AA, Brekhus SD, De Souza EC, Behnke EJ, Farahani K, Anzai Y, Lufkin R. Early postoperative appearance of radiofrequency lesions on magnetic resonance imaging. *Neurosurg* 1995; 36: 932–936.

181. Lee HK, Kwon HJ, Lee HB, Jin GY, Chung MJ, Lee YC. Radiofrequency thermal abla-tion of primary pleural synovial sarcoma. *Int J Thorac Med* 2006; 73: 250–252.

182. Benussi S, Pappone C, Nascimbene S, Oreto G, Caldarola A, Stefano PL, Casati V, Alfieri O. A simple way to treat chronic atrial fibrillation during mitral valve surgery: the epicardial radiofrequency approach. *Eur J Cardiothorac Surg* 2000; 17: 524–529.

183. Melo J, Adragão P, Neves J, Ferreira M, Timoteo A, Santiago T, Ribeiras R, Canada M. Endocardial and epicardial radiofrequency ablation in the treatment of atrial fibrilla-tion with a new intra-operative device. *Eur J Cardiothorac Surg* 2000; 18: 182–186.

184. Williams MR, Stewart JR, Bolling SF, Freeman S, Anderson JT, Argenziano M, Smith CR, Oz MC. Surgical treatment of atrial fibrillation using radiofrequency energy. *Ann Thorac Surg* 2001; 71: 1939–1944.

185. Thomas SP, Guy DJR, Boyd AC, Eipper VE, Ross DL, Chard RB. Comparison of epi-cardial and endocardial linear ablation using handheld probes. *Ann Thorac Surg* 2003; 75: 543–548.

186. Haissaguerre M, Jais P, Shah DC, Gencel L, Pradeau V, Garrigues S, Chouairi S, Hocini M, Le Metayer P, Roudaut R, Clementy J. Right and left atrial radiofrequency catheter therapy of paroxysmal atrial fibrillation. *J Cardiovasc Electrophysiol* 1996; 7: 1132–1144.

187. Jais R, Shah DC, Takahashi A, Hocini M, Haissaguerre M, Clementy J. Long-term follow-up after right atrial radiofrequency catheter treatment of paroxysmal atrial fibrillation. *Pacing Clin Electrophysiol* 1998; 21: 2533–2538.

188. Gaita F, Riccardi R. Lone atrial fibrillation ablation: transcatheter or minimally inva-sive surgical approaches? *J Am Coll Cardiol* 2002; 40: 481–483.

189. Guden M, Akpinar B, Sanisoglu I, Sagbas E, Bayindir O. Intraoperative saline-irrigated radiofrequency modified maze procedure for atrial fibrillation. *Ann Thorac Surg* 2002; 74: S1301–S1306.

190. Panescu D, Whayne JG, Fleischman SD, Mirotznik MS, Swanson DK, Webster JG. Three-dimensional finite element analysis of current density and temperature distribu-tions during radio-frequency ablation. *IEEE Trans Biomed Eng* 1995; 42: 879–890.

191. Jain MK, Wolf PD. A three-dimensional finite element model of radiofrequency ablation with blood flow and its experimental validation. *Ann Biomed Eng* 2000; 28: 1075–1084.

192. Melo, Adragão P, Neves J, Ferreira MM, Pinto MM, Rebocho MJ, Parreira L, Ramos T. Surgery for atrial fibrillation using radiofrequency catheter ablation: assessment of results at one year. *Eur J Cardiothorac Surg* 1999; 15: 851–855.

193. Sie HT, Beukema WP, Misier AR, Elvan A, Ennema JJ, Haalebos MMP, Wellens HJJ. Radiofrequency modified maze in patients with atrial fibrillation undergoing concomitant cardiac surgery. *J Thorac Cardiovasc Surg* 2001; 122: 249–256.

194. Sie HT, Beukema WP, Elvan A, Ramdat M, Anand R. Long-term results of irrigated radiofrequency modified maze procedure in 200 patients with concomitant cardiac surgery: six years experience. *Ann Thorac Surg* 2004; 77: 512–517.

195. Benussi S, Nascimbene S, Agricola E, Calori G, Calvi S, Caldarola A, Oppizzi M, Casati V, Pappone C, Alfieri O. Surgical ablation of atrial fibrillation using the epicardial radiofrequency approach: mid-term results and risk analysis. *Ann Thorac Surg* 2002; 74: 1050–1057.

196. Prasad SM, Maniar HS, Schuessler RB, Damiano R Jr. Chronic transmural atrial ablation by using bipolar radiofrequency energy on the beating heart. *J Thorac Cardiovasc Surg* 2002; 124: 708–713.

197. Santiago T, Melo J, Gouveia RH, Neves J, Abecasis A, Adragão P, Martins AP. Epicardial radiofrequency applications: in vitro and in vivo studies on human atrial myocardium. *Eur J Cardio-Thorac Surg* 2003; 4: 481–486.

198. Bonanomi G, Schwartzman D, Francischelli D, Hebsgaard K, Zenati, Marco A. A new device for beating heart bipolar radiofrequency atrial ablation. *J Thorac Cardiovasc Surg* 2003; 126: 1859–1866.

199. Wong JWW. Ensuring transmurality using irrigated radiofrequency modified maze in surgery for atrial fibrillation—a simple and effective way. *Heart Lung Circ* 2004; 13: 302–308.

200. Wisser W, Khazen C, Deviatko E, Stix G, Binder T, Seitelberger R, Schmidinger H, Wolner E. Microwave and radiofrequency ablation yield similar success rates for treatment of chronic atrial fibrillation. *Eur J Cardiothorac Surg* 2004; 25: 1011–1017.

201. Tai C-T, Liu T-Y, Lee P-C, Lin Y-J, Chang M-S, Chen S-A. Non-contact mapping to guide radiofrequency ablation of atypical right atrial flutter. *J Am Coll Cardiol* 2004; 44: 1080–1086.

202. Mokadam NA, McCarthy PM, Gillinov AM, Ryan WH, Moon MR, Mack MJ, Gaynor SL, Prasad SM, Wickline SA, Bailey MS, Damiano NR, Ishii Y, Schuessler RB, Damiano RJ. A prospective multicenter trial of bipolar radiofrequency ablation for atrial fibrillation: early results. *Ann Thorac Surg* 2005; 78: 1665–1670.

203. Geidel S, Ostermeyer J, Lass M, Betzold M, Duong A, Jensen F, Boczor S, Kuck K-H. Three years experience with monopolar and bipolar radiofrequency ablation surgery in patients with permanent atrial fibrillation. *Eur J Cardiothorac Surg* 2005; 27: 243–249.

204. Akpinar B, Sanisoglu I, Guden M, Sagbas E, Caynak B, Bayramoglu Z. Combined off-pump coronary artery bypass grafting surgery and ablative therapy for atrial fibrillation: early and mid-term results. *Ann Thorac Surg* 2006; 81: 1332–1337.

205. Haissaguerre M, Gencel L, Fischer B, Le Metayer P, Poquet F, Marcus FI, Clementy J. Successful catheter ablation of atrial fibrillation. *J Cardiovasc Electrophysiol* 1994; 5: 1045–1052.

206. Garg A, Finneran W, Mollerus M, Birgersdotter-Green U, Fujimura O, Tone L, Feld GK. Right atrial compartmentalization using radiofrequency catheter ablation for management of patients with refractory atrial fibrillation. *J Cardiovasc Electrophysiol* 1999; 10: 763–771.

207. Jais P, Shah Dc, Hocini M, Macle L, Choi K-J, Haissaguerre M, Clementy J. Radiofrequency ablation for atrial fibrillation. *Eur Heart J Suppl* 2003; 5: H34–H39.

208. Schmidt-Nowara WW, Coultas DB, Wiggins C, Skipper BE, Samet JM. Snoring in a Hispanic-American population. Risk factors and association with hypertension and other morbidity. *Arch Intern Med* 1990; 150: 597–601.

209. Schmidt-Nowara W, Lowe A, Wiegand L, Cartwright R, Perez-Guerra F, Menn S. Oral appliances for the treatment of snoring and obstructive sleep apnea. *Sleep* 1995; 18: 501–510.

210. NICE. Interventional procedures overview of radiofrequency ablation of the soft palate for snoring. *Intenational Procedures Programme*, UK, 2004.

211. Nevels RD, Arndt GD, Raffoul GW, Carl JR, Pacifico A. Microwave catheter design. *IEEE Trans Biomed Eng* 1998; 45: 885–890.

212. Brace CL, Laeseke F, van der Weide DW, Lee FT. Microwave ablation with a triaxial antenna: results in ex vivo bovine liver. *IEEE Trans Microw Theory Tech* 2005; 53: 215–220.

213. Brieger J, Pereira PL, Trubenbach J, Schenk M, Krober SM, Schmidt D, Aube C, Claussen CD, Schick F. In vivo efficiency of four commercial monopolar radiofrequency ablation systems: a comparative experimental study in pig liver. *Invest Radiol* 2003; 38: 609–616.

214. Jiao LR, Hansen PD, Havlik R, Mitry RR, Pignatelli M, Habib N. Clinical short-term results of radiofrequency ablation in primary and secondary liver tumors. *Am J Surg* 1999; 177: 303–306.

215. Goette A, Reek S, Klein HU, Geller JC. Case report: severe skin burn at the site of the indifferent electrode after radiofrequency catheter ablation of typical atrial flutter. *J Interv Card Electrophysiol* 2001; 5: 337–340.

216. Cha C, Lee FT Jr., Rikkers LF, Niederhuber JE, Nguyen BT, Mahvi DM. Rationale for the combination of cryoablation with surgical resection of hepatic tumors. *J Gastrointest Surg* 2001; 5: 206–213.

217. Buscarini L, Buscarini E, Di Stasi M, Quaretti P, Zangrandi A. Percutaneous radiofrequency thermal ablation combined with transcatheter arterial embolization in the treatment of large hepatocellular carcinoma. *Ultraschall Med* 1999; 20: 47–53.

218. de Baere T, Bessoud B, Dromain C, Ducreux M, Boige V, Lassau N, Smayra T, Girish BV, Roche A, Elias D. Percutaneous radiofrequency ablation of hepatic tumors during temporary venous occlusion. *Am J Roentgenol* 2002; 178: 53–59.

219. Curley SA, Marra P, Beaty K, Ellis LM, Vauthey JN, Abdalla EK, Scaife C, Raut C, Wolff R, Choi H, Loyer E, Vallone P, Fiore F, Scordino F, De Rosa V, Orlando R, Pignata S, Daniele B, Izzo F. Early and late complications after radiofrequency ablation of malignant liver tumors in 608 patients. *Ann Surg* 2004; 239: 450–458.

220. Rhim H, Dodd GD, Chintapalli KN, Wood BJ, Dupuy DE, Hvizda JL, Sewell PE, Goldberg SN. Radiofrequency thermal ablation of abdominal tumors: lessons learned from complications. *Radiographics* 2004; 24: 41–52.

221. Smith EH. Complications of percutaneous abdominal fine-needle biopsy. *Radiology* 1991; 178: 253–258.

222. Goldberg SN, Solbiati L, Halpern EF, Gazelle GS. Variables affecting proper system grounding for radiofrequency ablation in an animal model. *J Vasc Interv Radiol* 2000; 11: 1069–1075.

223. Livraghi T, Meloni F, Goldberg SN, Lazzaroni S, Solbiati L, Gazelle GS. Hepatocellular carcinoma: radio-frequency ablation of medium and large lesions. *Radiology* 2000; 214: 761–768.

224. Rhim H, Yoon K-H, Lee JM, Cho Y, Cho J-S, Kim SH, Lee W-J, Lim HK, Nam G-J, Han S-K, Kim YH, Park CM, Kim PN, Byun J-Y. Major complications after radiofrequency thermal ablation of hepatic tumors: spectrum of imaging findings. *Radiographics* 2003; 23: 123–134.

225. Buscarini B, Buscarini L. Radiofrequency thermal ablation with expandable needle of focal liver malignancies: complication report. *Eur Radiol* 2004; 14: 31–37.

226. Jansen MC, van Duijnhoven FH, van Hillegersberg R, Rijken A, van Coevorden F, van der Sijp J, Prevoo W, van Gulik TM. Adverse effects of radiofrequency ablation of liver tumours in the Netherlands. *Br J Surg* 2005; 92: 1248–1254.

227. Akahane M, Koga H, Kato N, Yamada H, Uozumi K, Tateishi R, Teratani T, Shiina S, Ohtomo K. Complications of percutaneous radiofrequency ablation for hepato-cellular carcinoma: imaging spectrum and management. *RadioGraphics* 2005; 25: S57–S68.

228. Climent V, Hurle A, Ho SW, Sanchez-Quintana D. Effects of endocardial microwave energy ablation. *Indian Pacing Electrophysiol J* 2005; 5: 233–243.

229. Garside R, Stein K, Wyatt K, Round A. Microwave and thermal balloon ablation for heavy menstrual bleeding: a systematic review. *BJOG* 2005; 112: 12–23.

230. Habash RWY, Alhafid HT. Key development in therapeutic applications of RF/micro-waves. *Int J Sci Res* 2006; 16: 451–455.

231. Rosen A, Greenspon AJ, Walinsky P. Microwave treat heart diseases. *IEEE Microw Mag* 2007; February: 70–75.

232. Organ LW. Electrophysiologic principles of radiofrequency lesion making. *Appl Neurophysiol* 1976; 39: 69–76.

233. Wonnel TL, Stauffer PR, Langberg JJ. Evaluation of microwave and radio-frequency catheter ablation in a myocardium-equivalent phantom model. *IEEE Trans Biomed Eng* 1992; 39: 1086–1095.

234. VanderBrink B, Gu Z, Rodriguez V, Link M, Homoud M, Estes AM, Rappaport C, Wang P. Microwave ablation using a wide-aperture antenna design in a porcine thigh muscle preparation: in vivo assessment of temperature profile and geometry. *J Cardiovasc Electrophysiol* 2000; 11: 193–198.

235. Hines-Peralta AU, Pirani N, Clegg P, Cronin N, Ryan TP, Liu Z, Goldberg SN. Micro-wave ablation: results with a 2.45-GHz applicator in ex vivo bovine and in vivo porcine liver. *Radiology* 2006; 239: 94–102.

236. Wright AS, Sampson LA, Warner TF, Mahvi DM, Lee FT. Radiofrequency versus microwave ablation in a hepatic porcine model. *Radiology* 2005; 236: 132–139.

237. Chiu HM, Mohan AS, Weily AR, Guy DJR, Ross DL. Analysis of novel expanded tip wire (ETW) antenna for microwave ablation of cardiac arrhythmias. *IEEE Trans Biomed Eng* 2003; 50: 890–899.

238. Wright AS, Lee FT, Mahvi DM. Hepatic microwave ablation with multiple antennae results in synergistically larger zones of coagulation necrosis. *Ann Surg Oncol* 2003; 10: 275–283.

239. Hurter W, Reinfold F, Lorenz WJ. A dipole antenna for interestial microwave hyper-thermia. *IEEE Trans Microw Theory Tech* 1991; 6: 1048–1056.

240. Labonte S, Blais A, Legault SR, Ali HO, Roy L. Monopole antennas for microwave catheter ablation. *IEEE Trans Microw Theory Tech* 1996; 44: 1832–1840.

241. Lin JC, Wang YJ. The cap-choke catheter antenna for microwave ablation treatment. *IEEE Trans Biomed Eng* 1996; 43: 657–660.

242. Lin JC. Catheter microwave ablation therapy for cardiac arrhythmias. *Bioelectromagnetics* 1999; 20(suppl 4): 120–132.

243. Gu Z, Rappaport M, Wang PJ, Vanderbrink BA. Development and experimental verification of the wide-aperture catheter-based microwave cardiac ablation antenna. *IEEE Trans Microw Theory Tech* 2000; 48: 1892–1900.

244. Pisa S, Cavagnaro P. Bernardi P, Lin JC. A 915-MHz antenna for microwave thermal ablation treatment: physical design, computer modeling and experimental measurement. *IEEE Trans Biomed Eng* 2001; 48: 599–601.

245. Reeves J, Birch M, Munro K, Collier R. Investigation into the thermal distribution of microwave helical antennas designed for the treatment of Barrett's oesophagus. *Phys Med Biol* 2002; 47: 3557–3564.

246. Longo I, Gentili GB, Cerretelli M, Tosoratti N. A coaxial antenna with miniaturized choke for minimally invasive interestial heating. *IEEE Trans Biomed Eng* 2003; 5: 82–88.

247. Shock SA, Meredith K, Warner TF, Sampson LA, Wright AS, Winter TC, Mahvi DM, Fine JP, Lee FT. Microwave ablation with loop antenna: in vivo porcine liver model. *Radiology* 2004; 231: 143–149.

248. Ahn HR, Lee K. Capacitive-loaded interstitial antennas for perfect matching and desirable SAR distributions. *IEEE Trans Biomed Eng* 2005; 52: 284–291.

249. Yu NC, Lu DSK, Raman SS, Dupuy DE, Simon CJ, Lassman C, Aswad BI, Ianniti D, Busuttil RW. Hepatocellular carcinoma: microwave ablation with multiple straight and loop antenna clusters—pilot comparison with pathologic findings. *Radiology* 2006; 239: 269–275.

250. Yang D, Bertram JM, Converse MC, O'Rourke AP, Webster JG, Hagness SC, Will JA, Mahvi DM. A floating sleeve antenna yields localized hepatic microwave ablation. *IEEE Trans Biomed Eng* 2006; 53: 533–537.

251. Matsukawa T, Yamashita Y, Arakawa A, Nishiharu T, Urata J, Murakami R, Takahashi M, Yoshimatsu S. Percutaneous microwave coagulation therapy in liver tumors. A 3-year experience. *Acta Radiol* 1997; 38: 410–415.

252. Lu MD, Chen JW, Xie XY, Liu L, Huang XQ, Liang LJ, Huang JF. Hepatocellular carcinoma: US-guided percutaneous microwave coagulation therapy. *Radiology* 2001; 221: 167–172.

253. Sato M, Watanabe Y, Kashu Y, Nakata T, Hamada Y, Kawachi K. Sequential percutaneous microwave coagulation therapy for liver tumor. *Am J Surg* 1998; 175: 322–324.

254. Shimada S, Hirota M, Beppu T, Matsuda T, Hayashi N, Tashima S, Takai E, Yamaguchi K, Inoue K, Ogawa M. Complications and management of microwave coagulation therapy for primary and metastatic liver tumors. *Surg Today* 1998; 28: 1130–1137.

255. Shibata T, Niinobu T, Ogata N, Takami M. Microwave coagulation therapy for multiple hepatic metastases from colorectal carcinoma. *Cancer* 2000; 89: 276–284.

256. Liang P, Dong B, Yu X, Yang Y, Yu D, Su L, Xiao Q, Sheng L. Prognostic factors for percutaneous microwave coagulation therapy of hepatic metastases. *Am J Roentgenol* 2003; 181: 1319–1325.

257. Liang P, Dong B, Yu X, Wang Y, Sheng L, Yu D, Xiao Q. Sonography-guided percutaneous microwave ablation of high-grade dysplastic nodules in cirrhotic liver. *Am J Roentgenol* 2005; 184: 1657–1660.

258. Seki T, Wakabayashi M, Nakagawa T, Itho T, Shiro T, Kunieda K, Sato M, Uchiyama S, Inoue K. Ultrasonically guided percutaneous microwave coagulation therapy for small hepatocellular carcinoma. *Cancer* 1994; 74: 817–825.

259. Murakami R, Yoshimatsu S, Yamashita Y, Matsukawa T, Takahashi M, Sagara K. Treatment of hepatocellular carcinoma: value of percutaneous microwave coagulation. *Am J Roentgenol* 1995; 164: 1159–1164.

260. Beppu T, Ogawa M, Matsuda T, Ohara C, Hirota M, Shimada S, Yamaguchi Y, Yamanaka T. Efficacy of microwave coagulation therapy (MCT) in patients with liver tumors. *Gan To Kagaku Ryoho* 1998; 25: 1358–1361.

261. Itamoto T, Asahara T, Kohashi T, Katayama S, Fukuda S, Nakatani T, Fukuda T, Yano M, Nakahara H, Okamoto Y, Katayama K, Dohi K. Percutaneous microwave coagulation therapy for hepatocellular carcinoma. *Gan To Kagaku Ryoho* 1999; 26: 1841–1844.

262. Seki T, Tamai T, Nakagawa T, Imamura M, Nishimura A, Yamashiki N, Ikeda K, Inoue K. Combination therapy with transcatheter arterial chemoembolization and percutaneous microwave coagulation therapy for hepatocellular carcinoma. *Cancer* 2000; 89: 1245–1251.

263. Kato T, Tamura S, Tekin A, Yamashiki N, Seki T, Berho M, Weppler D, Izumi N, Levi D, Khan F, Pinna A, Nery J, Tzakis AG. Use of microwave coagulation therapy in liver transplant candidates with hepatocellular carcinoma: a preliminary report. *Transplant Proc* 2001; 33: 1469.
264. Strickland AD, Clegg PJ, Cronin NJ, Swift B, Festing M, West KP, Robertson GSM, Lloyd DM. Experimental study of large-volume microwave ablation in the liver. *Br J Surg* 2002; 89: 1003–1007.
265. Dong BW, Zhang J, Liang P, Yu XL, Su L, Yu DJ, Ji XL, Yu G. Sequential pathological and immunologic analysis of percutaneous microwave coagulation therapy of hepatocellular carcinoma. *Int J Hyperthermia* 2003; 19: 119–133.
266. Shibata T, Iimuro Y, Yamamoto Y, Maetani Y, Ametani F, Itoh K, Konishi J. Small hepatocellular carcinoma: comparison of radio-frequency ablation and percutaneous microwave coagulation therapy. *Radiology* 2002; 223: 331–337.
267. D'Ancona FC, Francisca EA, Witjes WP, Welling L, Debruyne FM, de la Rosette JJ. High energy thermotherapy versus transurethral resection in the treatment of benign prostatic hyperplasia: results of a prospective randomized study with 1 year of follow up. *J Urol* 1997; 158: 120–125.
268. Sterzer F, Mendecki J, Mawhinney DD, Friedenthal E, Melman A. Microwave treatments for prostate disease. *IEEE Trans Microwave Theory Tech* 2000; 48: 1885–1891.
269. Ramsey EW, Dahlstrand C. Durability of results obtained with transurethral microwave thermotherapy in the treatment of men with symptomatic benign prostatic hyperplasia. *J Endourol* 2000; 14: 671–675.
270. Furukawa K, Miura T, Kato Y, Okada S, Tsutsui H, Shimatani H, Kajiwara N, Taira M, Saito M, Kato H. Microwave coagulation therapy in canine peripheral lung tissue. *J Surg Res* 2005; 123: 245–250.
271. Smith DL, Walinsky P, Martinez-Hernandez A, Rosen A, Sterzer F, Kosman Z. Microwave thermal balloon angioplasty in the normal rabbit. *Am Heart J* 1992; 123: 1516–1521.
272. Nardone DT, Smith DL, Martinez-Hernandez A, Consigny PM, Kosman Z, Rosen A, Walinsky P. Microwave thermal balloon angioplasty in the atherosclerotic rabbit. *Am Heart J* 1994; 127: 198–203.
273. Rappaport C. Treating cardiac disease with catheter-based tissue heating. *IEEE Microw Mag* 2002; 3: 57–64.
274. Morady F. Radio-frequency ablation as treatment for cardiac arrhythmias. *N Eng J Med* 1999; 340: 534–544.
275. Gillinov AM, Smedira NG, Cosgrove DM. Microwave ablation of atrial fibrillation during mitral valve operations. *Ann Thorac Surg* 2002; 74: 1259–1261.
276. Schuetz A, Schulze CJ, Sarvanakis KK. Surgical treatment of permanent atrial fibrillation using microwave energy ablation; a prospective randomized clinical trial. *Eur J Cardiothorac Surg* 2003; 24: 475–480.
277. Balkhy HH, Chapman PD, Arnsdorf SE. Minimally invasive atrial fibrillation ablation combined with a new technique for thoracoscopic stapling of the left atrial appendage: case report. *Heart Surg Forum* 2004; 7: 353–355.
278. Kabbani SS, Murad G, Jamil H, Sabbagh A, Hamzeh K. Ablation of atrial fibrillation using microwave energy early—experience. *Asian Cardiovasc Thorac Ann* 2005; 13: 247–250.
279. Molloy TA. Midterm clinical experience with microwave surgical ablation of atrial fibrillation. *Ann Thorac Surg* 2005; 79: 2115–2118.
280. Hemels MEW, Gu YL, Tuinenburg AE, Boonstra PW, Wiesfeld ACP, van den Berg MP, Van Veldhuisen DJ, Van Gelder IC. Favorable long-term outcome of maze surgery in patients with lone atrial fibrillation. *Ann Thorac Surg* 2006; 81: 1773–1779.

281. Lin JC, Beckman KJ, Hariman RJ, Bharati S, Lev M, Wang Y-J. Microwave ablation of the atrioventricular junction in open-chest dogs. *Bioelectromagnetics* 2005; 16: 97–105.
282. Gaynor SL, Byrd GD, Diodato MD, Ishii Y, Lee AM, Prasad SM, Gopal J, Schuessler RB, Damiano RJ. Microwave ablation for atrial fibrillation: dose–response curves in the cardioplegia-arrested and beating heart. *Ann Thorac Surg* 2006; 81: 72–76.
283. Jack AS, Cooper KG. Microwave endometrial ablation: an overview. *Rev Gynaecol Pract* 2005; 5: 32–38.
284. Downes E, O'Donovan P. Microwave endometrial ablation in the management of menorrhagia: current status. *Curr Opin Obstet Gynecol* 2000; 12: 293–296.
285. Jameel JKA, Ahmed T, Noble WL, Phillips K, Tilsed JVT. Microwave endometrial ablation (MEA) and bowel injury. *Gynecol Surg* 2005; 2: 131–133.
286. Skinner MG, Lizuka MN, Kolios MC, Sherar MD. A theoretical comparison of energy sources—microwave, ultrasound and laser—for interstitial thermal therapy. *Phys Med Biol* 1998; 43: 3535–3547.
287. Ryan TP. Comparison of six microwave antennas for hyperthermia treatment of cancer: SAR results for single antennas and arrays. *Int J Radiat Oncol Biol Phys* 1991; 21: 403–413.

Part III

Dosimetry and Imaging

11 Electromagnetic and Thermal Dosimetry

11.1 INTRODUCTION

EM dosimetry, i.e., measurement or calculation of the EM radiation absorbed by humans in radiation fields, has become increasingly important as the use of EM devices in our society has increased. Additionally, dosimetry considers the measurement or determination by calculation of induced current density, specific absorption (SA), or SAR distributions in objects like models (phantoms), animals, humans, or even parts of human body exposed to EM fields [1,2]. At lower frequencies (below ~100 kHz), many biological effects are quantified in terms of the current density in tissue, and this parameter is most often used as a dosimetric quantity. At higher frequencies, many (but not all) interactions are due to the rate of energy deposition per unit mass. This is why SAR is used as the dosimetric measure at those frequencies [3].

EM and thermal dosimetry, either theoretical or experimental, is based on modeling of the human body, which presents obvious differences between individuals. The variations are related to the size and shape of the body, to the distribution of biological tissues, and the various characteristics of each tissue [4]. In thermal therapy, the accuracy of dosimetry determines the precision of treatment and its role in treatment planning for patients.

In the literature, important techniques and areas of research in EM dosimetry [1,5–8], thermal dosimetry [6,9–16], and treatment planning [17] have been reviewed. The purpose of this chapter is to outline and discuss techniques which have been developed to ensure adequate EM and thermal dosimetry. Various models of heat transfer in living tissues with emphasis on Pennes' equation have been discussed. Knowledge about the temperature distributions achieved can be obtained through simulation of treatment process during thermal therapy by computer predictions and planning of patient therapy. This process is called thermal therapy planning system (TTPS), which is a large and complex system that has also been discussed.

11.2 EM INTERACTION WITH BIOLOGICAL MATERIALS

Interaction of EM energy with a biological material can be studied at two distinct levels:

1. Macroscopic level: objects and whole body
2. Microscopic level: cells, membranes, and molecules

Interaction phenomena at the two levels, however, cannot be regarded independently. One has to take into account the energy distribution that occurs within an object when placed under an EM field. The macroscopic level of interaction gives a short discussion of energy penetration and dissipation phenomena. The microscopic level is to study interaction mechanisms at smaller scales [18].

The effect of interaction of EM waves with biological tissues can be considered as the result of three phenomena [3]:

1. The penetration of EM waves into the living system and their propagation into it.
2. The primary interaction of the waves with biological tissues.
3. The possible secondary effects induced by the primary interaction.

It is clear from the above that the term interaction stresses the fact that end results not only depend on the action of the field but are also influenced by the reaction of the living system.

Electromagnetic waves propagate within tissues with reduced velocities and are refracted, diffracted, and reflected when encountering inhomogeneities. The specific electrical properties of each tissue govern the reduction of velocity, refraction, and diffraction. These properties, as well as the geometry of the inhomogeneities, determine the fraction of energy absorbed by tissues. The main parameters that describe EM waves are the frequency of oscillation, amplitude of the electric or magnetic field, and phase angle, which defines the instantaneous state of the oscillation.

It is very difficult to entirely characterize the propagation of EM fields in the human body, keeping in mind the complexity and nonhomogeneous character of biological tissues [1,2]. However, with the advent of computers, it is now possible to conduct highly accurate evaluations of dosimetry for the human body or part of the body. An EM wave involves both a varying electric field and a varying magnetic field. The propagation of EM is described by the differential form of the complex time-harmonic steady-state Maxwell's equations:

$$\nabla \times \mathbf{H} = J + \frac{\partial \mathbf{D}}{\partial t}$$

$$\nabla \times \mathbf{E} = -\frac{\partial \mathbf{B}}{\partial t} \tag{11.1}$$

$$\nabla \cdot \mathbf{B} = 0$$

$$\nabla \cdot \mathbf{D} = \rho$$

using the constitutive relationships

$$\mathbf{B} = \mu \mathbf{H}$$

$$\mathbf{D} = \varepsilon \mathbf{E} \tag{11.2}$$

$$J = \sigma \mathbf{E}$$

where $\mathbf{E}$ is the electric field in volts per meter, $\mathbf{H}$ the magnetic field in amperes per meter, $\mathbf{J}$ the current density in amperes per square meter (A/m^2), $\mathbf{B}$ the magnetic flux density in webers per square meter, $\mathbf{D}$ the electric displacement in coulombs per square meter, μ the permeability in henries per meter, ε the permittivity in farads per meter (F/m), and σ the conductivity in $\Omega^{-1}\text{m}^{-1}$.

Generally, three different quantities describe the permittivity of the medium: ε, ε_0, and a dimensionless quantity known as the relative permittivity ε_r or the dielectric constant, which is defined as the permittivity relative to that of free space ($\varepsilon_0 = 8.854 \times 10^{-12}$ F/m). The three quantities are related by

$$\varepsilon = \varepsilon_0 \varepsilon_r \tag{11.3}$$

The dielectric constant of free space is 1. This value is assumed for air in most applications. Values of the dielectric constant for most biological materials range from 1 (as for vacuum) to about 80 or so.

The term permeability refers to the magnetic property of any material. It is a measure of the flux density produced by a magnetizing current. The basic unit of permeability is henries/meter. Three different quantities describe the permeability of the medium: μ, μ_0, and a dimensionless quantity known as the relative permeability μ_r, which is defined as the permeability relative to that of free space ($\mu_0 = 4\pi \times 10^{-3}$ H/m). The three quantities are related by

$$\mu = \mu_0 \mu_r \tag{11.4}$$

In the special case of thermal therapy problems μ is constant, $\partial/\partial t$ is the equivalent of $j\omega$ where ω is the angular frequency (rad/s) at which the power is excited, ρ is zero, and j is $\sqrt{-1}$.

For isotropic, linear, and nonmagnetic media, Maxwell's equations in the steady-state form can be written in terms of Faraday's law

$$\nabla \times \mathbf{E} = -j\omega \mathbf{B} \text{ (Faraday's law)} \tag{11.5}$$

and Ampere's law with displacement current

$$\nabla \times \frac{\mathbf{B}}{\mu} = \mathbf{J} + j\omega\varepsilon \mathbf{E} \text{ (Ampere's law)} \tag{11.6}$$

Equations 11.5 and 11.6 allow the EM present in the biological system to be predicted. It is quite common to assume the constitutive parameters to be independent of the temperature, allowing the electric field to be predicted without knowledge of the temperature field. In ablation therapies, where temperatures may exceed 100°C, this assumption is no longer valid and the thermal and EM prediction problems become coupled [19].

To obtain the simplest solution for the EM, we first consider wave propagation in free space, i.e., no electric charges ($\rho = 0$) and no current ($\mathbf{J} = 0$). The solution is (arbitrarily) restricted to only one electric field component E_x spatially varying with

z only. By combining the set of four relations in Equation 11.1, a simplified form of the wave equation is obtained

$$\frac{\partial^2 E_x}{\partial z^2} + \frac{k^2}{\omega^2}\frac{\partial^2 E_x}{\partial t^2} = 0 \tag{11.7}$$

where the phase constant $k = \omega(\mu_0\varepsilon_0)^{1/2} = 2\pi/\lambda_0$ (λ_0 = wavelength in free space and ω = angular frequency). Solutions of this second-order differential equation correspond to plane traveling waves of the form:

$$E_x(z,t) = E_x e^{j(\omega t - kz)} \tag{11.8}$$

where E_x is the magnitude of the wave in the x direction and t the time. For propagation in a homogeneous dielectric medium, the plane wave expressions for E and H will include a complex propagation constant replacing a real-phase constant:

$$k^* = j\omega[\mu_0\varepsilon_0(\varepsilon' - \varepsilon'')]^{1/2} = \alpha + j\beta \tag{11.9}$$

where α is the attenuation constant and β the phase constant for a uniform plane wave. Expressions for α and β are

$$\alpha = \frac{2\pi}{\lambda_0}\left(\frac{\varepsilon'}{2}\right)^{1/2}\left\{\left[1 + \left(\frac{\varepsilon''}{\varepsilon'}\right)^2\right]^{1/2} - 1\right\}^{1/2} \quad \text{nepers/m} \tag{11.10}$$

$$\beta = \frac{2\pi}{\lambda_0}\left(\frac{\varepsilon'}{2}\right)^{1/2}\left\{\left[1 + \left(\frac{\varepsilon''}{\varepsilon'}\right)^2\right]^{1/2} + 1\right\}^{1/2} \quad \text{rad/m} \tag{11.11}$$

where $\varepsilon''/\varepsilon'$ is the loss tangent. The value of α decides the depth of penetration δ in tissues, which is the depth by which the electric field amplitude is reduced by e^{-1} of its original amplitude and can be calculated as

$$\delta = \frac{1}{\alpha} \tag{11.12}$$

Depth of penetration is important for radiative methods of heating.

11.3   MODELING POWER DEPOSITION

Living systems have a large capacity for compensating for the effects induced by external influences, in particular EM sources. This is very often overlooked and it is one more reason that conclusions derived from models have to be taken with precautions.

Physiological compensation means that the strain imposed by external factors is fully compensated and the organism is able to perform normally. Pathological compensation means that the imposed strain leads to the appearance of disturbances within the functions of the organism and even structural alterations may result. The borderline between these two types of compensation is obviously not always easy to determine [3].

11.3.1 TECHNIQUES FOR LOW FREQUENCIES

Several techniques have been developed for exposure from low-frequency sources such as power lines at 50/60 Hz, induction heaters, and other devices operating up to a few megahertz. These techniques include admittance and impedance methods, the FEM, the scalar potential finite difference (SPFD) method, and the FDTD method with frequency scaling. The impedance method has been found to be highly efficient as a numerical procedure for calculations of induced current densities and electric field for exposure to low-frequency EM fields [20]. Gandhi et al. [21] illustrated the use of the impedance method to calculate the electric fields and current densities induced in millimeter resolution anatomic models of the human body, namely an adult and 10- and 5-year-old children, for exposure to nonuniform magnetic fields typical of two assumed but representative electronic article surveillance (EAS) devices at 1 and 30 kHz, respectively.

11.3.2 TECHNIQUES FOR RADIOFREQUENCY RADIATION

To obtain the solution for the equations of EM deposition inside biological systems, it is required to choose a calculation method. Sometimes, the geometry of the model is simple enough (e.g., in one-dimensional models) and the equations can be solved by analytical methods. However, most models have a complex geometry (especially those based on a very realistic anatomy), with regions of different characteristics, and a numerical method has to be employed.

11.3.2.1 Analytical Techniques

Analytical techniques may be used to predict EM fields deposited inside modeled tissues by solving Maxwell's equations for general source configurations of canonical homogeneous bodies. However, for inhomogeneous bodies, one must resort to numerical analysis. Several early analytical studies have been carried out employing the plane wave transmission-line model approach to evaluate the EM fields and determine the energy deposited in a lossy, semi-infinite, and homogeneous target (man and animals) at high-frequency EM radiation [22,23]. Other models have also been employed, such as spheres [24], prolate spheroids [1,25,26], ellipsoids [27,28], and multilayer elliptic cylinders [29,30]. Values of field, absorbed energy in human body, and effect of layering on energy deposition have also been obtained [31–34].

11.3.2.2 Numerical Techniques

The use of numerical modeling techniques has improved the understanding of power deposition by EM energy in human bodies. Several numerical techniques have been investigated over the past several years. The FDTD method is extremely versatile for bioelectromagnetic problems. It has been used for modeling whole- or partial-body EM exposures. In this method, the time-dependent Maxwell's equations (Equation 11.1) are implemented for a lattice of subvolumes or Yee space cells that may be cubical or parallelepiped with different dimensions Δx, Δy, and Δz in the x, y, and z directions, respectively. The components of $\mathbf{E}$ and $\mathbf{H}$ are positioned about each of the cells at half-cell intervals and calculated alternately with half-time steps, $\Delta t/2$. The details of the FDTD and its implementation for bioelectromagnetic problems are available in several publications [35–51].

Another numerical technique that is usually applied to bioelectromagnetic problems is the FEM. It requires the complete volume of the configuration to be meshed, as opposed to surface integral techniques, which only require surfaces to be meshed. Each mesh element can have different material properties from those of neighboring elements. The corners of the elements are called *nodes*. The aim of the FEM analysis is to determine the field quantities at the nodes. The drawback of this method is that for complicated bodies it will be very difficult and sometimes impossible to carry out the integration procedure over the entire body. The details of the FEM and its implementation for bioelectromagnetic problems are available in several publications [52–64].

11.4 SPECIFIC ABSORPTION RATE MODELING

When considering EM interaction with biological systems, it is important to distinguish between levels of fields outside the body (the exposure) and field levels or absorbed energy within body tissues (the dose). The exposure is measured in terms of the $\mathbf{E}$ or $\mathbf{H}$ field strength, or power density incident on the body. The dose depends on the exposure, as well as on body geometry, size, its orientation with respect to the field, and other factors [65]. The central issue concerning the dosimetric assessment of the absorption of EM energy by biological bodies is how much is absorbed and where it is deposited [66]. This is usually quantified SAR, which is the mass-normalized rate at which EM energy is absorbed by the object at a specific location and thus is a good predictor of thermal effects. Mathematically, SAR is defined as

$$\text{SAR} = \frac{\sigma |\mathbf{E}|^2}{\rho} = c\frac{dT}{dt} \tag{11.13}$$

where dT/dt is the time derivative of the temperature in kelvin per second, σ the electrical conductivity in siemens per meter, ρ the mass density in kilogram per cubic meter, and c the specific heat in joules per kilogram per kelvin. The unit of SAR is watts per kilogram (W/kg).

It is clear from Equation 8.13 that the localized SAR is directly related to the internal electric field. Calculation of the internal field is, however, difficult to achieve because it is strongly dependent on many factors. These include the nature (near- or far-field zone) and frequency of the incident field, shape and dimension of the object, dielectric properties of the object, and whether or not the object is insulated from Earth [66]. SAR is a good dosimetric quantity between approximately 100 kHz and 10 GHz. At frequencies below 100 kHz, a more useful measure of dose is often the electric field strength in tissue, in units of volts per meter.

There are two major types of SAR: (1) whole-body average SAR and (2) local (spatial) peak SAR when the power absorption takes place in a confined body region, as in the case of a head exposed to a mobile phone. Whole-body SAR measurements are useful for estimating elevations of the core body temperature. As SAR increases, the possibility for heating and, therefore, tissue damage also rises. The whole-body SAR for a given organism will be highest within a certain resonant frequency range, which is dependent on the size of the organism and its orientation relative to the EMF vectors and the direction of wave propagation. For an average human the peak whole-body SAR occurs in a frequency range of 60–80 MHz, while the resonant frequency for a laboratory rat is about 600 MHz [67].

Both types of SAR are averaged over a specific period of time and tissue masses of 1 or 10 g (defined as a tissue volume in the shape of a cube). Averaging the absorption over a larger amount of body tissue gives a less reliable result. The 1-g SAR is a more precise representation of localized RF energy absorption and a better measure of SAR distribution. Local SAR is generally based on estimates from the whole-body average SAR. It incorporates substantial safety factors (e.g., 20).

11.4.1 THERMAL DOSE

A serious problem in thermal therapy is the definition of clinically meaningful dose. Thermal dose may be defined as what part of the body had which temperature for how long during a treatment. The actual temperature/heat-dose distribution in the tissue is one of the most important factors which determine the effectiveness of hyperthermic treatment [68]. Deposition of energy, usually stated in terms of SAR, although useful for quality control and cross-comparison of equipment, is not necessarily related to tissue temperature and, therefore, cytotoxicity.

Two key papers, published in the mid-1980s, attracted attention to the opportunity to assess efficacy of cell killing with heat [69,70]. These papers established the first concepts for thermal dosimetry and indicated that significant cell killing could occur if cells or tissues were heated to more than 42°C for 1 h or more. The effect of nonuniform temperature distributions on cytotoxicity is amplified by the temperature threshold effect, which may vary from tumor to tumor and from normal tissue to tissue.

The thermal dose is typically presented in equivalent minutes to 43°C. It is assumed that 43°C represents the so-called "break" point in the Arrhenius plot [71,72]. Every increase of temperature by 1°C above 43°C doubles the time in minutes equivalent to 43°C. Conversely, every decrease of temperature by 1°C below 43°C results in a reduction of equivalent time by a factor of ~4 (range from 2 to 6). These rules are consistent with laboratory data, proven for a variety of cell lines with a wide range of temperature sensitivities [16].

Thermal dosimetry is complicated by temperature heterogeneity within tumors and biologic variations and development of thermotolerance. This heterogeneity results from heterogeneous energy deposition and also from perfusion-related conductive cooling [70,73–75]. Moreover, the temperature heterogeneity is temporally dynamic [76] and heat effects are time dependent [77]. These issues have made development of a thermal dosimetry challenging.

Thermal dose formulations that have taken into account both the temperature distribution and time at various temperatures have shown good correlations with complete response rates [69,78] and duration of local tumor control [79,80].

11.4.2 Thermal Measurements

Thermal measurements are important, in particular on human beings. A comprehensive database is available on effects of a thermal nature, but it mainly concerns animal studies and *in vitro* studies. Several methods of biological effect determination are based on thermal measurements:

1. Calorimetric methods particularly suited for *in vitro* measurements, in which heating and cooling data can be analyzed to estimate the energy absorbed by an exposed sample.
2. Thermometric methods used to measure the temperature due to microwaves with particular types of nonperturbing thermometers, with only a few commercially available.
3. Thermographic techniques used to measure temperature with particular thermographic cameras.

The rate of temperature change in the subcutaneous tissue *in vitro* exposed to EM radiation is related to SAR as

$$\frac{\Delta T}{\Delta t} = \frac{(\mathrm{SAR} + P_m - P_c - P_b)}{C} \qquad (11.14)$$

where ΔT is the temperature increase, Δt the exposure duration, P_m the metabolic heating rate, P_c the rate of heat loss per unit volume due to thermal conduction, P_b the rate of heat loss per unit volume due to blood flow, and C the specific heat. If before the exposure a steady-state condition exists such as $P_m = P_c + P_b$, then during the initial period of exposure we have

$$\frac{\Delta T}{\Delta t} = \frac{\mathrm{SAR}}{C} \qquad (11.15)$$

and accordingly SAR can be determined from measurements of an increase in the tissue temperature over a short period of time following the exposure. For tissue phantoms and tissues *in vitro*, Equation 11.14 may be used as long as the thermal conductivity can be neglected, that is, for a short period of time. Several methods of SAR determination are based on thermal measurements and utilization of Equations 11.14 and 11.15. More generally, from a macroscopic point of view, thermal effects resulting from the absorption of EM waves inside biological materials are described in terms of bioheat equation [3].

11.5 BIOHEAT EQUATION

The temperature elevation within a biological system depends on the spatial distribution of the EM fields, the thermal constitutive parameters of the biological system, and the governing thermodynamics [81]. Knowledge of heat transfer in biological bodies has many therapeutic applications involving either raising or lowering of temperature and often requires precise monitoring of the spatial distribution of thermal histories that are produced during a treatment protocol [82]. Unlike the prediction of the electric field, for which an appropriate continuum physical model may exist, no clear compromise exists for a suitable mathematical model to predict heating patterns in biological objects [81].

Successful thermal treatment of tumors requires understanding the attendant thermal processes in both diseased and healthy tissue. Accordingly, it is essential for developers and users of thermal therapy equipment to predict, measure, and interpret correctly the tissue thermal and vascular response to heating. Modeling of heat transfer in living tissues is a means towards this end. Owing to the complex morphology of living tissues, such modeling is a difficult task and some simplifying assumptions are needed [83]. Modeling of the bioheat transfer requires as a first step mathematical techniques for solving Maxwell's equations for reasonably accurate representations of the actual objects. Because of the mathematical difficulties encountered in the process of calculation, a combination of techniques is used for the computation of the absorbed EM power distribution in the tissue. Each technique gives information over a limited range of parameters, depending on the chosen model. Such modeling is essential because it allows optimal source configurations and provides results that will serve as input data for developing thermal models. Various models such as blocks, spheroids, ellipsoids, and cylinders with suitable EM and thermal characteristics have been used in many studies [27,29,30,84–87] to represent different parts of the human body such as the head and limbs. Recently, MRI-based anatomically accurate models have been used in conjunction with FDTD-based solutions of Maxwell's equations [88–91].

11.5.1 PENNES MODEL

An extremely important study in the modeling of bioheat transfer was reported over half a century ago by Pennes [92]. Pennes developed a cylindrical model of a human limb to simulate first the human forearm but later generalized it to any limb. The model considered all the properties essential for the conduction, thermal storage, and environmental exchange terms for the tissue when he referred to the blood properties in the blood perfusion system. Pennes suggested a model in which the net heat transfer from blood to tissue was proportional to the temperature difference between the arterial blood entering the tissue and the venous blood leaving the tissue. Pennes' principal theoretical contribution was his suggestion that the rate of heat transfer between blood and tissue is proportional to the product of the volumetric perfusion rate and the difference between the arterial blood temperature and the local tissue temperature. When most researchers apply Pennes model, they assume that the temperature of venous blood is in equilibrium with the local tissue temperature, and that the arterial blood temperature T_a is constant. The Pennes model describes blood perfusion with acceptable accuracy, if no large vessels are nearby [83].

11.5.1.1 Bioheat Equation

Following Pennes' suggestion, the thermal energy balance for perfused tissue is expressed in the following form:

$$\rho c \frac{\partial T}{\partial t} = k\frac{\partial^2 T}{dx^2} + k\frac{\partial^2 T}{dy^2} + k\frac{\partial^2 T}{dz^2} + \omega_b c_b(T_a - T) + Q_m + Q_r(x,y,z,t) \quad (11.16)$$

where $T = T(x, y, z, t)$ is the temperature elevation (°C), ρ the physical density of the tissue (kg/m³), c the specific heat of the tissue (J/kg/°C), k the tissue thermal conductivity (W/m°C), ω_b the blood volumetric perfusion rate (kg/m³/s), c_b the specific heat of blood (J/kg/°C), and $T_a = T_a(x, y, z, t)$ the average temperature elevation of the arteries (°C). Q_m is the mechanism for modeling physiological heat generation (W/m³) and Q_r the regional heat delivered by the source (W/m³).

The term $\omega_b c_b(T_a - T)$, which is the perfusion heat loss (W/m³), is always considered in case of tissues with a high degree of perfusion, such as liver. Regarding RF cardiac ablation, the perfusion heat loss is incorporated in some models, but is generally ignored since its effect is negligible for cardiac ablation [93]. In general, ω_b is assumed to be uniform throughout the tissue. However, its value may increase with heating time because of vasodilation and capillary recruitment.

At the frequencies employed in RF ablation (300 kHz–1 MHz) and within the area of interest (it is known that the electrical power is deposited within a small radius around the active electrode), the tissues can be considered purely resistive because the displacement currents are negligible. For this reason, a quasi-static approach is usually employed to resolve the electrical problem. Then, Q_r may be given by

$$Q_r = JE \quad (11.17)$$

where J is the current density (A/m²) and E the electric field intensity (V/m). Equations 11.16 and 11.17 provide the solution of an electrical–thermal coupled problem, which generally represents adequately the ablation of biological tissues.

To build the complete theoretical model, the values of four physical characteristics have to be set for all the material of the model: mass density (ρ), specific heat (c), thermal conductivity (k), and electrical conductivity (σ). All the characteristics are normally considered to be isotropic. It is difficult to measure tissue thermal properties because they are spatially, temporally, and even thermally dependent [94]. The actual values of these physical properties are shown in Table 11.1 [95,96].

Computers are used to solve Equation 11.16 to obtain the temperature $T(x, y, z, t)$ time dependence and space distribution. Analytical solution of the three-dimensional (3D) Pennes equation is presented in Liu [97] using the multidimensional Green

TABLE 11.1

Approximate Value of Biological Tissue Constants

Properties	Value
Arterial temperature T_a (°C)	37
Thermal conductivity of tissue k (W/mK)	0.488
Mass density of tissue ρ (kg/m³)	1000
Specific heat capacity of tissue c (J/kg/K)	3590
Specific heat capacity of blood c_b (J/kg/K)	3840
Blood perfusion rate ω_b (kg/m³s)	0.5

function. Numerical techniques for solving the one-dimensional Pennes' equation are discussed in Zhao et al. [98].

11.5.1.2 Limitations

One advantage of Pennes' bioheat equation is its simplicity. Given the relevant properties and perfusion rates, it becomes fairly easy to solve for tissue temperature as a function of spatial location and time. It is well known that the Pennes perfusion source term overestimates the actual blood perfusion effect in tissue in two ways. The first limitation is, it considers that all the heat leaving the artery is absorbed by the local tissue and there is no venous rewarming [99]. Brinck and Werner [100] and Wissler [101] suggested a correction coefficient that is less than unity and accounts for venous rewarming that should multiply the perfusion term. A correction coefficient that is close to zero implies a significant countercurrent rewarming of the paired vein and a coefficient of unity implies no rewarming. Weinbaum et al. [102] showed that for most muscle tissues, the "correction coefficient" varies between 0.6 and 0.8. A second limitation of the Pennes perfusion source term is that the arterial temperature is assumed to be equal to the body core temperature. The alternative to the Pennes equation is to employ a decidedly more complex model that explicitly describes heat exchange between vessel pairs. Keller and Seiler [103] proposed such a model, which includes both countercurrent heat exchange between vessel pairs and thermal equilibration in the capillary bed.

Pennes' equation was further simplified to a first approximation by Goldberg et al. [104], who described the basic relationship guiding thermal ablation–induced coagulation necrosis as follows: coagulation necrosis = energy deposited × local tissue interactions − heat loss. On the basis of this equation, several strategies have been pursued to increase the amount of coagulation necrosis by improving tissue–energy interactions during thermal ablation, including increasing energy deposition or modulating tissue interactions or blood flow [105].

11.5.1.3 Analysis Based on Pennes' Equation

To better understand the heating performance of a heating probe on living tissues, analysis on the temperature response based on Pennes' equation may be necessary. For simplicity, the shape of the heating probe tip can be approximated as a sphere

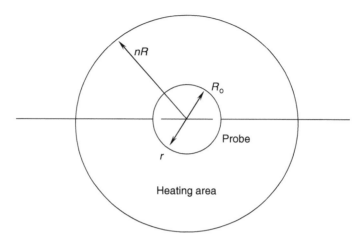

FIGURE 11.1 Geometry of the heating area of the tissue.

and the heat transfer geometry for the living tissues can be as shown in Figure 11.1. Equation 11.16 can be transformed as

$$\rho c \frac{\partial T}{\partial t} = \frac{k}{r} \frac{\partial^2 (rT)}{dr^2} + \omega_b C_b (T_a - T) + Q_m + Q_r(x, y, z, t) \qquad (11.18)$$

Considering the clinical situation, several assumptions may be made. First, the initial tissue temperature is treated as uniform at 37°C. Second, the heating area is n times the radius of the probe. Outside this range, the tissue temperature will not be affected by the heating and stays at a constant value of 37°C. Third, the temperature at the tip of the probe will be kept constant at the desired heating value, for example, at 100°C. Based on these assumptions, the boundary and initial conditions for Equation 11.18 can be expressed as [106]

$$\begin{aligned} T &= T_p & r &= R_o \\ T &= T_c & r &= nR_o \\ T &= T_c & t &= 0 \end{aligned} \qquad (11.19)$$

where R_o is the probe sphere radium and r the radial position.

11.5.2 WISSLER MODEL

An important feature of Pennes' approach is that his microscopic thermal energy balance for perfused tissue is linear, which means that the equation is amenable to analysis by various methods commonly used to solve the heat-conduction equation. Therefore, it has been adopted by many researchers who have developed mathematical models of heat transfer in the human body [107]. Wissler [108,109] modified the model of Pennes to obtain a model of the entire human body. This model subdivided the body into six elements: head, torso, two arms, and two legs. Each of these elements was assumed to have the following characteristics: (1) a uniformly distributed metabolic heat generation, (2) a uniformly distributed blood supply, (3) a composition of homogeneous materials, and (4) a geometry of isotropic cylinders. This model has been upgraded for active physiological factors in thermoregulation, such as regional perfusion rates [110].

11.5.3 STOLWIJIK MODEL

The entire human body was modeled by Stolwijik and associates at the John B. Pierce Foundation Laboratory [111]. The model was composed of three cylindrical segments, one each for the head, trunk, and extremities. The trunk was divided into three concentric layers: skin, muscle, and core. The head and extremities were divided into only two concentric layers: skin and core. For thermal modeling purposes, the authors suggested the concept of the body being composed of a controlled system and a controlling system. The controlled system can be modeled by a transient heat conduction model with internal heat generation (metabolism) and heat dissipation. The controlling system provides physiologically relevant thermal boundary conditions to maintain homeothermy. The heat transfer equation simulating this model is

$$\rho c \frac{\partial}{\partial t} T = \nabla \cdot k \nabla T + \left(\frac{1}{V}\right)(Q_m - Q_s - Q_{res}) \tag{11.20}$$

where Q_s represents the evaporative heat dissipation in the skin and Q_{res} is the respiratory heat loss in the lungs. The model consists of 15 cylindrical segments and a sphere for the head, with each segment divided into four concentric layers: core, muscle, fat, and skin. This model was later expanded by Stolwijik and Cunningham [112] and Stolwijik [113,114] to include six parts of the human body: head, trunk, arms, hands, legs, and feet.

11.5.4 WEINBAUM–JIJI MODEL

Weinbaum and Jiji [73] utilized the hypothesis that small arteries and veins are parallel and the flow direction is countercurrent, resulting in counterbalanced heating and cooling effects. This kind of tissue vascularization caused the isotropic blood perfusion term in the Pennes equation to be negligible and it causes the tissue to behave as an anisotropic heat transfer medium. Therefore, Weinbaum and Jiji [73] modified the thermal conductivity of the Pennes equation by means of an effective conductivity related quadratically to blood perfusion rate, which is affected by the dimensions and the directions of the vessels. The work of Weinbaum and Jiji [73] was utilized assuming a linear relation between the effective thermal conductivity and the blood perfusion rate to determine the increase in the thermal conductivity in a perfused tissue. They reported an 8% increase in the thermal conductivity. They suggested that in addition to a "temperature map," a "perfusion map" within the heated volume should be monitored routinely throughout the thermal therapy process since the local value of perfusion can vary substantially within a few centimeters. Song et al. [115] demonstrated that a tissue which exhibits only a small increase in thermal conductivity due to countercurrent convection in its vasoconstricted state (narrowing of the blood vessels) can exhibit more than a fivefold increase in thermal conductivity in its vasodilated state (during relaxation of the muscle).

Weinbaum et al. [102] developed a new model for muscle tissue heat transfer using Myrhage and Eriksson's [116] description of a muscle tissue cylinder surrounding secondary vessels as the basic heat transfer unit. This model provides a rational theory for the venous return temperature for the perfusion source term in a modified Pennes bioheat equation, and greatly simplifies the anatomical description of the microvascular architecture required in the Weinbaum–Jiji (W–J) model. An easy-to-use closed-form analytic expression has been derived for the difference between the inlet artery and venous return temperatures using a model for the countercurrent heat exchange in the individual muscle tissue cylinders. The perfusion source term calculated from this model is found to be similar in form to the Pennes source term except that there is a correction factor or efficiency coefficient multiplying the Pennes term, which rigorously accounts for the thermal equilibration of the returning vein. This coefficient is a function of the vascular cross-sectional geometry of the muscle tissue cylinder.

Wissler [117] pointed that the W–J model assumes the mean temperature in the neighborhood of an artery–vein to be the arithmetic mean of the arterial and venous blood at the point of entry and that the temperature of blood draining into veins from capillaries and small veins is equal to the temperature of venous blood at the point of entry, assuming there is very little heat transfer between thermally significant artery–vein pairs and the tissue. Wissler [117] indicated that these assumptions are questionable and the model suggested by Weinbaum and Jiji [73] was derived for a subcutaneous region (tissues under the skin). Wissler [117] noted that the muscle and skin are rather different and a formulation appropriate for one may not be applicable for another biological tissue.

11.5.5 Baish Model

Baish [118] presented a new bioheat transfer model for the perfused tissue. He considered simulation of a realistic vascular tree containing all thermally significant vessels in a tissue using a physiologically based algorithm. Baish's model is based on solving the convection of the blood coupled to the 3D conduction in the extravascular tissue while accounting for a statistical interpretation of the calculated temperature field. This model illustrates the dependence of the temperature distribution on the flow rate and the vascular geometry. Baish [118] also illustrates that the Pennes formulation accurately predicts the mean tissue temperature except when the arteries and veins are in closely spaced pairs. Baish's model is useful for fundamental studies of tissue heat transport.

11.5.6 Applications of Bioheat Transfer Models

Biomedical engineers have attempted to accurately model bioheat transfer in tissues since it is the basis for human thermotherapy [119] and the thermoregulation system [120]. The transfer of thermal energy in living tissues is a complex process involving multiple phenomenological mechanisms including blood perfusion, metabolic heat

TABLE 11.2
Summary of Bioheat Transfer Models

Bioheat Transfer Model	Characteristics
Pennes	Simple; based on uniform perfusion; not valid for all tissues
Weinbaum and Jiji	It is good when arteries and veins are close, leading to negligible blood perfusion; utilizes an effective conductivity as a function of the perfusion rate
Wissler	Avoids assumptions of the W–J model
Baish	Statistics-based model; considers simulation of a realistic vascular tree containing all thermally significant vessels

generation, conduction, convection, radiation, evaporation, and external interactions such as EM radiation from other sources. Table 11.2 summarizes the characteristics of the above bioheat transfer models.

Lang et al. [121] described an optimization process specially designed for regional hyperthermia of deep-seated tumors to achieve the desired steady-state temperature distributions. A nonlinear 3D heat transfer model based on temperature-dependent blood perfusion was applied to predict the temperature. Using linearly implicit methods in time and adaptive multilevel finite elements in space, the investigators were able to integrate efficiently the instationary nonlinear heat equation with high accuracy. Temperature distributions for two individual patients calculated on coarse and fine spatial grids and present numerical results of optimizations for a Sigma 60 Applicator of the BSD 2000 hyperthermia system were compared.

Liu et al. [122] used Pennes' bioheat transfer equation to model the transient heat transfer inside canine prostate during transurethral microwave thermal therapy. Incorporating the SAR of microwave energy in tissue, a closed-form analytical solution was obtained. Good agreement was found between the theoretical predictions and *in vivo* experimental results. Effects of blood perfusion and the cooling at the urethral wall on the temperature rise were investigated within the prostate during heating. The peak intraprostatic temperatures attained by application of 5, 10, or 15 W microwave power were predicted to be 38, 41, and 44°C. Zhu and Diao [123] used the Pennes equation to simulate the steady-state temperature distribution within the brain after head injury. Also, Deng and Liu [82] used the equation to study analytically the effect of pulsative blood perfusion on the tissue temperature. Wainwright [124] applied Pennes' thermal model and found the final steady-state temperature rise in the brain for a 0.25 W antenna at frequencies of 900 and 8100 MHz to be as high as 0.1°C. However, other EM devices could produce greater heating and there is the possibility that nonuniform heating could produce local higher temperature rises.

11.6 THERMAL THERAPY PLANNING SYSTEM

The accuracy of thermal therapy treatment simulation determines its role in prospective treatment planning and dosimetry for the individual patient. Today, a major limitation of thermal therapies is the lack of detailed thermal information available to guide the therapy [125–127]. Inadequate thermal doses received by the diseased tissue can cause failures in hyperthermic treatments. To compare different treatments and correlate the treatment data with the clinical results, it is mandatory to know what temperatures are reached in the target volume [68].

Because of limited thermometry, knowledge about the temperature distributions achieved can be obtained through simulation of treatment by computer predictions and planning of individual patient therapy. This process is called TTPS, which is a large and complex system that provides a complete 3D SAR and temperature distribution in the treatment area. The TTPS has to deal with a complex relation among the heating system, perfusion, discrete vasculature, and anatomy [128].

11.6.1 Objectives and Requirements

The aim of TTPS is to determine control parameters in such a way that a favorable temperature distribution is achieved. Such a distribution can be characterized by the requirements that the heating should be concentrated in the tumor and hot spots should be avoided in healthy tissues. Both the high-resolution FDTD code and the integral methods using FEM act as a core of absorbed power computations needed in the TTPS [129].

TTPS will ultimately provide information about the actual temperature distributions obtained and thus the tumor control probabilities to be expected. This will improve understanding of the clinical results of thermal therapy and will greatly help in both optimizing clinical heating technology and designing optimal clinical trials [128]. While a great deal of effort is applied toward solving the technical problems associated with modeling clinical thermal therapy treatments, especially in estimating the power deposition, effort should also be applied toward using the modeled power depositions as inputs to estimate the thermal therapy–induced 3D temperature distributions [130]. The type of treatment planning programs that have already been developed for radiotherapy must be developed for more complex requirements of both prospective and retrospective study of thermal dosimetry in clinical thermal therapy [6].

As a comprehensive process, treatment planning includes (1) methods for the determination of the target volume (target definition); (2) segmenting medical image data, generating 3D models of the target and normal tissue structures; (3) calculating the absorbed power distribution; (4) assigning tissue thermal properties; (5) virtually placing heat sources into the 3D structure; (6) measuring SAR patterns; (7) calculating heat transfer from the solution of bioheat equations during treatment from the power deposition to provide temperature distribution as a function of time; and (8) finally estimating 3D dose calculation [17,119,128]. An important feature of a thermal model must be its capability to describe the complex heat transfer related to the vasculature [128,131].

Based on the results of temperature calculation, optimal applicator parameters are determined, i.e., amplitudes and phases of the signals sent to the antennas. In case of the nonlinear bioheat equation, temperature calculation and optimization are coupled via a fixed-point iteration. An extensive set of visualization and evaluation tools must complete a treatment planning system [132]. For treatment planning or posttreatment evaluation of completed therapy, a more detailed study of the dielectric parameters, anatomical structures, and blood perfusion mechanism is necessary. Monitoring and control of temperatures during treatment requires advanced thermal imaging.

11.6.2 Developments in TTPS

The development of the first 2D TTPS to most advanced 3D models, having dynamic nonuniform grid generation and a conformal 3D FDTD scheme supporting high-resolution models at critical structures, is expected to allow *a priori* selection of the optimal energy deposition or temperature distribution [133]. Several treatment planning systems based on 3D patient anatomy have been developed for thermal therapy. Das et al. [134] and Paulsen et al. [135] have developed FEM-based treatment planning systems, while Nadobny et al. [136], Gellermann et al. [137], Van De Kamer et al. [138], and Van den Berg et al. [139] have developed FDTD-based system for predicting the SAR produced by the Sigma 60 applicator in the pelvic region of patient model.

Clegg et al. [130] presented a case report of a patient treated with thermal therapy at the Duke University Medical Center, where numerical modeling of the EM power deposition was used to prospectively plan the treatment. The modeled power was used as input to retrospectively reconstruct the transient 3D temperature distribution. The modeled power deposition indicated the existence of an undesirable region of high power in the normal tissue. Using the computed 3D transient temperature distribution, the thermal therapy thermal dose was computed.

Treatment planning systems for superficial thermal therapy are still lagging behind those for deep regional heating, although superficial thermal therapy is easier to control than deep heating due to the proximity of the heating applicator to the treatment object. Kumaradas and Sherar [62] presented a new numerical model of microwave heating, which is designed to aid in the development of new applicators for superficial heating. The model, which is based on FEM, was successfully verified against previously published measurements of heating from a modified water bolus attached to a conventional waveguide applicator.

Lagendijk [131] briefly described the state of the art in thermal therapy technology, followed by an overview of developments in TTPS. The review highlights the significant problems encountered with heating realistic tissue volumes and shows how treatment planning can help in designing better heating.

11.6.3 Thermal Monitoring

Although treatment planning can be used to prescribe the location of the heat source (electrode, antenna, etc.), it is unlikely to replace the need for active monitoring of thermal dose delivery during treatment. Deviations from predicted temperatures could be caused by a number of factors, including unpredictable or changing blood flow or changes in the electrical or thermal properties of tissue during coagulation, where these changes are not fully accounted for in the treatment plan [17]. Full 3D online thermal dosimetry would be the ideal; and of particular promise in this regard is the use of magnetic resonance thermometry [140].

11.7   STATUS AND TRENDS

Theoretical dosimetry offers several undeniable advantages over the experimental approach. Accordingly, it has become an essential tool to complement experimental studies on biomedical engineering. Not only it is less expensive and faster than experimental work, but it also allocates the time evolution and spatial distribution of physical variables to be analyzed. The objective of EM and thermal dosimetry is to advance the calculation to a level of sophistication where high-resolution SAR distributions and temperature profiles, generated graphically using computers, can be obtained and displayed with anatomical features for any part of the human body.

In response to radiation, rapid and reliable EM and thermal distribution estimates are crucial for risk assessment, and also for clinical planning of the treatment. Many clinical trials are being conducted to evaluate the effectiveness of thermal therapy. Despite positive outcomes, application of thermal therapy remains limited. This may partially relate to the lack of rigorous EM and thermal dosimetric data. The basic premise underlying the need for dosimetry is the ability to write a verifiable prescription for thermal therapy. As in any form of therapy, a sound dosimetric basis leads to unambiguous treatment, data reporting, and quality assurance [125].

Clinically, dosimetry offers valuable support in explaining the biophysical phenomena involved in the EM heating of biological tissues. For this reason, procedures are to be developed to allow modeling of the realistic treatment conditions due to EM energy. Effects will also be directed at improving thermal models of organs under treatment so that expected temperature distributions due to EM energy can be predicted and displayed graphically.

Much of the future success in dosimetry will be based on (1) accurate modeling of the electrical and thermal characteristics of biological tissues, (2) reliable techniques to quantify the thermal effect of the blood circulating in arteries and veins, and (3) development of fast computer simulation to develop better comparative thermal dosimetry that provides comparative evaluation of the potentials of different heating modes and configurations.

Although not all aspects of dosimetry are covered, the findings of this chapter give a rather comprehensive overview of the field. It is the strong belief of the author that a periodic review of this type is of benefit not only to the researchers but also to all workers in this field.

REFERENCES

1. Durney CH. Electromagnetic dosimetry for models of humans and animals: a review of theoretical and numerical techniques. *Proc IEEE* 1980; 68: 33–40.
2. Habash RWY. *Electromagnetic Fields and Radiation: Human Bioeffects and Safety.* New York: Marcel Dekker, 2001.
3. Vander Vorst A, Rosen A, Kotsuka Y. *RF/Microwave Interaction with Biological Tissues.* Hoboken, NJ: Wiley–IEEE Press, 2006.
4. Vecchia P. The approach of ICNIRP to protection of children. *Bioelectromagnetics* 2005; (Suppl 7): S157–S160.
5. Hudson RP, Marshak H, Soulen RJ Jr, Utton DB. Review paper: recent advances in thermometry below 300 mK. *J Low Temp Phys* 1976; 20: 1–120.

6. Conway J, Anderson AP. Electromagnetic techniques in thermal therapy. *Clin Phys Physiol Meas* 1986; 7: 287–381.
7. Fessenden P, Hand JW. Thermal therapy physics. In: Smith AR, Editor. *Medical Radiology: Radiation Therapy Physics*. Berlin: Springer-Verlag, pp. 315–363, 1995.
8. Adair ER, Petersen RC. Biological effects of radiofrequency/microwave radiation. *IEEE Trans Microw Theory Tech* 2002; 50: 953–962.
9. Cetas TC, Connor WG. Thermometry considerations in localized thermal therapy. *Med Phy* 1978; 5: 79–91.
10. Amemiya Y. Thermometry of thermal therapy. *Gan No Rinsho* 1986; 32: 1653–1660.
11. Foster KR, Cheever E. Microwave radiometry on biomedicine: a reappraisal. *Bioelectromagnetics* 1992; 13: 567–579.
12. Hand J, Machin D, Vernon C, Whaley J. Analysis of thermal parameters obtained during Phase III trials of hyperthermia as an adjunct to radiotherapy in the treatment of breast carcinoma. *Int J Hyperthermia* 1997; 13: 343–364.
13. Leroy Y, Bocquet B, Mamouni A. Non-invasive microwave radiometry thermometry. *Physiol Meas* 1998; 19: 127–148.
14. Denis De Senneville B, Quesson B, Moonen CTW. Magnetic resonance temperature imaging. *Int J Hyperthermia* 2005; 21: 515–531.
15. Jones E, Thrall D, Dewhirst MW, Vujaskovic Z. Prospective thermal dosimetry: the key to hyperthermia's future. *Int J Hyperthermia* 2006; 22: 247–253.
16. Wust P, Cho CH, Hildebrandt B, Gellermann J. Thermal monitoring: invasive, minimal invasive and non-invasive approach. *Int J Hyperthermia* 2006; 22: 255–262.
17. Sherar MD, Trachtenberg J, Davidson SR, Gertner MR. Interstitial microwave thermal therapy and its application to the treatment of recurrent prostate cancer. *Int J Hyperthermia* 2004; 20: 757–768.
18. Ponne CT, Bartels PV. Interaction of electromagnetic energy with biological material—relation to food processing. *Radiat Phys Chem* 1995; 45: 591–507.
19. Diller KR, Ryan TP. Heat transfer in living systems: current opportunities. *Trans ASME* 1998; 120: 810–829.
20. Gandhi OP. Electromagnetic fields: human safety issues. *Annu Rev Biomed Eng* 2002; 4: 211–234.
21. Gandhi OP, Kang G. Calculation of induced current densities for humans by magnetic fields from electronic article surveillance devices. *Phys Med Biol* 2001; 46: 2759–2771.
22. Hubing TH. Survey of numerical electromagnetic modeling techniques. Electromagnetic Compatibility Laboratory. Report No TR91-1-001.3, 1991.
23. Razansky D, Soldea DF, Einziger PD. Generalized transmission-line model for estimation of cellular handset power absorption in biological tissues. *IEEE Trans Electromag Compat* 2005; 47: 61–67.
24. Lin JC, Guy AW, Johnson CC. Power absorption in a spherical model of man exposed to 1–20 MHz electromagnetic field. *IEEE Trans Microw Theory Tech* 1973; 21: 791–797.
25. Johnson CC, Durney CH, Massoudi H. Long wavelength electromagnetic power absorption in prolate spheroid models of man and animals. *IEEE Trans Microw Theory Tech* 1975; 23: 739–747.
26. Barber PW. Electromagnetic absorption in prolate spheroidal models of man and animals at resonance. *IEEE Trans Biomed Eng* 1977; 24: 513–521.
27. Massoudi H, Durney CH, Johnson CC. Long wavelength analysis of plane wave irradiation of an ellipsoidal model of man. *IEEE Trans Microw Theory Tech* 1977; 25: 41–46.
28. Barber PW. Resonance electromagnetic absorption by non-spherical dielectric objects. *IEEE Trans Microw Theory Tech* 1977; 25: 373–381.
29. Caorsi S, Pastorino M, Raffetto M. Analytic SAR computation in a multilayer elliptic cylinder for bioelectromagnetic applications. *Bioelectromagnetics* 1999; 20: 365–371.

30. Caorsi S, Pastorino M, Raffetto M. Analytic SAR computation in a multilayer elliptic cylinder: the near-field line-current radiation case. *Bioelectromagnetics* 2000; 21: 473–479.
31. Livesay DE, Chen KM, Electromagnetic fields induced inside arbitrary shaped biological bodies. *IEEE Trans Microw Theory Tech* 1974; 22: 1273–1280.
32. Chen KM, Guru BS. Internal EM field and absorbed power density in human torso induced by 1–500 MHz EM waves. *IEEE Trans Microw Theory Tech* 1977; 25: 746–756.
33. Barber PW, Gandhi OP, Hagmann MJ, Chatterjee I. Electromagnetic absorption in a multilayered model of man. *IEEE Trans Biomed Eng* 1979; 26: 400–405.
34. King RWP. Electromagnetic field generated in model of human head by simplified telephone transceivers. *Radio Sci* 1995; 30: 267–281.
35. Yee KS. Numerical solution of initial boundary value problems involving Maxwell's equations in isotropic media. *IEEE Trans Antennas Propag* 1966; 14: 302–307.
36. Taflove A, Brodwin ME. Computation of the electromagnetic fields and induced temperatures within a model of the microwave irradiated human eye. *IEEE Trans Microw Theory Tech* 1975; 23: 888–896.
37. Taflove A, Brodwin ME. Numerical solution of steady state electromagnetic problems using the time dependent maxwell's equations. *IEEE Trans Microw Theory Tech* 1975; 23: 623–660.
38. Sullivan DM, Borup DT, Gandhi OP. Use of the finite difference time domain method in calculating absorption in human tissues. *IEEE Trans Bioem Eng* 1987; 34: 148–157.
39. Spiegel RJ, Fatmi MBA, Stuchly SS, Stuchly MA. Comparison of finite-difference time-domain SAR calculations with measurements in a heterogeneous model of man. *IEEE Trans Biomed Eng* 1989; 36: 849–855.
40. Taylor HC, Lau RWM. Evaluation of clinical thermal therapy treatment using time domain finite difference modeling technique. *ACES J* 1992; 7: 85–96.
41. Gandhi OP, Gu Y-G, Chen J-Y, Bassen HI. Specific absorption rates and induced current distributions in an anatomically based human model for plane-wave exposures. *Health Phys* 1992; 63: 281–290.
42. Kunz KS, Raymond JL. *The Finite Difference Time Domain Method for Electromagnetics*. Boca Raton, FL: CRC Press, 1993.
43. Watanabe S, Taki M, Kamimura Y. Frequency characteristics of energy deposition in human model exposed to near field of an electric or a magnetic dipole. *IEICE Trans Commun* 1994; E77-B6: 725–731.
44. Kuwano S, Kokubun K. Microwave power absorption in a cylindrical model of man in the presence of a flat reflector. *IEICE Trans Commun* 1995; E78-B: 1548–1550.
45. Taflove A. *Computational Electrodynamics: The Finite-Difference Time-Domain Method*. Norwood, MA: Artech House, 1995.
46. Taflove A. *Advances in Computational Electrodynamics: The Finite-Difference Time-Domain Method*. Norwood, MA: Artech House, 1998.
47. Lin JC, Hirai S, Chiang CL, Hsu WL, Su JL, Wang YJ. Computer simulation and experimental studies of SAR distributions of interstitial arrays of sleeved-slot microwave antennas for thermal therapy treatment of brain tumors. *IEEE Trans Microw Theory Tech* 2000; 48: 2191–2197.
48. Hamada L, Saito K, Yoshimura H, Ito K. Dielectric-loaded coaxial-slot antenna for interstitial microwave thermal therapy: longitudinal control of heating patterns. *Int J Hyperthermia* 2000; 16: 219–229.
49. Pisa S, Cavagnaro M, Piuzzi E, Bernardi P, Lin JC. Power density and temperature distributions produced by interstitial arrays of sleeved-slot antennas for hyperthermic cancer therapy. *IEEE Trans Microw Theory Tech* 2003; 51: 2370–2388.

50. Chiu H-M, Mohan AS, Weily AR, Guy DJR, Ross DL. Analysis of a novel expanded tip wire (ETW) antenna for microwave ablation of cardiac arrhythmias. *IEEE Trans Biomed Eng* 2003; 50: 890–899.

51. Kim J, Rahmat-Samii Y. Implanted antennas inside the human body: simulations, designs, and characterizations. *IEEE Trans Microw Theory Tech* 2004; 52: 1934–1943.

52. Jin JM. *The Finite Element Method in Electromagnetics*. Piscataway: Wiley, 1993.

53. Silvester PP, Pelosi G. *Finite Elements for Wave Electromagnetics*. New York: IEEE Press, 1994.

54. Shahidi AV, Savard P. A finite element model for radiofrequency ablation of the myocardium. *IEEE Trans Biomed Eng* 1994; 41: 963–968.

55. Kaouk Z, Khebir A, Savard P. A finite element model of a microwave catheter for cardiac ablation. *IEEE Trans Microw Theory Tech* 1996; 44: 8148–8154.

56. Labonte S, Blais A, Legault SR, Ali HO, Roy L. Monopole antennas for microwave catheter ablation. *IEEE Trans Microw Theory Tech* 1996; 44: 8132–8140.

57. Haemmerich D, Staelin ST, Tungjitkusolmun S, Lee, FT Jr, Mahvi DM, Webster JG. Hepatic bipolar radio-frequency ablation between separated multiprong electrodes. *IEEE Trans Biomed Eng* 2001; 48: 1145–1152.

58. Haemmerich D, Tungjitkusolmun S, Staelin ST, Lee FT, Mahvi DM, Webster JG. Finite element analysis of hepatic multiple probe radio-frequency ablation. *IEEE Trans Biomed Eng* 2002; 49: 836–842.

59. Haemmerich D, Wright AS, Mahvi DM, Webster JG, Lee FT. Hepatic bipolar radiofrequency ablation creates lesions close to blood vessels: a finite element study. *Med Biol Eng Comput* 2003; 41: 317–323.

60. Tungjitkusolmun S, Staelin S, Haemmerich D, Cao H, Tsai J-Z, Cao H, Webster JG, Lee FT, Mahvi DM, Vorperian VR. Three-dimensional finite element analyses for radio-frequency hepatic tumor ablation. *IEEE Trans Biomed Eng* 2002; 49: 3–9.

61. Siauve N, Nicolas L, Vollaire C, Marchal C. 3D modelling of electromagnetic fields in local thermal therapy. *Eur Phys J* 2003; 21: 243–250.

62. Kumaradas JC, Sherar MD. Optimization of a beam shaping bolus for superficial microwave thermal therapy waveguide applicators using a finite element method. *Phys Med Biol* 2003; 48: 1–81.

63. Berjano EJ, Hornero F. Thermal-electrical modeling for epicardial atrial radiofrequency ablation. *IEEE Trans Biomed Eng* 2004; 51: 1348–1357.

64. Wu L, McGough RJ, Arabe OA, Samulski TV. An RF phased array applicator designed for thermal therapy breast cancer treatments. *Phys Med Biol* 2006; 51: 1–20.

65. Ziskin MC. COMAR technical information statement: the IEEE exposure limits for radiofrequency and microwave energy. *IEEE Eng Med Biol Mag* 2005; 24: 114–117.

66. Spiegel RJ. A review of numerical models for predicting the energy deposition and resultant thermal response of humans exposed to electromagnetic fields. *IEEE Trans Microw Theory Tech* 1984; 32: 730–746.

67. Durney CH, Massoudi H, Iskander MF. Radiofrequency radiation dosimetry handbook. Brooks AFB, TX: USAF School of Aerospace Medicine, Aerospace Medical Division: USAFSAM-TR-85-73, 1986.

68. Baiotto B, Marini P. Thermometry: clinical aspects and perspectives. In: Baronzio GF, Hager ED, Editors. *Locoregional Radiofrequency-Perfusional and Whole-Body Hyperthermia in Cancer Treatment: New Clinical Aspects*. New York: Eurokah.com and Springer Science Business Media, 2005.

69. Field SB, Morris CC. The relationship between heating time and temperature: its relevance to clinical hyperthermia. *Radiother Oncol* 1983; 1: 179–186.

70. Sapareto SA, Dewey WC. Thermal dose determination in cancer therapy. *Int J Radiat Oncol Biol Phys* 1984; 10: 787–800.

71. Dewey WC. Arrhenius relationships from the molecule and cell to the clinic. *Int J Hyperthermia* 1994; 10: 457–483.
72. Dewhirst MW, LaRue SM, Gerweck L. Tumor physiology and cell kinetics. *Semin Vet Med Surg* 1995; 10: 148–157.
73. Weinbaum S, Jiji M. A new simplified bioheat equation for the effect of blood flow on local average tissue temperature. *J Biomech Eng* 1985; 107: 131–139.
74. Chen Z, Roemer R. The effects of large blood vessels on temperature distributions during simulated hyperthermia. *J Biomech Eng* 1992; 84: 473–481.
75. Gelvich E, Maxokhin V. Resonance effects in applicator water boluses and their influence on SAR distribution patterns. *Int J Hyperthermia* 2000; 16: 83–128.
76. Acker J, Dewhirst M, Honore G, Samulski T, Tucker J, Oleson J. Blood perfusion measurements in human tumours: evaluation of laser Doppler methods. *Int J Hyperthermia* 1990; 6: 287–304.
77. Dewey W, Hopwood L, Sapareto S, Gerweck L. Cellular responses to combinations of hyperthermia and radiation. *Radiology* 1977; 123: 4631–4674.
78. Oleson JR. Cumulative minutes with T90 greater than Tempindex is predictive of response to hyperthermia and radiation. *Int J Radiat Oncol Biol Phys* 1993; 25: 841–847.
79. Kapp DS, Cox R. Thermal treatment parameters are most predictive of outcome in patients with single tumor nodules per treatment field in recurrent adenocarcinoma of the breast. *Int J Radiat Oncol Biol Phys* 1995; 33: 887–899.
80. Thrall DE, LaRue SM, Yu D, Samulski T, Sanders L, Case B, Rosner G, Azuma C, Poulson J, Pruitt AF, Stanley W, Hauck ML, Williams L, Hess P, Dewhirst MW. Thermal dose is related to duration of local control in canine sarcomas treated with thermoradiotherapy. *Clin Cancer Res* 2005; 11: 5206–5214.
81. Kowalski ME, Jin J-M. A temperature-based feedback control system for electromagnetic phased-array thermal therapy: theory and simulation. *Phys Med Biol* 2003; 48: 633–651.
82. Deng Z-S, Liu J. Analytical study on bioheat transfer problems with spatial or transient heating on skin surface or inside biological bodies. *J Biomed Eng* 2002; 124: 638–649.
83. Arkin H, Xu LX, Holmes KR. Recent developments in modeling heat transfer in blood perfused tissues. *IEEE Trans Biomed Eng* 1994; 41: 97–107.
84. Joines WT, Spiegel RJ. Resonance absorption of microwaves by human skull, *IEEE Trans Biomed Eng* 1974; 21: 46–48.
85. Lin JC. Microwave properties of fresh mammalian brain tissues at body temperature. *IEEE Trans Biomed Eng* 1975; 22: 74–76.
86. Hagmann MJ, Gandhi OP. Numerical calculations of electromagnetic energy deposition in models of man with grounding and reflector effects. *Radio Sci* 1979; 14: 23–29.
87. Karimullah K, Chen K-M, Nyquist DP. Electromagnetic coupling between a thin-wire antenna and a neighboring biological body: theory and experiment. *IEEE Trans Microw Theory Tech* 1980; 28: 1281–1325.
88. Xu Li, Hagness SC. A confocal microwave imaging algorithm for breast cancer detection. *IEEE Microw Wirel Compon Lett* 2001; 11: 130–132.
89. Zhao H, Crozier S, Liu F. Finite difference time domain (FDTD) method for modeling the effect of switched gradients on the human body in MRI. *Magn Reson Med* 2002; 48: 1037–1042.
90. Liu F, Crozier S, Zhao H, Lawrence B. Finite-difference time-domain-based studies of MRI pulsed field gradient-induced eddy currents inside the human body. *Concepts Magn Resonan (Part B: Magn Reson Eng)* 2002; 15: 26–36.
91. Liu F, Beck BL, Xu B, Fitzsimmons JR, Blackband SJ, Crozier S. Numerical modeling of 11.1T MRI of a human head using a MoM/FDTD method. *Concepts in Magn Reson (Part B: Magn Reson Eng)* 2005; 24B: 28–38.

92. Pennes HH. Analysis of tissue and arterial blood temperatures in the resting human arm. *J Appl Physiol* 1948; 1: 93–122.
93. Haines DE, Watson DD. Tissue heating during radiofrequency catheter ablation: a thermodynamic model and observations in isolated perfused and superfused canine right ventricular free wall. *Pacing Clin Electrophysiol* 1989; 12: 962–976.
94. Liu YJ, Qiao AK, Nan Q, Yang XY. Thermal characteristics of microwave ablation in the vicinity of an arterial bifurcation. *Int J Hyperthermia* 2006; 22: 491–506.
95. Vrba J, Lapes M, Oppl L. Technical aspects of microwave thermotherapy. *Bioelectrochem Bioenerg* 1999; 48: 305–309.
96. Shen W, Zhang J. Modeling and numerical simulation of bioheat transfer and biomechanics in soft tissue. *Math Comput Model* 2005; 41: 1251–1265.
97. Liu J. Uncertainty analysis for temperature prediction of biological bodies subject to randomly special heating. *J Biomed* 2001; 34: 1637–1642.
98. Zhao J, Zhang J, Kang N, Yang F. A two level finite difference scheme for one dimensional Pennes' bioheat equation. *Appl Math Comput* 2002; 171: 320–331.
99. Zhu L, Xu LX, He Q, Weinbaum S. A new fundamental bioheat equation for muscle tissue—Part II: Temperature of SAV vessels. *ASME J Biomech Eng* 2002; 124: 121–132.
100. Brinck H, Werner J. Efficiency function: improvement of classical bioheat approach. *J Appl Physiol* 1994; 77: 1617–1622.
101. Wissler EH. Comments on Weinbaum-Jiji's discussion of their proposed bioheat equation. *ASME J Biomech Eng* 1988; 108: 355–356.
102. Weinbaum S, Xu LX, Zhu L, Ekpene A. A new fundamental bioheat equation for muscle tissue: Part I—blood perfusion term. *J Biomech Eng* 1997; 119: 278–288.
103. Keller KH, Seiler L. An analysis of peripheral heat transfer in man. *J App Physiol* 1971; 30: 779–786.
104. Goldberg SN, Gazelle GS, Mueller PR. Thermal ablation therapy for focal malignancy: a unified approach to underlying principles, techniques, and diagnostic imaging guidance. *AJR Am J Roentgenol* 2000; 174: 323–331.
105. Ahmed M, Goldberg SN. Thermal ablation therapy for hepatocellular carcinoma. *J Vasc Interv Radiol* 2002; 90: 272–289.
106. Yu T-H, Zhou Y-X, Liu J. Development of a new mini-invasive tumour thermal therapy probe using high-temperature water vapour. *J Med Eng Tech* 2004; 28: 167–177.
107. Wissler EH. Pennes' 1948 paper revisited. *J Appl Physiol* 1998; 85: 35–41.
108. Wissler EH. Steady-state temperature distribution in man. *J Appl Physiol* 1961; 16: 734–740.
109. Wissler EH. Steady-state temperature distribution in man. *Bull Math Biophys* 1964; 26: 147–166.
110. Wissler EH. *A Mathematical Model of the Human Thermoregulatory Behavior.* Houston, TX: Am Soc Mech Eng, 1981.
111. Stolwijik JAJ, Hardy JD. Temperature regulation in man—a theoretical study. *Pflugers Arch* 1966; 291: 129–162.
112. Stolwijik JAJ, Cunningham DJ. Expansion of a mathematical model of thermoregulation to include high metabolic rates. NASA CR-92443 (NTIS N69-16568) Washington, DC, pp. 133, 1968.
113. Stolwijik JAJ. Expansion of a mathematical model of thermoregulation to include high metabolic rates. NASA CR-102192 (NTIS NTD-195831). Washington, DC, 1969.
114. Stolwijik JAJ. Expansion of a mathematical model of physiological temperature regulation in man. NASA CR-1855 (NTIS N71-33401). Washington, DC, 1971.
115. Song CWM, Shakil A, Griffin RJ, Okajima K. Improvement of tumor oxygenation status by mild temperature thermal therapy alone or in combination with carbogen. *Semin Oncol* 1997; 24: 626–632.

116. Myrhage R, Eriksson E. Vascular arrangements in hind limb muscles of the cat. *J Anat* 1980; 131: 1–17.
117. Wissler EH. Comments on the new bioheat equation proposed by Weinbaum and Jiji. *ASME J Biomed Eng* 1987; 109: 226–232.
118. Baish JW. Formulation of the statistical model of heat transfer in perfused tissue. *ASME J Biomech Eng* 1994; 116: 521–527.
119. Sherar MD, Gladman AS, Davidson SRH, Trachtenberg J, Gertner MR. Helical antenna arrays for interstitial microwave thermal therapy for prostate cancer: tissue phantom testing and simulations for treatment. *Phys Med Biol* 2001; 46: 1905–1918.
120. Sayal DC, Maji NK. Thermoregulation through skin under variable atmospheric and physiological conditions. *J Theor Biol* 2001; 208: 451–456.
121. Lang J, Erdmann B, Seebass M. Impact of nonlinear heat transfer on temperature control in regional hyperthermia. *IEEE Trans Biomed Eng* 1999; 46: 829–838.
122. Liu J, Zhu L, Xu LX. Studies on the three-dimensional temperature transients in the canine prostate during transurethral microwave thermal therapy. *J Biomech Eng* 2000; 122: 372–379.
123. Zhu L, Dia C. Theoretical simulation of temperature distribution in the brain during mild hypothermia treatment for brain injury. *Med Biol Eng Comput* 2001; 39: 681–687.
124. Wainwright PR. Thermal effects of radiation from cellular telephones. *Phys Med Biol* 2002; 45: 2363–2372.
125. Dewhirst MW, Prosnitz L, Thrall D, Prescott D, Clegg S, Charles C, MacFall J, Rosner G, Samulski T, Gillette E, LaRue S. Hyperthermic treatment of malignant diseases: current status and a view toward the future. *Semin Oncol* 1997; 24: 616–625.
126. Myerson RJ, Strauble WL, Moros EG, Emami BN, Lee HK, Perez CA, Taylor ME. Simultaneous superficial hyperthermia and external radiotherapy: report of thermal dosimetry and tolerance to treatment. *Int J Hyperthermia* 1999; 15: 251–266.
127. Dewhirst MW, Sneed PK. Those in gene therapy should pay closer attention to lessons from thermal therapy. *Int J Radiat Oncol Biol Phys* 2003; 57: 597–600.
128. Lagendijk JJW. Thermal therapy treatment planning. *Phys Med Biol* 2000; 45: R61–R76.
129. Paulsen KD. Principles of power deposition models. In: Saegenschmiedt, Fessenden P, Vernon CC, Editors. *Thermoradiotherapy and Thermochemotherapy*. Vol 1. New York: Springer, pp. 399–423, 1995.
130. Clegg ST, Das SK, Fullar E, Anderson S, Blivin J, Oleson JR, Samulski TV. Thermal therapy treatment planning and temperature distribution reconstruction: a case study. *Int J Thermal therapy* 1996; 12: 65–76.
131. Lagendijk JJW. The influence of blood flow in large vessels on the temperature distribution in thermal therapy. *Phys Med Biol* 1982; 27: 17–23.
132. Wust P, Gellermann J, Beier J, Wegner S, Tilly W, Troger J, Stalling D, Oswald H, Hege HC, Deuflhard P, Felix R. Evaluation of segmentation algorithms for generation of patient models in radiofrequency thermal therapy. *Phys Med Biol* 1998; 43: 3295–3307.
133. Van Rhoon GC, Wust P. Introduction: non-invasive thermometry for thermotherapy. *Int J Hyperthermia* 2005; 21: 489–495.
134. Das SK, Clegg ST, Anscher MS, Samulski TV. Simulation of electromagnetically induced thermal therapy: a finite element gridding method. *Int J Hyperthermia* 1995; 11: 797–808.
135. Paulsen KD, Geimer S, Tang J, Boyse WE. Optimization of pelvic heating rate distributions with electromagnetic phased arrays. *Int J Hyperthermia* 1999; 15: 157–186.
136. Nadobny J. Sullivan D, Wust P, Seebass M, Deuflhard P, Felix R. A high-resolution interpolation at arbitrary interfaces for the FDTD method. *IEEE Trans Microw Theory Tech* 1998; 46: 1759–1766.

137. Gellermann J, Wust P, Stalling D, Seebass M, Nadobny J, Beck R, Hege H, Deuflhard P, Felix R. Clinical evaluation and verification of the thermal therapy treatment planning system hyperplan. *Int J Radiat Oncol Biol Phys* 2000; 47: 845–856.
138. Van de Kamer JB, De Leeuw AA, Hornsleth SN, Kroeze H, Kotte AN, Lagendijk JJ. Development of a regional thermal therapy treatment planning system. *Int J Hyperthermia* 2001; 17: 207–220.
139. Van den Berg CAT, Bartels LW, De Leeuw AAC, Lagendijk JJW, Van de Kamer JB. Experimental validation of thermal therapy SAR treatment planning using MR B_{1+} imaging. *Phys Med Biol* 2004; 49: 5029–5042.
140. Vitkin IA, Moriarty JA, Peters RD, Kolios MC, Gladman AS, Chen JC, Hinks RS, Hunt JW, Wilson BC, Easty AC, Bronskill MJ, Kucharczyk W, Sherar MD, Henkelman RM. Magnetic resonance imaging of temperature changes during interstitial microwave heating: a phantom study. *Med Phys* 1997; 24: 269–277.

12 Thermometry and Imaging

12.1 INTRODUCTION

Guidance and monitoring of therapy is, in fact, very important for general clinical acceptance. Accurate targeting allows precise delivery of a therapeutic dose to the diseased tissue while avoiding exposure to the adjacent normal tissue. Monitoring allows one to assess the tissue response to the dose. Therefore, a practical guidance and monitoring system will contain the following features: (1) pretreatment imaging of the site and surrounding tissue to identify and target the exact location of the abnormal tissue, (2) imaging of the treatment site during therapy to provide dynamic localization of the abnormal tissue, and (3) post treatment imaging to map the treated region for follow-up and or continued therapy [1].

Doctors have imaged human body using x-rays since the early years of the 1900s. However, x-ray has many disadvantages, including the exposure of the subject to ionizing radiation [2]. Given this fact and probably other issues related to the quality of x-ray images, the idea of thermal detection had obvious appeal. The first report of the use of temperature measurements to diagnose cancer was apparently published by Lawson [3].

In thermal therapy, the temperature at the treatment location must be controlled at certain levels depending on the type of therapy technique [4]. Accordingly, high quality thermometry is needed to (1) ensure safe delivery of adequate therapy and (2) provide the quantitative information needed to develop prognostic parameters which will aid research in planning and dosimetry [5].

Temperature measurement methods in the intraorganism are generally classified into invasive methods and noninvasive methods. Temperatures are routinely measured invasively, but only sparse measurements can be made. The limited number of measurements may result in less information than is necessary to produce satisfactory temperature distributions in order to assess thermal dosimetry properly [6,7]. This information in real time would considerably improve the ability to deliver consistently effective temperature distributions [8–11]. As an efficient thermometry method in thermal therapy, noninvasive methods for temperature measurement without inserting the sensor into the human body are more desirable. However, currently, technological means of measuring temperature accurately by noninvasive methods have not been well established [4].

The purpose of this chapter is to discuss invasive and noninvasive thermometry and imaging techniques necessary for clinical guidance and monitoring of the treatment. Various systems and their operations are described and future trends are speculated.

12.2   DEVELOPMENT OF THERMOMETRY

Temperature refers to a certain standard of reference. The use of hands to estimate heat emanating from the body remained well into the sixteenth and seventeenth centuries. Temperature is measured with thermometers that may be calibrated to a variety of temperature scales. A thermometer is a device with a measurable output that changes with temperature in a reproducible manner.

Thermometry developed slowly from Galileo's experiments. There were Florentine and Venetian glassblowers in Italy who made sealed glass containers of various shapes, which were tied onto the body surface. The rising or falling of small leads or seeds within the fluid inside the container assessed the temperature of an object. Such measurement was without a scale. It was the work of Huygens, Roemer, and Fahrenheit that proposed the need for a calibrated scale in the seventeenth and early eighteenth centuries. Celsius proposed a centigrade scale based on ice and boiling water. He suggested that on his scale boiling water should be zero, and melting ice should be 100. However, the Danish biologist Linnaeus in 1750 proposed the reversal of this scale, as it is known today [12].

Prof. Carl Wunderlich of Leipzig in 1868 advanced the use of thermometry in medicine with the first set of temperature charts on individual patients with a wide range of diseases. Clinical experience with this type of thermometer exceeds 130 years. This thermometer has a limited scale around the normal internal body temperature of 37°C or 98.4°C [12,13]. The 37°C was considered to be normal based on a study of axillary temperatures in adults, incorporating over 25,000 readings undertaken using mercury-in-glass thermometers in 1868 [14]. The advantages of using mercury-in-glass thermometers are that accuracy is verified by calibration, they do not rely on battery power, and they are capable of providing reliable clinical readings regardless of the environmental conditions, providing the clinical measurement technique is carefully implemented. The disadvantages of these thermometers are their long reading times, and they cannot be used orally in uncooperative patients or young children [13].

The use of liquid crystals became another technique of displaying skin temperature. Cholesteric esters can have the property of changing color with temperature, and this was established by Lehmann in 1877. The practical application involved the use of elaborate panels that encapsulated the crystals and were applied to the surface of the skin, but due to a large area of contact, they affected the temperature of the skin.

A major development in the early 1940s was the first electronic sensor for IR radiation that could be used for thermal imaging. This was made from indium antimonide, and was mounted at the base of a small Dewar vessel to allow cooling with liquid nitrogen. The first medical images taken with a British prototype system, the Pyroscan, were made at Middlesex Hospital in London and the Royal National Hospital for Rheumatic Diseases in Bath in 1959–1961 [12]. The basis for the above discovery was laid by the astronomer, Sir William Herschel, in Bath, who discovered the existence of IR radiation by trying to measure the heat of the separate colors of the rainbow spectrum cast on a table in a darkened room.

He found the highest temperature to fall beyond the red end, which he reported to the Royal Society as Dark Heat in 1800. His son, Sir John Herschel, who was interested in photography, recorded the heating rays on the IR side of red by creating an evaporograph image using a carbon suspension in alcohol. This image was named the thermogram.

Recently, there has been a move away from glass thermometers in many countries, giving rise to more disposable sterile thermocouples and radiometers for middle ear temperature [12].

12.3 INVASIVE TECHNIQUES

Clinical thermometry can be performed (minimally) invasively and noninvasively. Invasive thermometry methods require implantation of catheters in tissues. This ensures good thermal contact with tissues, but these methods were questioned over the years. The low acceptance by patients and physicians was a limiting factor, when large patient numbers were to be heated according to randomized studies. Problems encountered included time-consuming invasive placement of the catheters with the risk of hemorrhage or neurological complaints in the form of acute side effects. Additional toxicity such as infections and a variety of discomforts were observed [15].

The temperature meters used for invasive thermometry are characterized by high accuracy and high temporal and spatial resolution. However, to obtain high-quality thermometry the temperature probes must be placed at the critical locations [16,17]. Traditionally, invasive thermometry has been used to measure temperatures in target regions. However, it is time-consuming, uncomfortable, and risky for the patient [17]. Invasive thermometry can be accomplished generally by three types of electrodes: thermocouple sensors, thermistors, and optical fiber thermometers [4]. For hyperthermia, international guidelines recommend invasive intratumoral temperature measurements, ideally along two to three orthogonal scanning lines [18,19]. It is recommended to register temperature position scans every 5–10 min. Either index temperatures averaged over time or thermal dose parameters accumulated over time are derived from these data [15]. These intratumoral measurements have been successfully correlated with clinical endpoints, in particular with response [20–22].

12.3.1 THERMOELECTRIC THERMOMETRY

A thermocouple is a sensor that measures temperature. It consists of two different types of metals, joined together at one end. When the junction of the two metals is heated or cooled, a voltage is created that can be correlated back to the temperature. Thermocouples are normally made from special thermocouple alloy wire that is joined at one end by a weld or other mechanical connection. The thermocouple has been used widely to measure temperature in various applications. This thermometry principle is based on the Seebeck effect, discovered by Thomas Johann Seebeck in 1821.

Thermocouples are most useful where low mass or differential temperature measurements are required. They must be calibrated *in situ* because the entire length of the wire contributes to the output voltage if it traverses a temperature gradient. Variations in wire composition, homogeneity, or even mechanical strain can affect the temperature reading [23].

There are two types of thermocouples: a sheath type and a protected-tube type. Sheathed thermocouple probes are available with one of three junction types: grounded, ungrounded, or exposed. At the tip of a grounded junction probe, the thermocouple wires are physically attached to the inside of the probe wall. This results in good heat transfer from the outside, through the probe wall to the thermocouple junction. In an ungrounded probe, the thermocouple junction is detached from the probe wall. Response time is slower than with the grounded style, but the ungrounded offers electrical isolation. The thermocouple in the exposed junction style protrudes out of the tip of the sheath and is exposed to the surrounding environment. This type offers the best response time, but is limited in use to dry, noncorrosive, and nonpressurized applications.

The thermocouple of the protected-tube type consists of a protected tube, a terminal box, and a glass that insulates the thermocouple wire. The outside dimension is on the order of 3–30 mm. In general, the sheath type has rapid response with respect to temperature change because the sheath diameter is relatively narrow and the inside of the sheath is filled with inorganic insulation material when compared with the protected-tube type [4].

An advantage of thermocouples is the possibility of combining multiple sensors in one probe. A disadvantage of thermocouples is their susceptibility to EM disturbances. Thermocouples are very difficult to use as low-temperature thermometers in the presence of magnetic fields, as the thermoelectric power depends on both the temperature and the magnetic field [23,24].

12.3.2 THERMISTOR

The most popular and widely available temperature sensor for low temperature is a resistor. A temperature sensor called a thermistor is a thermally sensitive resistor that exhibits a change in electrical resistance with a change in its temperature. There are two main resistor classifications: positive temperature coefficient (PTC) and negative temperature coefficient (NTC). PTC resistors are typically a pure metal such as platinum, copper, or nickel, or a pure metal with small impurities such as rhodium–iron or platinum–cobalt. Semiconductors such as germanium have NTC behavior [23]. Thermistors typically work over a relatively small temperature range, compared with other temperature sensors, and can be very accurate and precise within that range [25].

Commonly the resistance falls exponentially with increasing the temperature, so they are very sensitive to changes over a short temperature range. Electronic circuitry is therefore essential both for measuring the resistance and using stored calibration data, describing the nonlinear changes of resistance with temperature, to convert this into a displayed temperature reading [13].

12.3.3 OPTICAL FIBER THERMOMETER

Sometimes, it is better to use noninductive optical fiber to measure temperature in a strong EM field environment such as for thermal therapy treatments. In 1987, the first laser-based emissivity measuring IR thermometer was introduced. This instrument is currently in worldwide use in industrial and research applications. In 1990 a fiber optic sensor version was developed; this provided broader temperature measurement ranges, smaller target sizes, lower cost, and most importantly flexibility of sensor head size, shape, and materials. The optical fiber thermometer has a simple thermosensor attached to the tip of an optical fiber, which is composed of a phosphor capable of excitation by a light-emitting diode (LED). The tip of the optical fiber is attached to the measured object and a pulse of the IR excitation light at a wavelength of 940 nm is applied. This applied pulse is converted into visible light, at a wavelength of 550 nm, while at the same time it is modulated by the temperature. After the IR pulse is applied, there is an afterglow for a while, even if the exciting light is cut off. There is a temperature dependency of this afterglow quantity. Therefore, the temperature is measured by the variation of afterglow. By carrying out the sequential sampling of this afterglow quantity in a time series and summing it, after the search of the afterglow integral luminance, the temperature is calculated [4].

12.3.4 APPLICATIONS AND COMPARISON

Currently, temperature sensors placed on the skin surface and inside invasively placed catheters within the treatment volume are the only reliable means available for acquiring detailed thermometry data. Manual mapping of various types of temperature sensors through phantoms, animal, and human tissues has been employed to characterize temperature distributions during treatments and to determine applicator SAR patterns [5,26]. Commercially available thermometry equipment is inadequate in terms of its ability to provide, at a reasonable cost, the thermometry information needed to properly control these applicators. One method of increasing the amount of accessible temperature data is by spatially multiplexing the available thermometry by automatically scanning the sensors through catheters placed within the treatment field. Several investigators have used invasive techniques to measure temperature elevation during thermal therapy [17,24]. A list of invasive temperature measuring devices is given in Table 12.1.

TABLE 12.1
Invasive Thermometry Methods

Type	Description
Thermistors	Strong interaction with EM fields. Accurate when not used in EM fields.
Fiber optics	No interaction with EM fields. Frequent calibration required.
Thermocouples	Multiple junction probes possible. Filtering and shielding required. Microjunction preferable. Multiple junction probes possible.

12.4   NONINVASIVE TECHNIQUES

Noninvasive measurement of the temperature distribution within the body is an attractive concept with the potential to visualize the 3D temperature distribution during thermal therapy. Some techniques are currently in clinical use, while others are still in the preclinical or experimental stage [27]. Thermal imaging is classified into two main types: active and passive. Active methods for thermal imaging expose the region of interest to energy. The energy is modulated by the tissue temperature and analyzed to retrieve information on the temperature within the body. Passive methods estimate the temperature within the body by analyzing the spontaneously radiated energy from the human body [28].

In general, noninvasive thermometry in clinical thermal therapy remains a distant goal, although developments in microwave radiometry may lead to systems with suitable spatial, temporal, and temperature resolutions for use in superficial treatments. Today, noninvasive thermometry can be achieved using several different physical approaches: impedance tomography [29], active and passive microwave imaging [30], CT, laser, IR, ultrasound, and MR techniques [31,32].

Table 12.2 summarizes the noninvasive thermometry and imaging techniques. Of all these different techniques, ultrasound and MRI are the most advanced technologies for acquiring functional information and are widely used clinically, mainly in experimental settings for thermal therapy. However, morphological information is widely acquired by using x-ray imaging and MRI. Therefore, each modality has its own characteristics as regards the information acquired. As a result, these modalities nowadays compete and complement each other.

The ultimate goal for the thermometry engineer working in clinical thermal therapy is to develop a noninvasive 3D method with a spatial resolution of 5–10 mm^3, temperature accuracy and resolution of 0.1–0.2°C, and a temporal resolution of less than 1 s [33–35]. This goal remains elusive, although progress is being made so far.

TABLE 12.2
Noninvasive Thermometry and Imaging Techniques

Type	Description
Ultrasound	Depth limited by reflection at tissue–air interfaces. Good spatial distribution. Velocity sensitive to tissue composition.
MRI	Able to visualize temperature changes dynamically. Expensive, nonportable, and uncomfortable for patients.
Microwaves	Measurement depth restricted to 2 or 3 cm in muscle. Improved spatial resolution with multi-frequency or correlation techniques. Good for imaging superficial tissues.
Terahertz	Able to image inside most dielectric materials. The system is expensive and large.
Computer tomography	High image quality. Difficult to interface with heating systems.

12.4.1 ULTRASOUND

The history of ultrasound imaging is much more recent than that of x-ray imaging. After the pioneering work of Wild and Reid in the 1950s [36], the image quality of medical ultrasound has advanced slowly from low-resolution, bistable images to images with much greater detail. Currently, ultrasound image quality is sufficient to make it an important and often indispensable imaging modality in disease diagnosis and in obstetrics [37]. Ultrasound imaging is now a mature technology, to the extent that it has a well-established place in clinical practice, as confirmed by the fact that it currently accounts for about one in four of all imaging procedures worldwide. However, this does not mean that the pace of development, either of the understanding of the physics of the interaction between ultrasound and tissue or of innovation in techniques, has slowed down. Indeed, the opposite is true [38].

12.4.1.1 Apparatus

Methods for using ultrasound as a noninvasive thermometer fall into three categories: (1) those based on echo-shifts due to changes in tissue thermal expansion and speed of sound (SOS), (2) those that use the measurement of the acoustic attenuation coefficient, and (3) those that exploit the change in backscattered energy (CBE) from tissue inhomogeneities [39].

Ultrasound uses a nonionizing pressure wave generated by acoustic transducers usually placed on the skin of the patient to transmit sound into the body. This represents a convenient and inexpensive modality with relatively simple signal processing requirements. During its transit through the body, the pressure wave loses energy due to both scattering and absorption. Sound scattered out of the main beam may be used to form images; absorbed energy gives rise to tissue heating. Accordingly, ultrasound applications in medicine fall into two principal classes, diagnostic imaging and therapy, which differ in the power, intensity, and duration of the ultrasound. Medical ultrasound is perhaps best known for its diagnostic use in obstetrics. An ultrasound scan is now routinely offered to women early in pregnancy. Ultrasound imaging is used in many other fields of medicine, because it gives effective diagnostic information from a number of anatomical sites. Figure 12.1 shows an ultrasound imaging plane.

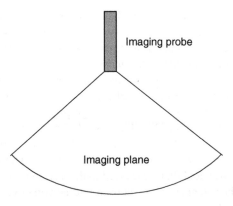

FIGURE 12.1 Ultrasound imaging plane.

The transducer is the most critical component in any ultrasonic imaging system. The trend for many years has been toward broader bandwidth transducers with more elements, since these will provide superior resolution at multiple depths by allowing the best possible compromise between penetration/resolution and attenuation to be made [40]. Nowadays, the transducers that are in clinical use almost exclusively use a piezoelectric material, of which the artificial ferroelectric ceramic, lead zirconate titanate (PZT), is the most common. The ideal transducer for ultrasonic imaging would have characteristic acoustic impedance perfectly matched to that of the human body, and have high efficiency as a transmitter and high sensitivity as a receiver, a wide dynamic range, and a wide frequency response for pulse operation [38].

Temperature dependence of ultrasonic tissue parameters has been reported extensively from *in vitro* analyses of ultrasonic tissue characteristics [41–44]. These early investigators looked at changes in tissue characteristics with temperature in order to evaluate thermal errors in tissue characterization.

12.4.1.2 Advantages and Limitations

Benefits claimed for ultrasound include the real-time visualization of applicator placement, portability of the technology, nearly universal availability, improved image quality, low cost, and ability to target and guide therapy with intracavitary endoluminal transducers (for transrectal or transgastric energy application to the prostate and abdominal organs). Because of its ability to obtain blood flow and perfusion information via the Doppler effect, ultrasound is progressively achieving a broader role in radiology, cardiology, and image-guided surgery and therapy.

Ultrasound's limitations come mainly from its rapid attenuation by both bone and gas at the frequencies used, commonly 1–20 MHz. Other limitations of ultrasound include occasional poor lesion visualization as a result of overlying bone- or gas-containing structures [45]. These attributes make it an attractive method to use for temperature estimation, if an ultrasonic parameter, which is dependent on temperature, can be found, measured, and calibrated.

12.4.1.3 Two- to Three-Dimensional Ultrasonography

For more than a decade one major goal in transducer development has been the construction of a fully electronic 2D array, which would allow for complete beam steering in 3D space (axial, lateral, and azimuthal) [46]. Ultrasound systems that use 2D arrays keep the transducer stationary and use electronic scanning to sweep the ultrasound beam over the volume of interest to produce 3D images in real time. Investigators have described a number of 2D-array designs, but the one developed at Duke University for real-time 3D echocardiography is the most advanced and has been used for clinical imaging [47]. The transducer is composed of a 2D phased array of elements that are used to transmit a broad beam of ultrasound that diverges away from the array and sweeps out pyramidal volumes. The returned echoes are detected by the 2D array and then processed to display, in real time, multiple planes from the volume. These planes can be chosen interactively to allow the user to view the desired region under investigation.

In conventional 2D ultrasonography, an experienced diagnostician manipulates the ultrasound transducer and mentally transforms the 2D images into a 3D comprehension of the lesion or anatomical volume necessary for the diagnosis or the interventional procedure. An alternative to the use of 2D arrays is the use of a 1D array, which is manipulated mechanically or manually to sweep out the desired volume of interest. As the transducer is moved over the anatomy, a series of 2D images is recorded rapidly and then reconstructed into a 3D image. If mechanical means are used to move the conventional transducer in a precise predefined manner, the relative position and angulation of each 2D image can be accurately determined. The angular or spatial interval between the digitized 2D images is usually made adjustable to minimize the scanning time while optimally sampling the volume.

Over the past two decades, many investigators have focused their efforts on the development of various types of 3D imaging techniques by taking advantage of ultrasound positioning flexibility and data acquisition speed [37]. These approaches have focused on reconstructing a 3D image by integrating transducer position information with the 2D ultrasound image. Because of the enormous demands on the computers needed to produce nearly real-time and low-cost systems, most attempts have not succeeded. It is only in the last few years that computer technology and visualization techniques have progressed sufficiently to make 3D ultrasound imaging viable.

It is now recognized that 3D ultrasound imaging has an important role to play in ultrasound-guided therapies such as prostate cryosurgery and brachytherapy, in addition to other clinical applications such as in diagnosing facial abnormalities and assessment of blood flow in various organs. Its role could be greatly expanded if a number of advances were achieved in coupling the 3D image acquisition and display to therapy planning and monitoring [37,40].

12.4.2 MAGNETIC RESONANCE IMAGING

MRI is a relatively new imaging technique that offers several advantages. It produces no ionizing radiation and provides superior tissue discrimination, lesion definition, an improved anatomic context for surrounding vessels and nerves, and excellent spatial resolution at close to or in real time. MRI also provides the capability of characterizing functional and physiological parameters of tissues, including diffusion, perfusion, flow, and temperature. However, high costs are associated with MRI; it also requires a special environment that can hinder patient accessibility [1].

MRI is based on the principles of NMR, a spectroscopic technique used by scientists to obtain microscopic chemical and physical information about molecules. The technique was called magnetic resonance imaging rather than NMR imaging (NMRI) because of the negative connotations associated with the word nuclear in the late 1970s. MRI started out as a tomographic imaging technique; that is, it produced an image of the NMR signal in a thin slice through the human body. MRI has advanced beyond a tomographic imaging technique to a volume imaging technique. In 2003, there were approximately 10,000 MRI units worldwide, and approximately 75 million MRI scans per year performed. As the field of MRI continues to grow, so do the opportunities in MRI [48].

12.4.2.1   Operation

MR thermometry has been in use since the 1990s for controlling interventional ther-moablative procedures [49]. MRI relies on the relaxation properties of excited hydro-gen nuclei in tissue water. The object to be examined is positioned in a static external magnetic field, whereupon the spins of the protons align in one of two opposite directions: parallel or antiparallel. The protons process with a frequency determined by the strength of the magnetic field and the gyromagnetic ratio. The object is then exposed to EM pulses with a frequency identical to the precession frequency in a plane perpendicular to the external magnetic field. For a 1-Tesla (T) scanner, a pulse frequency of 42.58 MHz is used. The pulses cause some of the magnetically aligned hydrogen nuclei to assume a temporary nonaligned high-energy state. As the nuclei realign, they emit energy, which can be detected by a receiver coil [27]. Figure 12.2 shows the main components of a magnetic resonance imaging system.

The mechanical integration of any applicator for thermotherapy with MR tomo-graphs is generally easy to realize. Conversely, interfaces with other methods for non-invasive thermometry (e.g., ultrasound or microwave imaging) are problematic [50]. A particular advantage of MRI is that it not only allows temperature mapping, but it can be used as well for target definition and may provide an early evaluation of thera-peutic efficacy [51]. A promising technique for noninvasive thermometry using NMR with CT has been proposed and studied by Kamimura and Amemiya [52].

Implementing noninvasive monitoring for RF/microwave thermal therapy using MR technique must solve the problem of EM compatibility: the interference between MR tomography (typically receiving and analyzing low-power signals of microwatts at 63.9 MHz) and thermal therapy RF applicator (transmitting power signals at therapeutic levels of kilowatts at hundreds of hertz). Both of these systems must be operated simultaneously and without any interaction. In particular, the MR measure-ments must not be disturbed by any radiation from the thermal therapy system [53].

Much of the current research in MRI guidance is directed toward thermal dosim-etry. The high correlation of lesion formation with temperature provides a means

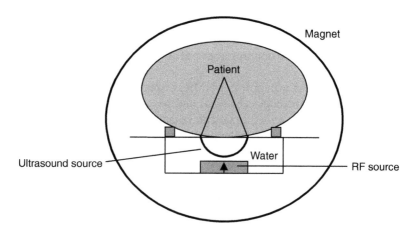

FIGURE 12.2   Magnetic resonance imaging.

to measure the treatment volume and quantify tissue damage. Several investigators have used MRI to measure temperature elevation during thermal therapy [53–61].

12.4.2.2 Advantages

MRI is attractive in clinical medicine because it provides images with exquisite soft tissue contrast and it is completely noninvasive [62]. MRI has demonstrated advantages over other imaging modalities in localizing tissue abnormalities and determining apparent tumor margins. It is therefore ideal for guiding various biopsies and tumor resections. Noninvasive MRI during thermal therapy treatments provides the capability to monitor changes in perfusion, temperature, necrosis, and chemistry. It is unique as an imaging modality in its ability to visualize temperature changes dynamically, therefore providing a mechanism through which thermal therapy can be monitored and controlled. Using the MRI in conjunction with thermal therapy allows the surgeon to view the deposition of energy within the tissues while proceeding with therapy [63,64]. However, high costs are associated with MRI; it also requires a special environment that can hinder patient accessibility; and minimal use of metal parts in the therapy assembly is necessary to prevent distortion of the MRI trends [1].

Major current topics of study include the improvement of image quality in fast imaging, improvement of the accuracy of fMRI, clinical applications of diffusion/perfusion imaging, and the development of ultrahigh magnetic field devices with magnetic field intensities above 10 T [65].

12.4.3 Microwave Radiometric Imaging

Biomedical imaging techniques for the human body using microwave technology have been of interest for many years. Microwave images are maps of the electrical property distributions in the body. The electrical properties of various tissues may be related to their physiological state [66]. Because EM radiation can be detected over distance, microwave thermometry can be used to estimate a temperature at depth even if the surface temperature is low. Near-field microwave radiometry and radiometric imaging are noninvasive techniques that are able to provide temperature information at a depth of up to several centimeters in subcutaneous tissues. They are based on the measurement of microwave thermal noise [67]. The principal behind the use of the microwave radiometer as a tool for biomedical imaging is the possibility of monitoring a thermal noise produced by objects with temperatures above absolute zero. Figure 12.3 shows the principle of imaging by microwave radiometer.

The advantage of the microwave radiometer is the ability to see the temperature increase under the surface of human body. Its main attraction is the innocuous nature of this type of energy at low levels, the relatively low cost of even complex microwave systems compared with the computer-assisted tomography (CAT) and MRI, and the distinctly different permittivity of tumor tissue compared with normal tissue [68,69]. Excellent reviews of the subject are those of Foster and Cheever [70] and Rosen et al. [69].

Since the 1970s, several research groups have carried out clinical evaluations with microwave radiometry (passive, hybrid, and active approaches) for noninvasive thermometry [68,71–90]. The most important work was done by Barret et al. [73] in the

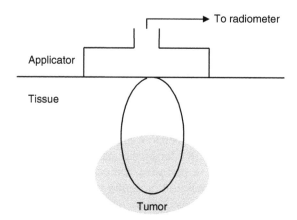

FIGURE 12.3   Principle of imaging by microwave radiometer.

field of breast cancer screening. One thousand patients were examined at the Faulkner Hospital in Boston with microwave radiometry (operating at 1.3, 3.3, and 6 GHz) and IR thermography. Breast cancer was confirmed by both methods for 39 patients. Microwave imaging has been explored as a new modality for breast cancer diagnosis since tissue physical properties are unique to the microwave spectrum, namely, the translucent nature of normal breast tissues and the significant contrast in the dielectric properties of normal tissue and malignant tumors [91,92]. Although the specific contrasts vary with frequency and among the results from different groups, there is now a general belief that these contrasts are substantial, especially near 800 MHz [66,91–96].

Other clinical evaluations were made with radiometers for measuring changes in lung water [75], cerebral temperatures [76], measurement of blood flow [78], and inflammatory arthritis [81].

Current microwave imaging systems image biomedical objects of various sizes, sometimes even the full body. However, despite its unique capabilities, microwave radiometry has so far received only limited acceptance by the medical community, and little commercial success. The chief reasons, we suggest, are the shallow depth of sensing and the difficulty of extracting imaging information from radiometry signals emitted by electrically heterogeneous media. A secondary factor has been the difficulty of validating many proposed clinical applications for the method—in particular, cancer detection. The implementation of a clinically viable microwave imaging system is a technically daunting task since high-resolution imaging requires a sophisticated scanned antenna array. On the signal processing side, it should be noted that the classical projection-type tomography algorithms are not applicable at microwave frequencies [70,97]. Microwave radiometry is a viable method of thermal sensing, but its successful applications are likely to be quite different than those that were originally conceived for the technique [70].

12.4.4   TERAHERTZ TECHNOLOGY

Terahertz (THz) radiation, which falls between microwaves and IR light of the EM spectrum, occupies the region between approximately 0.3 and 20 THz. This region of the EM spectrum is sometimes called the "THz-gap" [98]. It is one of the least explored ranges of the EM spectrum. Radiation at these wavelengths is nonionizing and subject to far less Rayleigh scatter than visible or IR wavelengths, making it suitable for medical applications. THz technology is gaining attention from researchers because it shows great promise for applications to the life sciences, including medical imaging or even clinical treatment and chemical sensing. The energy levels of this band are very low (1–12 meV); therefore, damage to cells or tissue would be limited to generalized thermal effects, i.e., strong resonant absorption seems unlikely [99–101].

12.4.4.1   Characteristics of THz Radiation

THz-ray imaging has several advantages when compared to other sensing and imaging techniques. While microwave and x-ray imaging modalities produce density pictures, THz-ray imaging also provides spectroscopic information within the THz range. The unique rotational, vibrational, and translational responses of materials (molecular, radicals, and ions) within the THz range provide information that is generally absent in optical, x-ray and NMR images [102]. THz-ray can also easily penetrate and image inside most dielectric materials, which may be opaque to visible light and low contrast to x-ray, making THz-rays a useful and complementary imaging source in this context. The distinctive rotational and vibrational responses of biological tissues within the THz range provide information that cannot be offered by optical, x-ray, or MRI techniques. THz-rays can also easily penetrate and image inside most dielectric materials, which are opaque to visible light and low contrast to x-ray, making THz-ray a practical imaging source in the context.

One of the hopes for THz applications in the medical area is in the detection and early characterization of disease. The first use of this technology in this area has been in the identification of dental caries [103] and in the examination of skin to assess the magnitude and depth of burns [104]. Recently, THz imaging was used to detect the extent of subdermal carcinomas [101].

The excitement about THz imaging stems in part from its degree of penetration. Unlike x-rays, THz radiation is nonionizing. Unlike ultrasound, THz waves can image without contact, and they can go deeper than IR radiation. THz radiation puts much less energy into biological tissue than the above techniques, which are inadequate. In addition, x-rays raise safety concerns due to the use of ionizing radiation in regular screening. One advantage of THz is the ability to perform spectroscopic measurements at each pixel in an image. This would allow, for example, the use of spectroscopy of tissue to identify regions of disease. THz medical imaging systems can be tuned to highlight specific types of tissue such as skin cancers. Because THz waves can penetrate plastic and cloth, they can be used to detect concealed objects. THz radiation is also capable of detecting chemicals such as toxic gases and explosives. Among the challenges to making THz sensing and imaging applications more practical is finding ways to direct the waves to specific targets. Researchers are working to develop THz waveguiding devices that are similar to the waveguides used to channel microwaves and light waves.

12.4.4.2 THz-Ray System

Until relatively recently, it was difficult to efficiently generate and detect THz radiation. At frequencies up to approximately 0.5 THz, EM radiation may be generated by electronic devices including resonant tunneling diodes, Gunn devices, and field effect or bipolar transistors. A second approach is to use lasers to produce THz radiation [98]. Most THz sources are either low-brightness emitters with power output inversely related to the square of the frequency, or cumbersome, single-frequency molecular vapor lasers with limited operation [99,100,105].

Detection usually relies on bolometers cooled by liquid helium, which require cryogenic operation and generally provide low sensitivity due to background radiation. These devices measure only the intensity of the radiation and do not provide any phase information. For these reasons, direct and coherent measurement of the THz electric field in the time domain is preferred [98].

The challenges in THz imaging appear to lie primarily in the difficulties of fabricating solid-state THz sources. Researchers have focused attention on all-optical techniques of producing THz radiation employing visible/near-IR lasers. Currently, most systems produce THz emissions either by frequency upconversion from the radio wave regime or by frequency downconversion from optical wavelengths. Common downconversion methods include photomixing, notably using semiconductor lasers typical for telecom applications, operating around 1.5 μm. An alternative is to irradiate a semiconductor microantenna with the IR output, typically from a titanium-doped sapphire (Ti: Sapphire) laser with the output wavelength centered around 800 nm [98,99,105].

The first THz imaging systems were based on CW THz radiation. The setup is less expensive than conventional time-domain imaging systems that comprise femtosecond lasers. CW imaging affords a compact, simple, fast, and relatively low-cost system. The system uses a two-color external-cavity laser diode. Hence it is much more compact as compared with systems based on optically pumped solid-state lasers. The coherent detection scheme is phase sensitive and operates at room temperature. These low-cost, compact systems have image capture rates comparable with those from state-of-the-art pulsed THz systems.

Terahertz time-domain spectroscopy (THz-TDS) based on femtosecond lasers is one of the first and most interesting techniques to generate and detect THz radiation, which is based on frequency conversion using nonlinear optics (Figure 12.4). Using THz-TDS, the phase and amplitude of the THz pulse at each frequency can be determined. Like radar, THz-TDS also provides time information that allows us to develop various 3D THz tomographic imaging modalities. The key components of a THz-TDS system are a femtosecond laser and a pair of specially designed transducers. By gating these transducers with ultrafast optical pulses, one can generate bursts of THz radiation and subsequently detect them with high signal-to-noise ratio (SNR). These THz transients consist of only one or two cycles of EM field, and they span a very broad bandwidth. Bandwidths extending from 100 GHz to 5 THz can be obtained. By placing an object at the focus of the THz beam, it is possible to measure the waveform that has traversed through the object. By translating the object, and measuring the transmitted THz waveform for each position of the object, one can build an image pixel by pixel. To form images in a reasonable time, the waveforms must be digitized and the desired information extracted on the fly. This can be accomplished using a

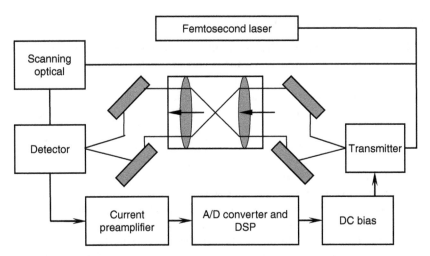

FIGURE 12.4   Schematic diagram of a THz system.

commercial digital signal processor in a computer, which synchronizes the motion of the object through the focal spot with the waveform acquisition [99,106].

12.4.4.3   Challenges

The THz region of the EM spectrum was very difficult to explore until recent advances made the generation and detection of the radiation possible [98]. Sensing and imaging with THz frequency for biomedical applications faces many challenges. These challenges include SNR, high absorption rate of water, scattering, acquisition rate and resolution, and the need for a spectroscopic database for biological tissues. Solutions to the problem of SNR are sought in improving the THz-ray hardware. THz sources have very low average output power and THz sensors have relatively low sensitivity compared with sources and sensors operating in the optical range. Both of these aspects of THz-ray systems are foci of current research and continue to improve [102].

Scattering is a common problem for many imaging modalities. THz-rays exhibit significantly reduced scattering in human tissue compared with near-IR optical frequencies due to the increased wavelength. Pearce and Mittleman [107] investigated this issue using Teflon spheres and scattering-related dispersion. This may allow the scattering process to be accurately modeled to aid the future development of diffusion imaging algorithms, such as those adopted for near-IR imaging.

Perhaps one of the most restrictive challenges facing THz imaging in biomedical engineering is the high absorption rate of water and other polar liquids. This strong absorption limits the sensing and imaging in water-rich samples and prohibits transmission-mode imaging through a thick tissue. For this reason, current biomedical THz research has primarily focused on skin conditions [102,108].

Other disadvantages of THz systems are the size and cost. Current THz-ray imaging systems require areas of a few square meters, most of which is dominated by the ultrafast laser. In addition, the high cost of ultrafast laser ($100,000–$200,000) may impede THz imaging in a number of application settings [102].

12.4.5   X-Ray Computed Tomography

A CT scan, also known as "CAT scanning" (computer-assisted tomography), was developed in the early to mid-1970s and is now available throughout the world. The now ubiquitous CT uses x-rays to make detailed pictures of structures inside of the body. CT is fast; patient friendly; and has the unique ability to image a combination of soft tissue, bone, and blood vessels. X-ray CT provides cross-sectional images of the chest, including the heart and great vessels. A CT scan can be used to study many parts of your body such as the chest, belly, pelvis, or an arm or leg. It also can take pictures of body organs such as the liver, pancreas, intestines, kidneys, adrenal glands, lungs, and heart. It also can study blood vessels, bones, and the spinal cord.

By spinning the x-ray source and the sensor/detectors around the patient, data are collected from multiple angles. A computer then processes this information to create an image on the video screen. These images are called sections or cuts because they appear to resemble cross-sections of the body. This technique eliminates the problem of conventional x-rays, where all the shadows overlap. Because it does use x-rays to form the image, this computerized technique has some limitations that are similar to those for plain film radiographs.

The first successful CT images were produces at the Atkinson Morley Hospital in London in 1972, based on the achievement of the English engineer G. N. Hounsfield, who is now generally recognized as the inventor of CT [109]. In 1979 Hounsfield and Allan M. Cormack, an engineer and a physicist, were awarded the Nobel Prize for Medicine in recognition of their outstanding achievements [110]. Three main types of CT scanners are currently used in routine clinical practice. These include conventional, spiral, and multislice scanners.

12.4.5.1   Conventional CT Scanners

In first generation (conventional) scanners, the tube produces a narrow beam of x-rays that passes through the patient and is picked up by a row of detectors on the other side. The tube and detectors are positioned on opposite sides of a ring that rotates around the patient. After each rotation the scanner must stop and rotate in the opposite direction. Each rotation acquires an axial image, typically with a slice thickness of 1 cm, taking approximately 1 s per rotation. The table moves the patient a set distance through the scanner between each slice. Conventional scanners have some limitations; for example, the first clinical scanners were slow, allowing for the acquisition of single images in 300 s. Such scanners are prone to artifacts caused by movement or breathing. They have a poor ability to reformat in different planes, studies of dynamic contrast are impossible, and small lesions between slices may be missed [110,111].

12.4.5.2   Spiral (Helical) CT Scanners

The basics for modern CT and its success are the fact that the increase in speed does apply not only to the acquisition of single images, but also to the acquisition of image data complete volumes [110]. The incorporation of slip ring technology into the design of scanners in the late 1980s removed the need for a rigid mechanical linkage between the power cables and the x-ray tube. This "simple" development, by enabling the tube to rotate in one direction indefinitely, has reestablished CT at the forefront of imaging. While the tube is rotating, the table supporting the patient also moves continuously so that a volume of tissue rather than individual slices is scanned. The data are then reformatted automatically to display the images as axial slices. High-quality reconstructed (reformatted) images in coronal, sagittal, and oblique planes can be readily acquired on a workstation. Spiral scanning has several advantages. Closely spaced scans are readily obtained, allowing good quality reconstructions in different planes. Lesions can be evaluated during different phases of contrast enhancement. Spiral CT is a powerful diagnostic tool. A spiral scanner is not as fast as a multislice scanner but is considerably cheaper [111]. The first clinical trials of spiral CT scanner were already completed in 1989; however, it took about 3 years for this scanner to receive wider acceptance. Spiral CT scanners provide scan times down to 2 s [110].

12.4.5.3   Multislice CT Scanners

Since 1992, an amazing technical development has been observed, providing huge increases in x-ray power, computer capacities, and further technical improvements. But it was not only technical parameters and increased scan speed; it was the improvement of image quality: the potential for improved 3D resolution and lesion detection. These potentials became clinical reality with the introduction of the multislice CT system and rotation times of 0.5 s in the year 1998 [110]. A multislice (multidetector) CT scanner can be considered as a "turbocharged" spiral scanner. Conventional and spiral scanners use a single row of detectors to pick up the x-ray beam after it has passed through the patient. Multislice scanners currently have up to eight active rows of detectors, and scanners under development will use direct digital detectors on flat panels. The increased number of detectors and tube rotation times that take a fraction of a second combine to give faster coverage of a given volume of tissue [111]. The first years of the new millennium showed direct continuation of the development trends of the previous decade. Image quality has reached a very high level, which can be guaranteed even at the shorter examination times. Coronary angiography, for example, can be performed easily and noninvasively with 64-slice CT and with scan times of less than 10 s with impressive results [110].

12.4.6   THz-Ray CT

THz CT is based on geometrical optics and inspired by x-ray CT. Like radar, based on the phase and amplitude of the THz pulse at each frequency, THz waves provide temporal and spectroscopic information that allows us to develop various 3D THz tomographic imaging modalities. The hardware is a relatively simple extension of modern transmission-mode THz imaging systems. THz-ray CT extends THz imaging to enable the mapping of 3D objects. It provides sectional images of objects in a manner analogous to conventional CT techniques such as x-ray CT. The interaction between a coherent THz pulse and an object provides rich information about the object under study; therefore, 3D THz imaging is a very useful tool to inspect or characterize dielectric and semiconductor objects.

THz pulse imaging is used to obtain images of the target at multiple projection angles, and the filtered back-projection algorithm enables the reconstruction of the object's frequency-dependent refractive index. THz-ray CT directly measures the transmitted amplitude and phase of broadband pulses of THz radiation at multiple projection angles. The filtered back-projection algorithm then allows a wealth of information to be extracted from the target object, including both its 3D structure and its frequency-dependent far-IR dielectric properties.

The applicability of the THz-ray CT technique is limited by two important restrictions: the THz power available and approximations made by the reconstruction algorithm. As THz-ray CT operates in transmission mode, it is only suitable for objects that do not attenuate or scatter the THz radiation too severely. This is a particular limitation for biomedical applications where the absorption of moist tissue is prohibitive. In addition, the current simple reconstruction algorithm does not describe the full interaction of THz radiation with complex structures, and more sophisticated methods are required before strongly diffracting objects can be imaged accurately [112].

12.5   STATUS AND TRENDS

The last four decades have witnessed an innovative development in the field of thermometry and diagnostic imaging. Related techniques and modalities, which were only in the experimental research phase in the early 1970s and 1980s, have now become worldwide-accepted clinical procedures. They include CT, MRI-based thermometry, ultrasound-based thermometry, microwave-based thermometry, THz imaging, etc.

The choice of the modality should be based on robust evidence that it fits the purpose with regard to the accuracy and reliability of the temperature reading in the clinical setting for which it is intended [13]. The consistent measurement of the temperature distribution inside living tissue is still the primary problem of thermometry, although the measurement of other parameters, such as tissue properties, blood perfusion, or heat flux, is also of enormous importance. Important developments in this field are those on noninvasive thermometry. This thermometry is used to visualize full 3D temperature distribution, a tool that contributes to an easier and better-controlled application of thermal therapy [113]. Commonly, temperature measurement techniques require the insertion of several temperature monitoring probes into the tumor and normal surrounding tissues. Currently, invasive thermometry is an absolute necessity to determine the temperature distributions achieved [114]. This invasive thermometry is, besides the problems with the extremely limited information about highly inhomogeneous thermal dose distributions, a major clinical problem in the acceptance of thermal therapy [16]. Efforts to establish noninvasive thermometry techniques with thermal therapy have been conducted in recent years [24,115]. However, there are two issues that must be solved to implement noninvasive thermometry efficiently. First, the EM compatibility problem of interference between thermometry device, such as MR tomography and thermal therapy applicators must be solved. Second, the acquisition process for a particular method of thermography must be carefully validated at first in a phantom under experimental conditions representative of a clinical setting [24,53].

MRI could become the most widely used medical imaging modality if several development variables such as reducing the actual cost of an exam and designing smaller MRI systems come to realization.

Potential biomedical applications in THz imaging have emerged recently, spanning fields as diverse as contraband detection and tumor recognition. It provides spectroscopic information about the chemical composition as well as the shape and location of the targets they pass through or scatter from. THz rays are nonionizing, since they have low photon energies; for example, typical x-ray photon energy is in the range of keV, which is one million times higher than that of a THz-ray photon. Biologically, this means THz radiation is noncarcinogenic. However, there remains a critical need for new initiatives and advanced technology development in the THz band, especially the development of solid-state sources and detectors. The relatively unexplored THz band must remain a focus for future research.

Techniques for noninvasive thermometry and imaging have been discussed in detail. Results presented in the literature have shown MRI, x-ray CT, and ultrasonic imaging to be adequate thermometry modalities. Other modalities including microwave and THz-based imaging have a promising future. Speaking for all thermometry and imaging techniques, the future is exciting and challenging for biomedical engineering; the prospects are certainly brighter than ever before. Future research will indicate whether the promise evolves into reliable clinical techniques.

REFERENCES

1. Vaezy A, Andrew M, Kaczkowski P. Image-guided acoustic therapy. *Annu Rev Biomed Eng* 2001; 3: 375–390.
2. Foster KR. Thermographic detection of breast cancer. *IEEE Eng Med Biol Mag* 1998; Nov/Dec: 10–14.
3. Lawson RN. Implications of surface temperature in the diagnosis of breast cancer. *Can Med Assoc J* 1956; 75: 309–310.
4. Vorst VA, Rosen A, Kotsuka Y. RF/microwave interaction with biological tissues. Hoboken, NJ: Wiley-IEEE Press, 2006.
5. Hand JW. Heat delivery and thermometry in clinical thermal therapy. *Recent Results Cancer Res* 1987; 104: 1–23.
6. Myerson RJ, Perez CA, Emami B, Straube W, Kuske RR, Leybovich L, Von Gerichten D. Tumor control in long-term survivors following superficial hyperthermia. *Int J Radiat Oncol Biol Phys* 1990; 81: 823–829.
7. Myerson RJ, Strauble WL, Moros EG, Emami BN, Lee HK, Perez CA, Taylor ME. Simultaneous superficial hyperthermia and external radiotherapy: report of thermal dosimetry and tolerance to treatment. *Int J Hyperthermia* 1999; 15: 251–266.
8. Underwood HR, Burdette EC, Ocheltre KB, Magin RL. A multielement ultrasonic hyperthermia applicator with independent element control. *Int J Hyperthermia* 1987; 3: 257–267.
9. Samulski TV, Grant WJ, Oleson JR, Leopold KA, Dewhirst MW, Vallario P, Blivin J. Clinical experience with a multi-element ultrasonic hyperthermia system: analysis of treatment temperatures. *Int J Hyperthermia* 1990; 6: 909–922.
10. Stauffer PR, Rossetto F, Leoncini M, Gentilli GB. Radiation patterns of dual concentric conductor microstrip antennas for superficial hyperthermia. *IEEE Trans Biomed Eng* 1998; 45: 605–613.

11. Novak P, Moros EG, Straube WL, Myerson RJ. SURLAS: a new clinical grade ultra-sound system for sequential or concomitant thermoradiotherapy of superficial tumors: applicator description. *Med Phys* 2005; 32: 230–240.

12. Ring EFJ. The historical development of thermometry and thermal imaging in medicine. *J Med Eng Technol* 2006; 30: 192–198.

13. Crawford DC, Hicks B, Thompson MJ. Which thermometer? Factors influencing best choice for intermittent clinical temperature assessment. *J Med Eng Tech* 2006; 30: 199–211.

14. Wunderlich C. *On the Temperature in Diseases: A Manual of Medical Thermometry.* Translated from the 2nd German edition by W.B. Woodman. London: New Sydenham Society, 1871.

15. Wust P, Cho CH, Hildebrandt B, Gellermann J. Thermal monitoring: invasive, minimal invasive and non-invasive approach. *Int J Hyperthermia* 2006; 22: 255–262.

16. Van der Zee, Peer-Valstar JN, Rietveld PJ, de Graaf-Strukowska L, Van Rhoon GC. Practical limitations of interstitial thermometry during deep hyperthermia. *Int J Radiat Oncol Biol Phys* 1998; 40: 1205–1212.

17. Wust P, Gellermann J, Harder C, Tilly W, Rau B, Dinges S, Schlag P, Budach V, Felix R. Rationale for using invasive thermometry for regional thermal therapy of pelvic tumors. *Int J Radiat Oncol Biol Phys* 1998; 41: 829–837.

18. Hand JW, Lagendijk JJ, Bach Andersen J, Bolomey JC. Quality assurance guidelines for ESHO protocols. *Int J Hyperthermia* 1989; 5: 421–428.

19. Dewhirst M. *Thermal Dosimetry: Thermo-Radiotherapy and Thermochemotherapy.* Berlin: Springer-Verlag; 1995.

20. Oleson JR, Dewhirst MW, Harrelson JM, Leopold KA, Samulski TV, Tso CY. Tumor temperature distributions predict hyperthermia effect. *Int J Radiat Oncol Biol Phys* 1989; 16: 559–570.

21. Issels RD, Prenninger SW, Nagele A, Boehm E, Sauer H, Jauch KW, Denecke H, Berger H, Peter K, Wilmanns W. Ifosfamide plus etoposide combined with regional hyperthermia in patients with locally advanced sarcomas: a phase II study. *J Clin Oncol* 1990; 8: 1818–1829.

22. Leopold K, Dewhirst M, Samulski T, Dodge RK, George SL, Blivin JL, Prosnitz LR, Oleson JR. Cumulative minutes with T90 greater than Tempindex is predictive of response to hyperthermia and radiation. *Int J Radiat Oncol Biol Phys* 1993; 25: 841–847.

23. Yeager CJ, Courts SS. A review of cryogenic thermometry and common temperature sensors. *IEEE Sens J* 2001; 1: 325–360.

24. Van Haaren PM, Kok HP, Zum Vorde Sive Vording PJ, van Dijk JD, Hulshof MC, Fockens P, van Lanschot JJ, Crezee J. Reliability of temperature and SAR measurements at oesophageal tumour locations. *Int J Hyperthermia* 2006; 22: 545–561.

25. Shantesh H, Naresh T, Mekala, Nagraj H. Thermometry studies of radio-frequency induced hyperthermia on hydrogel based neck phantoms. *J Can Res Ther* 2005; 1: 162–167.

26. Fessenden P, Lee ER, Samulski TV. Direct temperature measurement. *Cancer Res* 1984; 44: 4799S–4804S.

27. Frich L. Non-invasive thermometry for monitoring hepatic radiofrequency ablation. *Minim Invas Ther Allied Technol* 2006; 15: 18–25.

28. Miyakawa M, Bolomey JC. *Non-Invasive Thermometry of the Human Body.* Boca Raton, FL: CRC Press, 1995.

29. Paulsen K, Moskowitz M, Ryan T, Mitchell S, Hoopes P. Initial in vivo experience with EIT as a thermal estimator during thermal therapy. *Int J Therm Ther* 1996; 12: 573–591.

30. Meaney P, Paulsen K, Hartov A, Crane R. Microwave imaging for tissue assessment: initial evaluation in multitarget tissue-equivalent phantoms. *IEEE Trans Biomed Eng* 1996; 43: 878–890.

31. Conway J, Anderson AP. Electromagnetic techniques in thermal therapy. *Clin Phys Physiol Meas* 1986; 7: 287–318.
32. Hynynen K, Chung A, Fjield T, Buchanan M, Daum D, Colucci V, Lopath P, Jolesz F. Feasibility of using ultrasound phased arrays for MRI monitored noninvasive surgery. *IEEE Trans Ultrason Ferroelectr Freq Control* 1996; 43: 1043–1125.
33. Christensen DA. Thermometry and thermography. In: Storm FK, Editor. *Thermal Therapy in Cancer Therapy*. Boston: GK Hall Medical Publishers, pp. 223–232, 1983.
34. Shrivastava PN, Saylor TK, Matloubieh AY, Paliwal BR. Thermal therapy thermometry evaluation: criteria and guidelines. *Int J Radiat Oncol Biol Phys* 1988; 14: 327–335.
35. Kapp DS, Cox R. Thermal treatment parameters are most predictive of outcome in patients with single tumor nodules per treatment field in recurrent adenocarcinoma of the breast. *Int J Radiat Oncol Biol Phys* 1995; 33: 887–899.
36. Wild JJ, Reid JM. Application of echo-ranging techniques to the determination of the structure of biological tissues. *Science* 1952; 115: 226–230.
37. Fenster A, Downey DB. 3-D ultrasound imaging: a review. *IEEE Eng Med Biol* 1996; 15: 41–51.
38. Wells PNT. Ultrasound imaging. *Phys Med Biol* 2006; 51: R83–R98.
39. Arthur RM, Straube WL, Trobaugh JW, Moros EG. Non-invasive estimation of thermal therapy temperatures with ultrasound. *Int J Hyperthermia* 2005; 21: 589–600.
40. Forsberg F. Ultrasonic biomedical technology; marketing versus clinical reality. *Ultrasonics* 2004; 42: 17–27.
41. Jansson F, Sundmar E. Determination of the velocity of ultrasound in ocular tissues at different temperatures. *Acta Ophthalmol* 1961; 39: 899–910.
42. Gammell PMP, LeCroissette DH, Heyser RC. Temperature and frequency dependence of ultrasonic attenuation in selected tissues. *Ultrasound Med Biol* 1979; 5: 269–277.
43. Shore D, Miles CA. Attenuation of ultrasound in homogenates of bovine skeletal muscle and other tissues. *Ultrasonics* 1988; 26: 218–222.
44. McCarthy RN, Jeffcort LB, McCartney RN. Ultrasound speed in equine cortical bone: effects of orientation, density, porosity and temperature. *J Biomech* 1990; 23: 1139–1143.
45. Goldberg SN, Gazelle GS, Mueller PR. Thermal ablation therapy for focal malignancy: a unified approach to underlying principles, techniques, and diagnostic imaging guidance. *Am J Roentgenol* 2000; 174: 323–331.
46. Light ED, Davidsen RE, Fiering JO, Hruschka TA, Smith SW. Progress in 2-D arrays for real time volumetric imaging. *Ultrason Imag* 1998; 20: 1–16.
47. Smith SW, Trahey GE, von Ramm OT. Two-dimensional arrays for medical ultrasound. *Ultrason Imag* 1992; 14: 213–233.
48. Hornak JP. *The Basics of MRI*, 1996. http://www.cis.rit.edu/htbooks/mri.
49. Quesson B, de Zwart JA, Moonen CTW. Magnetic resonance temperature imaging for guidance of thermotherapy. *J Magn Reson Imag* 2000; 12: 525–533.
50. Van Rhoon GC, Wust P. Introduction: non-invasive thermometry for thermotherapy. *Int J Hyperthermia* 2005; 21: 489–495.
51. De Senneville DB, Quesson B, Moonen CTW. Magnetic resonance temperature imaging. *Int J Hyperthermia* 2005; 21: 515–531.
52. Kamimura Y, Amemiya Y. *Automedica*. Vol 8. New York: Gordon and Breach, pp. 295–313, 1987.
53. Gellermann J, Wlodarczyk W, Ganter H, Nadobny J, Fahling H, Seebass M, Felix R, Wist P. A practical approach to thermography in thermal therapy/magnetic resonance hybrid system: validation in a heterogeneous phantom. *Int J Radiat Biol Phys* 2005; 61: 267–277.
54. Cline HE, Hynynen K, Watkins RD, Adams WJ, Schenck JF, Ettinger RH, Freund WR, Vetro JP, Jolesz FA. Focused US system for MR imaging-guided tumor ablation. *Radiology* 1995; 194: 731–737.

55. Fjield T, Hynynen K. The combined concentric-ring and sector-vortex phased array for MRI guided ultrasound surgery. *IEEE Trans Ultrason Ferroelectr Freq Control* 1997; 44: 1157–1167.

56. Carter DL, MacFall JR, Clegg ST, Wan X, Prescott DM, Charles HC, Samulski TV. Magnetic resonance thermometry during thermal therapy for human high-grade sarcoma. *Int J Radiat Oncol Biol Phys* 1998; 40: 815–822.

57. McDannold NJ, Hynynen K, Wolf D, Wolf G, Jolesz FA. MRI evaluation of thermal ablation of tumors with focused ultrasound. *J Magn Reson Imag* 1998; 8: 91–100.

58. Sokka SD, Hynynen K. The feasibility of MRI-guided whole prostate ablation with a linear aperiodic intracavitary ultrasound phased array. *Phys Med Biol* 2000; 45: 3373–3383.

59. Smith NB, Merilees NK, Hynynen K, Dahleh M. Control system for an MRI compatible intracavitary ultrasound array for thermal treatment of prostate disease. *Int J Hyperthermia* 2001; 17: 271–282.

60. Marguet CH, Melo de Lima D, Fakri-Bouchet L, Favre B, Cathignol D, Brigu A. NMR antenna for an interstitial ultrasound applicator. *Eur Phys J* 2003; 23: 213–216.

61. Arora D, Cooley D, Perry T, Guo J, Richardson A, Moellmer J, Hadley R, Parker D, Skliar M, Roemer RB. MR Thermometry-based feedback control of efficacy and safety in minimum-time thermal therapies: phantom and *in-vivo* evaluations. *Int J Hyperthermia* 2006; 22: 29–42.

62. Hu X, Norris DG. Advances in high-field magnetic resonance imaging. *Annu Rev Biomed Eng* 2004; 6: 157–184.

63. Bleier A, Jolesz FA, Cohen M, Weisskoff R. Real-time magnetic imaging of laser heat deposition in tissue. *Magn Reson Med* 1991; 21: 132–137.

64. Higuchi N, Bleier AR, Jolesz FA, Colucci VM, Morris JH. MRI of the acute effects of interstitial neodymium: YAG laser on tissues. *Investig Radiol* 1992; 27: 814–821.

65. Endo M. Recent progress in medical imaging technology. *Sys Comput Jpn* 2005; 36: 1–17.

66. Fear EC, Meaney PM, Stuchly MA. Microwaves for breast cancer detection. *IEEE Potentials* 2003; 22: 12–18.

67. Leroy Y, Bocquet B, Mamouni A. Non-invasive microwave radiometry thermometry. *Physiol Meas* 1998; 19: 127–148.

68. Rosen A, Rosen HD. *New Frontiers in Medical Device Technology.* New York: Wiley, 1995.

69. Rosen A, Stuchly MA, Vander Vorst A. Applications of RF/microwaves in medicine. *IEEE Trans Microw Theory Tech* 2002; 50: 963–974.

70. Foster KR, Cheever E. Microwave radiometry on biomedicine: a reappraisal. *Bioelectromagnetics* 1992; 13: 567–579.

71. Enander B, Larson G. Microwave radiometric measurements of the temperature inside a body. *Electron Lett* 1974; 10: 315–317.

72. Edrich J, Hardee PC. Thermography at millimeter wavelength. *Proc IEEE* 1974; 62: 1391–1392.

73. Barret AH, Myers PC, Sadowski NL. Detection of breast cancer by microwave radiometry. *Radioscience* 1977; 12: 167–171.

74. Edrich J, Jobe WE, Hendee WR, Cacak HK, Gautherie M. Imaging thermograms at cm and mm wavelength. *Ann NY Acad Sci* 1980; 335: 154–160.

75. Iskander MF, Durney CH. Microwave methods of measuring changes in lung water. *J Microw Power* 1983; 18: 265–275.

76. Gustov AV, Troitskii VS, Gorbachev VP, Arzhanov NI, Tseitlina VN. Investigation of craniocerbral temperature by decimeter radiothermometry. *Hum Physiol* 1985; 8: 69–72.

77. Leroy Y, Mamouni A, Van de Velde JC, Bocquet B, Dujardin B. Microwave radiometry for non-invasive thermometry. *Automedia* 1987; 8: 88–202.

78. Gabrielian ES, Khachatrian LA, Nalbandian SG, Grigorian FA. Microwave method of determining cerebral blood flow (in Russian). *Biull Eksp Biol Med* 1987; 103: 625–627.

79. Bocquet B, Van de Velde JC, Mamouni A, Leory Y, Giaux G, Delannoy J, Delvallee D. Microwave radiometric imaging at 3 GHz for the exploration of breast tumors. *IEEE Trans Microw Theory Tech* 1990; 38: 791–792.

80. Giaux G, Delannoy G, Delvalle D, Leroy Y, Mamouni A, Van de Velde JC, Bocquet B. Microwave radiometric imaging: characterization of breast tumours. *J Photogr Sci* 1991; 39: 164–165.

81. MacDonald AG, Land DV, Sturrock RD. Microwave thermography as a noninvasive assessment of disease activity in inflammatory arthritis. *Clin Rheumatol* 1994; 13: 589–592.

82. Bri S, Bellarbi L, Habibi M, ELKadiri M, Mamouni A. Experimental evaluation of new thermal inversion approach incorrelation microwave thermometry [tumour detection]. *Electro Lett* 2000; 36: 439–440.

83. Hand JW, Mizushina JMJ, Van de Kamer JB, Maruyama K, Sugiura T, Azzopardi DV, Edwards AD. Monitoring of deep brain temperature in infants using multi-frequency microwave radiometry and thermal modeling. *Phys Med Biol* 2001; 46: 1885–1903.

84. Mouty S, Bocquet B, Ringot R, Rocourt N, Devos P. Microwave radiometric imaging (MWI) for the characterisation of breast tumours. *Eur Phys J* 2000; 10: 73–78.

85. Meaney PM, Fanning MW, Li D, Poplack P, Paulsen KD. A clinical prototype for active microwave imaging of the breast. *IEEE Trans Microw Theory Tech* 2000; 48: 1841–1853.

86. Jacobsen S, Stauffer P, Neuman D. Dual-mode antenna design for microwave heating and non-invasive thermometry of superficial tissue disease. *IEEE Trans Biomed Eng* 2000; 47: 1500–1509.

87. Jacobsen S, Stauffer PR. Multi-frequency radiometric determination of temperature profiles in a lossy homogeneous phantom using a dual-mode antenna with integral water bolus. *IEEE Trans Microw Theory Tech* 2002; 50: 1737–1746.

88. Davis SK, Tandradinata H, Hagness SC, Van Veen BD. Ultrawideband microwave breast cancer detection: a detection-theoretic approach using the generalized likelihood radio test. *IEEE Trans Biomed Eng* 2005; 52: 1237–1250.

89. Fear EC. Microwave imaging of the breast. *Technol Cancer Res Treat* 2005; 4: 69–82.

90. Hashemzadeh, Fhager A, Persson M. Experimental investigation of an optimization approach to microwave tomography. *Electromagn Bio Med* 2006; 25: 1–12.

91. Hagness SC, Taflove A, Bridges JE. Two-dimensional FDTD analysis of a pulsed microwave confocal system for breast cancer detection: fixed-focus and antenna-array sensors. *IEEE Trans Biomed Eng* 1998; 45: 1470–1479.

92. Hagness SC, Taflove A, Bridges JE. Three-dimensional FDTD analysis of a pulsed microwave confocal system for breast cancer detection: design of an antenna-array element. *IEEE Trans Antennas Propagat* 1999; 47: 783–791.

93. Joines WT, Zhang Y, Li C, Jirtle RL. The measured electrical properties of normal and malignant human tissues from 50 to 900 MHz. *Med Phys J* 1994; 21: 547–550.

94. Caorsi GL, Gragnani L, Pastorino M. An electromagnetic imaging approach using a multi-illumination technique. *IEEE Trans Biomed Eng* 1994; 41: 406–409.

95. Meaney PM, Paulsen KD, Hartov A, Crane RK. An active microwave imaging system for reconstruction of 2-D electrical property distributions. *IEEE Trans Biomed Eng* 1995; 42: 1017–1025.

96. Fear EC, Stuchly MA. Microwave detection of breast cancer. *IEEE Trans Microw Theory Tech* 2000; 48: 1854–1863.

97. Huo Y, Bansal R, Zhu Q. Modeling of noninvasive microwave characterization of breast tumors. *IEEE Trans Biomed Eng* 2004; 51: 1089–1094.

98. Smye SW, Chamberlain JM, Fitzgerald AJ, Berry E. The interaction between terahertz radiation and biological tissue. *Phys Med Biol* 2001; 46: R101–R112.
99. Mittleman DM, Gupta M, Neelamani R, Baraniuk RG, Rudd JV, Koch M. Recent advances in terahertz technology. *Appl Phys B* 1999; 68: 1085–1094.
100. Fitzgerald AJ, Berry E, Zinoveev EE, Walker GC, Smith MA, Chamberlain JM. An introduction to medical imaging with coherent terahertz frequency radiation. *Phys Med Biol* 2002; 47: 67–84.
101. Siegel HS. Terahertz technology in biology and medicine. *IEEE Trans Microw Theory Tech* 2004; 52: 2438–2447.
102. Zhang X-C. Terahertz wave imaging: horizons and hurdles. *Phys Med Biol* 2002; 47: 3667–3677.
103. Crawley DA, Longbottom C, Cole BE, Ciesla CM, Arnone D, Wallace VP, Pepper M. Terahertz pulse imaging: a pilot study of potential application in dentistry. *Caries Res* 2003; 37: 352–359.
104. Mittleman D. Terahertz imaging. In: Mittleman D, Editor. *Sensing with Terahertz Radiation*. Berlin, Germany: Springer-Verlag, pp. 117–153, 2003.
105. Davies AG, Linfield EH, Johnston MB. The development of terahertz sources and their applications. *Phys Med Biol* 2002; 47: 3679–3689.
106. Wang S, Zhang X-C. Pulsed terahertz tomography. *J Phys D Appl Phys* 2004; 37: 1–36.
107. Pearce J, Mittleman DM. Propagation of single-cycle terahertz pulses in random media. *Opt Lett* 2001; 6: 2002–2004.
108. Loffler T, Bauer T, Siebert KJ, Roskos HG, Fitzgerald A, Czasch S. Terahertz dark-field imaging of biomedical tissue. *Opt Exp* 2001; 9: 616–621.
109. Hounsfield GN. Computerized transverse axial scanning (tomography): I. Description of system. *Br J Radiol* 1973; 46: 1016–1022.
110. Kalender WA. X-ray computed tomography. *Phys Med Biol* 2006; 51: R29–R43.
111. Garvey CJ, Hanlon R. Computed tomography in clinical practice. *BMJ* 2002; 324: 1077–1080.
112. Ferguson B, Wang S, Gray D, Abbot D, Zhang X-C. T-ray computed tomography. *Optics Lett* 2002; 27: 1312–1314.
113. Wust P, Hildebrandt B, Sreenivasa G, Rau B, Gellermann J, Riess H, Felix R, Schlag PM. Hyperthermia in combined treatment of cancer. *Lancet Oncol* 2002; 3: 487–497.
114. Lagendijk JJW, Hofman P, Schipper J. Perfusion analysis in advanced breast carcinoma during hyperthermia. *Int J Hyperthermia* 1998; 4: 479–495.
115. Chen JC, Moriarty JA, Derbyshire JA, Trachtenberg J, Bell SD, Doyle J, Arrelano R, Wright GA, Henkelman RM, Hinks RS, Lok S-Y, Toi A, Kucharczyk W. Prostate cancer: MR imaging and thermometry during microwave thermal ablation—initial experience. *Radiology* 2000; 214: 290–297.

Acronyms and Abbreviations

1D	1-dimensional
2D	2-dimensional
3D	3-dimensional
1G	first generation
2G	second generation
3G	third generation
AC	alternating current
AD	Alzheimer's Disease
AF	atrial fibrillation
ALL	acute lymphocytic leukemia
ALS	amyotrophic lateral sclerosis
AM	amplitude modulation
AML	acute myeloid leukemia
ANSI	American National Standards Institute
APC	adaptive power control
ARPANSA	Australian Radiation Protection and Nuclear Safety Agency
ASA	American Standard Association
AV	atrioventricular
BBB	blood–brain barrier
BCS	breast-conserving surgery
BMR	basal metabolic rate
BPH	benign prostatic hyperplasia
BTS	base transceiver station
CAT	computer-assisted tomography
CENELEC	European Committee for Electrotechnical Standardization
CDMA	code division multiple access
CGS	centimeter-gram second
CLL	chronic lymphocytic leukemia
CLM	colorectal liver metastases
CNS	central nervous system
CRT	cathode ray tube
CT	computed tomography
CUA	Catholic University of America
CW	continuous wave
dB	decibel
DCS	Digital Communication Services
DECT	Digital European Cordless Telephone

DNA	deoxyribonucleic acid
DOE	Department of Energy
EAS	electronic article surveillance
ECG	electrocardiogram
EEG	electroencephalography
ELF	extremely low frequency
EM	electromagnetic fields
EMC	electromagnetic compatibility
EMF	electric and magnetic field
EMF RAPID	Electric and Magnetic Fields Research and Public Information Dissemination
ETW	expanded tip wire
EMI	electromagnetic inference
EMIT	electromagnetic interference toolbox
ENU	eurocarcinogen ethylnitrosoura
EPA	Environmental Protection Agency
ES	electrical sensitivity
ETSI	European Telecommunications Standards Institute
EU	European Union
eV	electron volt
FCC	Federal Communications Commission
FDTD	finite difference time domain
FDA	Food and Drug Administration
FEM	finite element method
FEHRM	Framework for Environmental Health Risk Management
FM	frequency modulation
fMRI	functional magnetic resonance imaging
GM	geometric mean
GFD	generalized finite difference
GICs	geomagnetically induced currents
GPS	global positioning system
GSM	global system for mobile communication
HAPS	high altitude atmosphere platform station
HCC	hepatocellular carcinoma
HF	high frequency
HIFU	high-intensity focused ultrasound
HSP	heat-shock protein
Hz	Hertz, originally cycles per second
ICES	International Commission for Electromagnetic Safety
IEBCM	iterative extended boundary condition method
IEEE	Institute of Electrical and Electronics Engineers

IEGMP	Independent Expert Group on Mobile Phones
ICNIRP	International Commissions on Non-Ionizing Radiation Protection
INIRC	International Nonionizing Radiation Committee
IR	infrared
IRPA	International Radiation Protection Association
ISM	industrial, scientific, and medical
ITS	intelligent transport systems
LCD	liquid crystal display
LED	light-emitting diode
LF	low frequency
MBA	microwave balloon angioplasty
MEA	microwave endometrial ablation
MFH	magnetic fluid hyperthermia
MPE	maximum permissible exposure
MPT	Ministry of Posts and Telecommunications (Japan)
MR	magnetic resonance
MRI	magnetic resonance imaging
MRI/MRS	magnetic resonance imaging and spectroscopy
MRS	magnetic resonance spectroscopy
NICE	National Institute for Clinical Excellence
NIEHS	National Institute of Environmental Health Sciences
NMR	nuclear magnetic resonance
NMT	Nordic Mobile Telephone
NRC	National Research Council
NRPB	National Radiological Protection Board
NTC	negative temperature coefficient
ODC	ornithine decarboxylase
Oe	oersted
OR	odds ratio
OSA	obstructive sleep apnea
PACS	Personal Access Communications System
PCS	Personal Communication Services
PHS	Personal Handyphone System
PTC	positive temperature coefficient
PZT	lead zirconate titanate
RF	radiofrequency
RFID	radiofrequency identification
RFR	radiofrequency radiation
RIF	radiation-induced fibrosarcoma
RITA	RF interstitial tumor ablation

RMS	root mean square
RNA	ribonucleic acids
ROW	rights-of-way
SAD	specific absorption per day
SAR	specific absorption rate
SCE	sister chromatid exchange
SD	standard deviation
SF	shielding factor
SIR	standardized incidence ratio
SMR	standardized mortality ratio
SNR	signal-to-noise ratio
SP	slow brain potentials
SPFD	scalar potential finite difference
SPECT	single photon emission tomography
TACS	Total Access Telecommunication System
TDMA	time division multiple access
TER	thermal enhancement ratios
TETRA	Terrestrial Trunked Radio
TNF	tumor necrosis factor
TTPS	thermal therapy planning system
TUMT	transurethral microwave thermotherapy
TV	television
TWA	time-weighted average
UHF	ultra high frequency
UK	United Kingdom
US	United States
USAF	U.S. Air Force
USASI	United States of America Standard Institute
UV	ultraviolet
VDT	video display terminal
VEGF	vascular endothelial growth factor
VHF	very high frequency
VLF	very low frequency
WBH	whole-body hyperthermia
WCDMA	wide code division multiple access
WHO	World Health Organization

Index

A

B

Milton Keynes UK
Ingram Content Group UK Ltd.
UKHW021823071024
449327UK00021B/1405